Contents

Preface

The incidence and prevalence of anabolic steroid abuse, especially by adolescents, carries with it significant social as well as health-risk concerns. There are a number of questions regarding this misuse that need to be addressed. Do results from well-controlled studies support the efficacy of anabolic steroids in increasing muscle mass and augmenting performance? What information is available on the health consequences of misuse of anabolic steroids at suprapharmacological doses over extended periods of time? Do steroids have the potential for development of tolerance and dependence, and do they meet the criteria for abuse potential as defined in strict pharmacological terms? Are adolescents at particular risk? These are among the questions that prompted the National Institute on Drug Abuse to undertake this review on anabolic steroid abuse in an effort to understand the extent and scope of the problem and to identify research priorities in this area.

The contents of this monograph encompass a wide range of topics beginning with the important question of whether anabolic steroids possess abuse potential and whether they play a role in the abuse of other substances. There follows an historical overview of the discovery and development of anabolic steroids, a critical evaluation of the performance-enhancing effects of anabolic steroids, and an ethnographic study of anabolic steroid abuse in New York City. Next is a summary of the epidemiological evidence on the incidence and prevalence of steroid use. To better understand the health consequences of abuse, the normal endocrine physiology and pharmacology, as well as molecular and receptor mechanisms underlying the actions of anabolic steroids, are presented, followed by an appraisal of the health risks associated with abuse. Since adolescents are of special concern, a detailed account of the endocrinological effects of anabolic steroids in this special population is included. Finally, this review is completed with a discussion of the behavioral aspects of anabolic steroid use including indications of psychological dependence and evidence for steroid-induced mental status changes and aggressive behavior.

This monograph represents a "state-of-the-art" information resource concerning anabolic steroid abuse and suggests future directions for research. It is hoped that this monograph will serve to stimulate further research in this area. The monograph should be valuable to members of the scientific community who are involved in drug abuse research; to those interested in the field of anabolic steroids, including professionals in sports medicine, endocrinology, psychiatry, and education; and to government agencies with regulatory responsibility, drug enforcement responsibility, or both.

The editors would like to express their thanks to the authors of the chapters in this monograph and to all the participants in the technical review on which this monograph is based. We would especially like to thank Dr. Marvin Snyder, Director, Division of Preclinical Research, for his role in initiating and supporting this effort.

Geraline C. Lin, Ph.D.
Lynda Erinoff, Ph.D.

Division of Preclinical Research
National Institute on Drug Abuse

Abuse Liability of Anabolic Steroids and Their Possible Role in the Abuse of Alcohol, Morphine, and Other Substances[1]

Theodore J. Cicero and Lynn H. O'Connor

INTRODUCTION

The purpose of this chapter is to discuss the possible abuse potential of anabolic steroids in man and animals. A second major goal is to provide an overview of the relevant literature concerning the possible involvement of steroids in the acute and chronic actions of more commonly abused drugs, such as opiates and alcohol.

At the outset, several considerations should be borne in mind. First, there seems to be little doubt that steroids are misused and that such use has significant adverse effects, particularly when steroids are used by prepubertal and pubertal adolescents, who are unusually susceptible to the disruptive effects of steroids (Haupt and Rovere 1984; Lombardo, this volume; Taylor 1987; Wilson 1988). However, the issue of whether these compounds have abuse liability in the classical, pharmacological sense of that term remains a matter of debate and will be the primary focus of this chapter.

Second, there is a paucity of data relevant to the abuse potential of anabolic steroids in humans, and even less information is at hand utilizing animal models. Moreover, the absence of well-controlled, double-blind studies utilizing placebo controls severely limits the conclusions that can be drawn. Specifically, as will be elaborated below, it is virtually impossible to distinguish between "expectancy" effects of steroid use and the immediate reinforcing properties of the drugs from the studies currently available.

Finally, steroid abusers rarely if ever abuse only a single steroid. Rather, taking a number of steroids, other illicit and prescription drugs, and hormones (growth hormone), a practice often referred to as "stacking," appears to be the normal pattern of use (Taylor 1987; Wilson 1988). Compounding this problem, the patterns of steroid use by regular users, including doses and frequency of administration, are highly variable, which makes well-controlled studies in an experimental situation difficult at best and, perhaps, of somewhat limited value vis-à-vis an examination of "normal" steroid misuse in humans, Moreover, since these compounds are generally obtained illicitly on the black market, their purity is frequently suspect, which makes self-reported estimates of the doses and types of compounds administered of questionable validity. For these reasons, it has proven to be extremely difficult to assess the dependence liability of a given steroid in polydrug-abusing individuals with highly irregular patterns of self-administration.

This chapter is divided into several sections: first, an overview of the actions of steroids in the brain; second, a discussion of the widely accepted pharmacological criteria necessary to establish the abuse liability of drugs; third, a critical evaluation of the extent to which steroids meet these criteria in humans and animals; and, finally, the potential role of steroids in the abuse liability of other substances. Discussion is confined to the abuse liability of gonadal steroids, since there is little indication that users of steroids self-administer other steroids, such as those secreted by the adrenal gland.

STEROID ACTIONS ON THE BRAIN

Clearly, steroids affect numerous target organs, including the secondary sex organs, muscles, liver, and brain, through specific steroid receptors. In this chapter the effects of steroids on only the brain will be considered, as the primary focus is to examine the motivating factors that lend to the self-administration of steroids and, hence, their abuse liability. Since drug-seeking behavior is undoubtedly mediated by the brain, as has been unequivocally demonstrated with all other psychoactive compounds with significant abuse potential, a detailed discussion of the effects of steroids in nonneuronal tissues is not pertinent to the current discussion. In the course of the discussion of the abuse liability of steroids, however, we will briefly address the issue of the mechanisms by which steroids may enhance muscular development and athletic performance, both of which appear to represent the driving force behind the self-administration of steroids in humans.

Organizational vs. Activational Effects of Steroids

Just as certain muscles are acutely sensitive to the effects of steroid hormones, during certain stages of development the growth and differentiation of the brain is also responsive to steroid hormones. These irreversible actions of steroid hormones on the development of the structure and function of the brain, which occur either prenatally or very early in postnatal life (before neural systems are fully developed), are generally referred to as

2

"organizational" effects of steroid hormones. The word "activational" is reserved for those effects of steroids that occur during adulthood and involve short-term, reversible activation of previously established neural pathways. The activational effects of hormones are dependent upon the nature of the particular organizational effects of steroids that occurred earlier in life.

The utility of the terms "organizational" and "activational" has been supported by a wealth of experimental data, and these terms are now used more generally to describe not only hormone effects on behavior, as they were initially used (Phoenix et al. 1959; Young et al. 1964), but also a variety of hormonally mediated structural and functional dimorphisms of the nervous system. Recently, a number of significant exceptions to the criteria distinguishing organizational from activational effects have been described (Arnold and Breedlove 1985). Of particular interest is the finding that steroid hormones can cause long-lasting and sometimes permanent changes in brain morphology and behavior even when administered to adult animals. For example, in adult animals, androgen influences the size of the somas and nuclei of androgen-sensitive motor neurons of the spinal nucleus of the bulbocavemosus in rats (Breedlove and Arnold 1981). Androgen influences the volume of cell nuclei in the preoptic hypothalamic area of adult mongolian gerbils (Commins and Yahr 1984a; Commins and Yahr 1984b). In adult female canaries and zebra finches, androgen influences the size of two nuclei involved in song production (Gurney and Konishi 1980; Gurney 1981; Gurney 1982; Nottebohm 1980). In the arcuate nucleus, estrogen or testosterone increases neuronal membrane exo-endocytotic pits (Garcia-Segura et al. 1987). Also, estrogen injection or testosterone deficiency promotes the formation of whorl bodies in the arcuate that are suggestive of neuronal damage (Price et al. 1976; Brawer et al. 1980; Garcia-Segura et al. 1986). Estrogen influences synaptic morphology in the midbrain central gray (Chung et al. 1988), and progesterone changes neuronal ultrastructure in the ventromedial hypothalamic nucleus (Meisel and Pfaff 1988). In adult rats, androgen influences regeneration of the hypoglossal nerve (Yu and Srinivasan 1981), and estrogen promotes lesion-induced sprouting in the arcuate nucleus (Matsumoto and Arai 1979; Matsumoto and Arai 1981) and hippocampus (Scheff et al. 1988). Estrogen also causes changes in the tuberoinfundibular dopamine neurons that persist for 22 months after hormone exposure (Steger et al. 1989).

In addition to changes in brain morphology, brief periods of exposure to steroid hormones in adulthood can cause long-lasting changes in behavioral responsiveness. For example, in female rodents, short periods of hormonal exposure can have long-lasting effects that facilitate behavioral responsiveness to a subsequent hormone injection (Collins et al. 1938; Whalen and Nakayama 1965; Beach and Orndoff 1974; Gerall and Dunlap 1973; Parsons et al. 1979). Similarly, in castrated rats and doves, restoration of sexual behavior by hormone administration becomes increasingly more difficult as the time since castration increases, unless small maintenance doses of hormones are given (Davidson 1972; Damassa and Davidson 1973; Hutchinson 1978). These studies suggest that sensitivity to a steroid is partly regulated by the steroid itself and that, typically, prior exposure to estrogen or androgen increases sensitivity to that steroid. In contrast, prior exposure to other compounds with abuse potential, as well as most psychoactive drugs, generally produces a period of tolerance.

Mechanisms of Steroid Action

A primary mechanism of steroid hormone action in the brain is through interaction of hormone-specific receptor complexes with acceptor sites on DNA. Through this interaction, steroids influence the synthesis of specific messages and the production of proteins by cells. Actions of steroids that involve changes in protein synthesis are slow changes requiring hours or even days to produce observable physiological effects. For example, after estradiol injection, a minimum of 11 to 18 hours is required for estradiol to prime the nervous system for display of rodent sexual behavior (Eaton et al. 1975; Feder et al. 1977; Walker and Feder 1977), and optimal displays of behavior do not occur until 36 to 40 hours after estradiol exposure.

Steroids also have direct actions on cell membranes mediated either by specific receptors for steroids on cell membranes (Ramirez and Dluzen 1987; Robel et al. 1987; Simmonds et al. 1984; Towle and Sze 1983) or by interactions with neurotransmitter receptors (LaBella et al. 1978; Su et al. 1988). Membrane effects of steroids appear to be rapid and of relatively short duration.

Clearly, the existence of two separate and distinct mechanisms of steroid action in the nervous system, one extremely rapid and the other quite slow, needs to be taken into account when interpreting experiments designed to elucidate the abuse potential of steroids.

CRITERIA TO ASSESS WHETHER A SUBSTANCE HAS ABUSE POTENTIAL

It is widely accepted (Brady 1988; Brady and Lucas 1984) that, before any substance can be classified as having abuse liability, the following criteria must be met.

Self-Administration

The drug must be self-administered for its immediate reinforcing properties, e.g., euphoria, feeling of well-being. Furthermore, it must be shown that the drug is self-administered for sustained periods of time and that it is voluntarily ingested in preference to alternative substances. Operant conditioning paradigms have proved to be an extremely valuable tool in meeting this criterion in humans and animals. An illustrative example of a standard technique used in animals to assess whether a drug is self-administered and, hence, has reinforcing properties is provided below.

Subjects are fitted with appropriate catheters or are otherwise permitted access to the drug, e.g., delivery of aqueous drug solutions for oral consumption, and are then required to perform some task or goal-oriented behavior to obtain the drug. For example, a common procedure used with many substances of abuse is to insert an intravenous catheter through which specified doses of drugs can be administered. The subject is required to depress one of several levers that will deliver the active compound, placebo, or, in many instances, other alternatives as well. If the drug has immediate reinforcing properties, the active lever will be uniformly selected after a training or acquisition period; various techniques can be employed to assess the strength of the drug as a reinforcer (fixed- or variable-ratio schedules). Using these methods, the experimenter can easily manipulate all experimental variables, determine the amount of "work" the subject will perform to obtain the drug, and, most important, objectively determine the relative reinforcing properties of the drug when compared to other more commonly abused drugs, which are often used as standards.

Obviously, the example given is based on an animal preparation, but well-established paradigms have been developed in recent years that have permitted the same rigorous experimental analysis of drug-seeking behavior in humans (Fischman and Mello 1989). The most important point to be gleaned from this discussion is that it must be shown, under standardized, well-controlled conditions, that any drug is self-administered for its reinforcing properties and that such behavior is robust and strongly motivated.

Drug Discrimination

The abused substance must be easily identified when the user is provided the opportunity to discriminate his drug of choice from a variety of alternatives, including, most significantly, a placebo. Numerous procedures have been developed to permit an assessment of drug-discrimination behavior. Perhaps the most common technique is to first establish a strong pattern of self-administration and then abruptly change the drug-appropriate operant response by, for example, substituting the delivery of the active compound with placebo or another compound devoid of activity, in which case self-administration should cease. Alternatively, the operant conditioning paradigms used during the training and acquisition of self-administration behavior can be changed such that the subject will now have to modify its behavior to seek out the active compound under a new set of experimental conditions. Either of these techniques has been highly successful in assessing the discriminative properties of a variety of psychoactive substances.

Tolerance

Tolerance typically develops to all abused drugs such that more drug is required to produce the desired pharmacological effect. The mechanisms involved in tolerance may, in some cases, be an enhanced metabolism of the drug or, most often, a diminished response of the central nervous system (CNS) to the effects of the drug by as yet unknown mechanisms. Tolerance must be clearly shown to occur by demonstrating that more drug is required to produce a specific effect. Tolerance is often inferred in self-selection paradigms by noting increased patterns of drug administration with time, but it can be assessed more directly by administering the drug at various doses in tolerant and naive animals and measuring its subsequent behavioral or physiological effects. Generally, a parallel shift in the do&-response curve to the right, indicating that more drug is required in tolerant animals to produce the same effect as in drug-naive animals, is considered as a prerequisite to definitively establish whether long-term drug use has in fact produced tolerance.

Physical Dependence

A withdrawal syndrome should rapidly ensue upon abrupt withdrawal of the drug, which, in most cases, serves as a strong stimulus to continue to self-administer the drug. Typically, physical dependence or the withdrawal syndrome is characterized by signs and symptoms opposite to those produced acutely by the drug. This criterion is satisfied relatively easily, as, in most cases, the withdrawal syndrome is striking and uniquely characteristic for each drug.

DO ANABOLIC STEROIDS SATISFY THE CRITERIA FOR ABUSE POTENTIAL?

The question of whether anabolic steroids satisfy the criteria for abuse liability has not been unequivocally answered in large measure because of the factors outlined in the introduction, particularly the absence of well-controlled, double-blind studies utilizing placebo controls. Some investigators have concluded that double-blind studies cannot be carried out to assess the efficacy of steroids, since those assigned to the treatment group uniformly break the code because of some discriminative "beneficial" effects of the steroids (mood enhancement, relief of fatigue) or possibly their unwanted and adverse side effects (Crist et al. 1983; Freed et al. 1975; Taylor 1987; Wilson 1988). This issue will be discussed in detail, but there appears to be significant controversy regarding the discriminative properties of steroids and whether in fact subjects can truly discriminate between placebo and steroid administration. Even if one assumes that steroids can be easily discriminated by users, these discriminative properties should be exploited to examine whether the criteria described above can be met. Specifically, if these drugs can readily be identified by chronic users, then it should be possible to examine whether they are self-administered in a free-choice situation, whether they can be discriminated from placebo or other steroids, and, finally, whether tolerance and physical dependence actually develop. Unfortunately, we are unaware of any properly designed studies that have attempted to take advantage of the presumed discriminative properties of the steroids, which, it is claimed, render double-blind studies impossible to carry out, to assess the abuse liability of these compounds.

There are, however, numerous other problems with many of the studies reported to date, even in those that *can* be considered well designed and double-blind. For example, subject selection criteria have been particularly troublesome in terms of providing definitive conclusions. In all studies, only those persons already using steroids can be employed as research subjects for obvious ethical reasons. Because of this necessary consideration, the investigator has, at the outset, self-selected subjects who are highly motivated to enhance their performance and, significantly, fully anticipate, in most instances, that steroids will facilitate their exercise program. This variable poses sufficient problems by itself, but, in some studies, (Johnson and O'Shea 1969) subjects were assigned to treatment groups (active compound or placebo) on the basis of their willingness to take steroids. Those who believed that the steroid was too dangerous to take or feared its side effects based upon past history were assigned to the placebo group, whereas those expressing no concerns were assigned to the steroid group. Since both groups were athletes in training, it was assumed that motivational factors were therefore controlled. This appears to be a specious argument, since the regular users of steroids obviously expected that they would benefit from their use, whereas those who rejected the use of steroids knew that they were assigned to a placebo group and, hence, would be denied the real or perceived beneficial effects of the steroids. Under these conditions, it is perhaps not surprising that differences were shown between those assigned to steroid administration vs. placebo administration.

Finally, most investigators have focused exclusively on the issue of whether steroids enhance athletic performance or muscular development and, in some cases, have even made an attempt to discriminate between expectancy effects and the physiological actions of the steroid. However, the design of these studies does not lend itself to addressing the essential criteria necessary to establish abuse liability, since the studies were chronic in nature and did not use voluntary self-administration paradigms, which would be necessary to establish abuse liability as defined by the four criteria previously outlined.

Reported Effects of Steroids

Before assessing the extent to which the use of steroids satisfies the criteria for abuse liability, it is necessary to consider the pharmacological and physiological effects of steroids, the motivating factors responsible for the use and misuse of these compounds by regular users, and the numerous problems that have been encountered in examining these issues under well-controlled experimental conditions.

Steroids are reported by regular users to produce euphoria, a sense of well-being, increased libido, aggression, improved self-image, and, most commonly, an enhancement of athletic performance and muscular development (Haupt and Rovere 1984; Lombardo, this volume; Taylor 1987; Wilson 1988; Wilson and Griffin 1980). It is difficult to assess whether these self-reports represent immediate, discernible effects of the steroids or the expectation that the use of the steroid over time will produce these effects, because of the inherent limitations in the design of most studies carried out to date.

Despite the absence of a substantial data base regarding the real or perceived effects of steroids, there can be little question that the general public and, particularly, many young athletes are convinced that steroids enhance physique and athletic performance. Nonetheless, the results of the relatively few available double-blind studies using placebo controls indicate that there may be little scientific basis for this staunchly held belief. Although several studies have shown, under appropriately designed conditions, that steroids enhance athletic performance and that subjects can distinguish steroids from a placebo over an extended time period, an equal or perhaps greater number of studies have failed to demonstrate such effects (Haupt and Rovere 1984; Lamb 1984; Wilson 1988; Wilson and Griffin 1980). The literature supporting each position is illustrated in table 1. While not exhaustive, this listing of positive and negative studies represents those experiments in which reasonable designs were employed with appropriate numbers of subjects. The studies represented by an asterisk in this table represent well-controlled, double-blind studies. As can be seen from this extensive review of the literature, there are at least the same number, if not more, of negative studies as there are positive ones. Moreover, in many studies, the actual improvement in performance was so negligible that the efficacy of the steroids can be legitimately questioned, and it remains to be determined whether larger numbers of subjects would have produced statistically and biologically significant differences between groups. Nevertheless, on the basis of this review, it would seem reasonable to conclude that there is little compelling scientific evidence to support the concept that steroids enhance athletic performance.

The latter conclusion is heavily underscored by the results of a particularly important, well-controlled study by Ariel and Saville carried out in 1972, the results of which have not been challenged in the intervening 18 years. It was shown that subjects who were informed that they would receive daily injections of an anabolic steroid but instead received placebo could not recognize the difference and, notably, showed enhanced performance equivalent to that observed in those receiving the active compound. These

8

TABLE 1. *A Summary of studies that have reported that steroid use improved athletic performance or, conversely, had no effect*

Positive Studies	Negative Studies
O'Shea 1971*	Crist et al. 1983*
Johnson et al. 1972*	Fowler et al. 1965*
Freed et al. 1975	Hervey et al. 1976*
Ward 1973*	Holma 1977
Ariel 1973*	Ariel and Saville 1972
Ariel 1974*	Loughton and Ruhling 1977*
Win-May and Mya-Tu 1975*	Fahey and Brown 1973*
Hervey et al. 1981*	Stomme et al. 1974*
Johnson and O'Shea 1969	Johnson et al. 1975*
O'Shea 1974	Golding et al. 1974*
O'Shea and Winkler 1970	Samuels et al. 1942*

*Well-controlled, double-blind studies.

striking results not only indicate the need for rigorously controlled double-blind studies, but also point out the difficulty in documenting the primarily anecdotal reports that steroids enhance muscular development or athletic performance. If steroids do indeed enhance performance, a commonly held belief that is supported by intuitive and anecdotal evidence (Lombardo, this volume), then it should be possible to design appropriate studies to distinguish between expectancy effects and the demonstrable physiological effects of the steroids on athletic performance. Thus far, such studies are generally lacking.

Finally, it should be noted that the mechanism by which steroids enhance muscular development or athletic performance is not clear, if indeed steroids have such effects at all (Wilson 1988). The results of many studies examining this issue have been inconclusive, but it has been suggested that the effects of steroids in relieving fatigue may be more important in a vigorous training program than any known physiological effects of the steroids, e.g., direct effects on muscle mass. Moreover, it should be noted that, at the doses commonly employed by steroid misusers, all androgen receptors in brain and other androgen-sensitive organs are completely saturated (Wilson 1988), indicating that the full spectrum of their androgenic and anabolic effects should be expressed. Thus, the supraphysiological and suprapharmacological doses commonly used by steroid misusers may indicate either that the drugs are ingested for actions other than their normal physiological effects or that the subjects assume, perhaps incorrectly, that excessive doses of steroids will produce greater effects. There are insufficient data on hand to discriminate between these possibilities.

As a result of the factors discussed above, there is good reason to question whether the most frequently stated reasons for steroid use in chronic steroid misusers, i.e., enhancement of physique and athletic performance, is supported by any compelling scientific evidence concerning their efficacy in this regard. Most important, however, these experiments stress the need for reliance on well-controlled studies rather than anecdotal self-reports in assessing the efficacy of steroid use and in distinguishing between expectancy effects and the actual pharmacological or physiological actions of steroids.

Aside from the desired effect, a number of undesirable side effects follow ingestion of suprapharmacological doses of steroids (Haupt and Rovere 1984; Pope and Katz 1988; Taylor 1987; Wilson 1988). These include, most prominently, endocrine disturbances, particularly in adolescents; cardiac and liver problems; stunted growth; testicular atrophy; psychiatric disturbances; and violent expressions of hostility, frequently termed "roid rage" by chronic misusers. Despite the alarming incidence of these side effects, chronic users are still apparently willing to risk them to obtain what they believe will be a long-term desirable effect. Conversely, many users take steps to avoid the side effects of the steroids by ingesting other substances to counteract some of these adverse reactions, such as growth hormone and various prescription drugs, legally or illicitly obtained. Regrettably, however, the results of several recent surveys of a large number of steroid abusers indicated that, although many were aware of the side effects of steroid misuse, substantial numbers had little appreciation for the possible adverse consequences of chronic misuse (Fuller and LaFountain 1987; Johnson et al. 1989; Wilson 1988).

Additionally, because steroids are taken at doses that can only be described as suprapharmacological, well above the dose range necessary to produce therapeutic or "beneficial" physiological effects, the side effects are so readily discernible that, as discussed, double-blind studies may be very difficult to carry out. It is extremely important to note that the difficulty in carrying out double-blind studies may be owing to the users' ability to distinguish between the effects of the steroid and placebo based upon the side effects of chronic misuse rather than any perceived beneficial effects. This problem can easily be avoided if studies are carried out using dose ranges below those that produce a constellation of undesirable side effects but that would still be well within the range known to produce significant physiological effects, therapeutic effects, or both. These studies would be particularly important in terms of assessing whether steroid users ingest these compounds for their physiological effects or for some other reasons that have yet to be defined.

One final factor, which must be considered in evaluating the effects of steroids and determining their abuse liability, is the reasons most often given by individuals taking them on a regular basis. Several recent studies have examined this issue (Fuller and LaFountain 1987; Johnson et al. 1989; Taylor 1987; Wilson 1988). Not surprisingly, most users reported that, with a regular program of exercise and proper diet, steroids improved their physique and athletic performance and, thereby, their self-image, despite the fact that their efficacy in this regard is not altogether clear. Interestingly, some steroid misusers stated that even though they were not sure that the steroid had any direct athletic-enhancing performance effects, they used them because others against whom they were competing were suspected of using them, and, hence, they could not risk the possibility of losing the competitive edge. In addition, a relatively large number of adolescents reported that peer pressure was a significant factor in their decision to use steroids, and some reported that other presumed actions of the steroids, e.g., enhanced sexual performance, were strong motivating factors. These data clearly point out the need for educational efforts, as regular users are apparently not well versed on the full spectrum of the actions of steroids, including their efficacy in producing a desired effect, and, most important, the side effects associated with such misuse. Indeed, in all surveys examining the factors responsible for the use of steroids, the individuals uniformly reported that virtually all of their information concerning the efficacious effects of steroids and their side effects came from friends, magazines, information provided by "experts" at gyms, and, unfortunately, their coaches, in many instances.

It is apparent that most studies have focused on the long-term use of steroids by athletes. We are unaware of a single study in which the short-term, rewarding effects of steroids have been examined. The absence of these data make it virtually impossible to distinguish expectancy effects of the steroids from the immediate reinforcing properties of the drugs. Consequently, conclusions concerning their abuse liability, as defined pharmacologically by the four abuse-potential criteria discussed previously, are difficult at the present time.

Pharmacological Criteria for Assessing Abuse Potential

In discussing the available evidence regarding the extent to which steroids satisfy the pharmacological criteria for abuse liability there are very few studies that have directly examined this issue; much of the evidence represents self-reports, case histories, and anecdotal reports rather than systematic, well-controlled studies.

Self-Administration. Without question, human males self-administer steroids. Whether the drugs are self-administered for their immediate effects or the expectation of long-term gain is, as mentioned above, unresolved. As techniques are readily available to examine whether steroids have reinforcing properties, as discussed in the section on criteria to assess whether a substance has abuse potential and elsewhere (Brady 1988; Brady and Lucas 1984; Fischman and Mello 1989), it is difficult to understand the complete lack of attention to this critical issue. This paucity of data suggests either that negative results have been obtained or, most likely, that the issue has not been examined because investigators have correctly or incorrectly assumed that steroids are misused only for their long-term effects. Even if one assumes that steroids have only long-term effects, it would be extremely important to determine whether they have sufficient discriminative properties to permit an evaluation of self-administration behavior. Clearly, however, these studies should be carried out under well-controlled conditions consisting of at least the following: first, the use of doses within the physiological or therapeutic range rather than the suprapharmacological doses frequently taken by chronic users, which provide easily recognized side effects; and, second, permitting the subjects to voluntarily select their drug of choice from a variety of alternatives. These studies would be particularly important in determining whether steroids are self-administered for their direct immediate physiological or pharmacological effects or for some other reason.

As a particularly useful adjunct to human studies, the development of animal models would satisfactorily answer this question, since animals self-administer drugs solely for their immediate rewarding effects rather than for some long-term benefit. Unfortunately, no studies have shown that animals will self-administer steroids, and, in fact, there are reports (Louis Harris, personal communication) that rats could not be induced to self-administer steroids under a variety of conditions known to be optimal for other abused substances. However, unlike other abused substances, the most prevalent mechanism of steroid action is a genomic one that occurs at an extended time after steroid injection (see discussion of steroid actions on the brain). If the rewarding effects of steroids are mediated by genomic actions of steroids in brain, they might not occur until hours or days after the injection. This protracted period between injection and rewarding effects would render self-administration paradigms in humans and, particularly, animals useless. If, on the other hand, the rewarding effects of steroids were mediated by interactions with neurotransmitter receptors, then perhaps these effects could be discriminable. Nevertheless, it should be stressed that relatively little attention has been paid to the development of appropriate animal models, which would be extremely valuable in assessing the abuse potential of anabolic steroids, as they have been in the case of most commonly abused substances (Brady 1988; Brady and Lucas 1984).

Drug Discrimination. There have been no studies demonstrating that those persons abusing steroids can discriminate between their steroid of choice vs. other steroids or drugs or, for that matter, a placebo when given acutely. There are, however, conflicting reports regarding the issue of whether steroid abusers can detect differences between steroids and placebo in terms of the long-term physical or athletic performance-enhancing properties of these compounds. Some studies have shown that differences can be discerned (Crist et al. 1983; Freed et al. 1975) but only after extended periods, while other reports suggest that subjects cannot discriminate steroids from other compounds or even placebo (e.g., Ariel and Saville 1972). Moreover, in most studies, only placebo has been used as an alternative. To appropriately address whether steroids have discriminative properties, it would be necessary to offer structurally related steroids, with different pharmacological or physiological properties, as possible alternative choices. Of perhaps greater concern, there are no drug-discrimination studies available in which the subjects were actually allowed to voluntarily choose between their steroid of choice, placebo, or other compounds. Rather, all studies have simply involved randomly assigning subjects into drug or placebo groups and then determining at long-term intervals (weeks or months) whether they could appropriately identify the treatment group to which they were assigned. Aside from the fact that such studies have produced equivocal results, as discussed earlier, they do not appropriately address the issue of the discriminative properties of the drugs, as the studies have involved passive, nonvolitional administration, and the issue of what is being discriminated, e.g., side effects or therapeutic effects, has not been addressed. Appropriately designed self-selection paradigms seem to be the only way in which the discriminative properties of the steroids can be assessed. As for the criterion of self-administration of steroids, should the discriminative effects of steroids involve slow, genomic mechanisms of steroid action, the difficulties involved in appropriately designing self-selection paradigms might be insurmountable.

We are unaware of any studies demonstrating that animals can discriminate steroids from other drugs, which is not surprising, since there is no evidence that they are self-administered.

Tolerance. It has been reported that the use of steroids increases in frequency and amount in chronic users (Taylor 1987). While this has been interpreted as evidence of tolerance, there is no pharmacological evidence suggesting that tolerance actually develops, i.e., that more of the steroid is required to produce a specified pharmacological effect. Rather, the literature seems to be more consistent with the view that steroid abusers increase their usage under the assumption that more steroid use will have long-term advantages. As discussed previously, estrogen or androgen administration to animals is associated with enhanced behavioral sensitivity, not tolerance. If the misuse of steroids involves classical steroid hormone-receptor mechanisms, it is unlikely that tolerance would be demonstrable.

Physical Dependence. There is anecdotal evidence that the abrupt cessation of chronic steroid abuse leads to what has been termed a withdrawal syndrome (Taylor 1987). In general, the reported signs and symptoms (depression, decreased sexual desire, fatigue) seem to be the opposite of those observed during steroid administration, a finding that apparently satisfies the requirements for this criterion. However, it must be stressed that in all cases the subjects either abruptly withdrew themselves from steroids or their supply was suddenly terminated; hence, it is difficult to determine what role expectancy may play in these self-reports. Once again, double-blind studies would be required to address the important issue of the dependence liability of anabolic steroids.

Summary

From the brief review provided above, it seems clear that the use of steroids is a goal-oriented behavior, which some claim provides evidence that they are drugs of abuse (Taylor 1987). It remains to be determined whether steroid self-administration is based on their intrinsic pharmacological or reinforcing properties, or rather for some anticipated effect, real or perceived. As a result, it is unclear whether chronic users simply misuse these compounds or whether steroids have significant abuse liability as appropriately defined in a strict pharmacological sense.

In the preceding discussion, great pains have been taken to distinguish between abuse liability and the misuse of drugs. Although to many observers this distinction may be a matter of semantics. there is an important distinction. Many compounds or drugs are misused for a variety of reasons, such as the belief they may have some beneficial effect, but there is no clear indication that they have immediate pharmacological or therapeutic effects that would lead to their increased self-administration. By definition, the misuse of a drug should be restricted to describe a pattern of use that may or may not appear to be compulsive, for which there is no demonstrable therapeutic or otherwise beneficial effect. Since chronic users clearly do not use the suprapharmacological doses of steroids for their limited therapeutic value, and it is questionable whether the compounds have any substantive beneficial effects, it seems clear that they are misused substances like so many other drugs. On the other hand, abuse liability must be rigorously defined by the four abuse-potential criteria previously outlined. On the basis of the foregoing review of the litemture, it is apparent that there is insufficient information to determine whether steroids possess intrinsic abuse liability. It is hoped that this chapter will stimulate the necessary research in humans to unequivocally answer this question, but, at this time, it is extremely important that the casual use of the term "drug abuse" to refer to the misuse of steroids is not only pharmacologically inappropriate, but may lead to further confusion in an area of research already clouded by inconclusive experiments and excessive reliance on self-reports and anecdotal accounts.

Whether or not one chooses to conclude that the current literature supports the concept that steroids have abuse liability, this interpretation should not minimize the fact that the misuse of steroids is becoming an increasing social problem and that such use carries with it significant biomedical complications. Recent reviews (Fuller and LaFountaine 1987; Johnson et al. 1989) suggest an ever-growing use of anabolic steroids, particularly in adolescents, and little knowledge concerning the efficacious effects of the compounds, if any, or the potentially harmful side effects of long-term misuse. Consequently, this apparent epidemic of steroid use is a serious problem of drug misuse, which should be examined. It is not entirely clear how this problem should be tackled. Certainly, educational efforts must be made, but rigorous scientific inquiries should be undertaken to examine, under well-controlled, double-blind conditions, the prevalence of misuse, whether users are truly dependent on the drugs or rather are motivated to use the drugs by expectancy effects or other factors, and, ultimately, whether there is evidence of true abuse liability as defined pharmacologically. With this information in hand, both users of steroids and those who legally or illicitly prescribe them may be able to make better informed decisions.

Finally, it seems clear that animal models of steroid use and abuse must be developed, since they will ultimately provide valuable insights into the mechanisms involved in the abuse liability of steroids. Animal models have proven to be extremely useful tools in studies of the abuse potential of other drugs and their development in this area would be extremely valuable.

ROLE OF STEROIDS IN THE ABUSE OF OTHER SUBSTANCES

Steroid Modulation of the Acute Pharmacological Effects of Substances of Abuse

There is increasing evidence that steroids may participate in the acute and chronic effects of many abused substances.

It has been postulated that drug-induced alterations in the levels of testosterone may contribute to the mood changes associated with the acute effects of drugs, particularly alcohol (Mendelson and Mello 1974; Mendelson and Mello 1976; Mendelson and Mello 1979). These conclusions have not gained widespread acceptance for several reasons. For example, alcohol intoxication in some individuals produces aggression or hostility, whereas in others it generates passivity. In both groups of individuals, alcohol reduces serum testosterone levels; hence, there appears to be essentially no correlation between the mood-altering effects of alcohol and serum testosterone levels. In addition, it has been difficult to establish correlations between testosterone levels and mood shifts or passive-aggressive behavior under normal, drug-free conditions in humans or animals (Bancroft 1978; Doering et al. 1974; Mayer-Bahlburg et al. 1974; Persky et al. 1971; Sturup 1968). Despite these reservations and somewhat contradictory evidence against a relationship between alcohol-induced changes in serum testosterone levels and the behavioral effects of the drug, it would be unwise to dismiss the possibility of a link between steroids and alcohol's mood-altering properties.

Specifically, because of the slow onset and genomic effects of the steroids, poor correlations between the acute behavioral effects of alcohol and drug-induced modifications in steroid levels might be expected. Rather, it might be more profitable to focus on long-term correlations between serum testosterone levels and behavioral disturbances induced by chronic alcohol abuse. However, it should be noted that recent studies (Winslow and Miczek 1988; Winslow et al. 1988) have shown that there is, in fact, a strong positive correlation between acute changes in serum testosterone levels and mood shifts (passive-aggressive behavior) in nonhuman primates, but that these effects were dependent upon several factors, such as social context and endocrine status at the time of alcohol administration. These latter observations are particularly important, since they demonstrate not only that steroids may mediate at least some of alcohol's effect on behavior but that they may also help to explain the somewhat controversial nature of this relationship in humans reported in earlier studies.

In the female, attempts have been made to ask a somewhat different question: Do the marked alterations in sex steroids throughout the menstrual (human) or estrous (animal) cycle modify the acute response to abused drugs? The literature is now replete with evidence that the effects of opiate agonists and antagonists on reproductive hormones are markedly influenced by the stage of the estrous cycle in which they are administered (Cicero 1980a; Cicero 1980c; Cicero 1984; Cicero 1987). Similarly, the effects of alcohol on reproductive hormones are also affected by the stage of the estrous or menstrual cycle (Dees et al. 1985; Dees and Kozlowski 1984; Mello 1988; Mello et al. 1985; Mello et al. 1986a; Mello et al. 1986b; Mendelson et al. 1989). However, there is virtually nothing known about whether other pharmacological or physiological actions of alcohol or opiates are affected or whether the effects of other commonly abused drugs (marijuana, cocaine) are modulated by intrinsic fluctuations in female sex hormones.

As to whether there are alterations in drug-seeking behavior as a function of the menstrual or estrous cycle, there is little information at hand. While not conclusive, a limited number of studies suggest that the use of marijuana (Mello and Mendelson 1985) and alcohol (Belfer and Shader 1976, Belfer et al. 1971; Podolsky 1963) may increase during various phases of the menstrual cycle that appear to correlate with changes in mood swings. Clearly, these findings should be extended to determine whether a causal relationship exists between the self-administration of marijuana, alcohol, or both, and normal fluctuations in ovarian and pituitary hormones during the menstrual cycle in humans. At present, the data suggest a correlation, but cause-effect relationships are unclear, since an enhanced self-administration of a psychoactive compound at various points in the menstrual cycle could simply be related to alterations in mood, independent of steroid fluctuations per se. Nevertheless, these are exciting findings, and it would be of substantial interest to determine whether the self-administration of other drugs is similarly affected during the menstrual cycle.

We are aware of no systematic reports in the literature that would suggest that the self-administration of drugs of abuse is influenced by the menstrual cycle in nonhuman primates or the estrous cycle in animals. This paucity of data is difficult to understand, since such studies are clearly feasible and would provide valuable insights into the role of steroids in the abuse liability of commonly used drugs. Animal models would permit a degree of control of experimental variables that is clearly not feasible in humans and would, in the long run, provide much more definitive data.

In the male, the role of steroids in mediating the effects of substances of abuse has also been examined. There is now considerable evidence that steroids modulate the endocrine responses to opiates and to alcohol (Cicero 1980c, Cicero 1982a; Cicero 1982c; Cicero 1984; Cicero 1987). For example, recent studies in this laboratory have shown that in the testosterone-depleted, castrated male rat, the effects of morphine and alcohol on serum luteinizing hormone (LH) levels are diminished such that the normally suppressive effect of the drugs on serum LH levels was virtually abolished in long-term castrated male rats (Cicero et al. 1982b; Cicero et al. 1990). Interestingly, in these studies, we found that the castration-induced insensitivity to morphine and alcohol appeared to be selective to LH secretion because long- and short-term castrated and sham-operated rats were equally or more sensitive to other CNS effects of the two drugs. However, it should be noted that we have not assessed the full pharmacological profiles of morphine or alcohol in the castrated animal. It would be of substantial interest to determine whether other acute effects of these two drugs are affected in animals in which steroid concentrations are systematically altered. Given the discrete localization of steroids in the CNS, it should be possible to design studies to examine the effects of alcohol and morphine in castrated animals in which specified steroid levels are maintained and to examine how specific behavioral or physiological measures thought to be mediated by brain areas richly innervated by steroid-containing neuronal systems are affected.

The results discussed above clearly indicate that, in male animals, steroids may mediate at least some of the acute effects of alcohol and opiates. This area of research is in very early stages of development, but it promises to be. rewarding in terms of defining the possible role of steroids in mediating the actions, and consequently the use, of psychoactive compounds.

We are unaware of any studies in human males in which the possible role of steroids in mediating the effects of psychoactive compounds have been investigated. This is undoubtedly due to the absence in the human male of the very large and prominent rhythms in serum steroid levels that are observed in females. In addition, there are relatively few physiological conditions in which persistent increases or decreases in serum testosterone levels are observed, a fact that imposes restrictions on the types of experiments that can be. carried out. Nevertheless, there are circadian rhythms in testosterone release in the male, and, consequently, it should be possible to determine whether these fluctuations in any way modify the acute effects of a variety of commonly abused substances. At the present time, however, the castrated male rodent seems to provide an extremely valuable model to examine the role of testosterone in mediating the acute and chronic effects of abused substance-s, as the investigator has complete control of circulating serum testosterone levels throughout the course of the experiments.

Although the foregoing results suggest that steroids may play an important role in the acute effects of alcohol and opiates on reproductive function in the male rat, several extremely interesting questions remain to be examined: Do steroids participate in the nonendocrine effects of alcohol and morphine? Are the effects of other abused substances similarly affected by manipulations in the steroid milieu? Is the development of tolerance and physical dependence to morphine and alcohol altered by steroids? Are the reinforcing properties of these drugs affected by steroids? We are unaware of any systematic studies addressing these important issues. This is clearly an important area of research that deserves much greater attention.

One extremely interesting question, not discussed above, should be singled out for immediate, intensive study in view of the currently available evidence regarding an interaction between steroids and the effects of abused substances. Specifically, does the misuse of steroids by young athletes for prolonged periods of time result in any modifications in the effects of alcohol or other commonly abused drugs and, of perhaps greater interest, does the use of steroids lead to an enhanced self-administration of other abused substances? The literature reviewed in this section suggests that this possibility should be explored, but at the present time we are unaware of any literature relevant to this extremely important question. Clearly, this should be investigated and such studies can be easily carried out, initially by appropriately designed epidemiological studies.

Role of Steroids in the Development of Tolerance to Alcohol and Morphine

As discussed above, there is very limited information concerning the issue of whether steroids participate in the development of tolerance to and physical dependence on substances of abuse. However, there have been several recent attempts to examine whether drug-induced depressions in serum testosterone levels might be involved in the development of tolerance to these drugs (Cicero 1980a; Cicero 1980b; Cicero 1982a; Cicero 1982b; Cicero 1982c; Cicero 1984; Cicero 1985; Cicero 1987).

One particularly promising line of investigation has been an examination of the possibility that testosterone mediates the development of metabolic tolerance to alcohol, which is in part reflected by increases in the alcohol dehydrogenase (ADH)-dependent metabolism of alcohol. This system was initially selected for study, because it has been shown that testosterone modulates liver ADH activity. For example, castration leads to immediate increases in the ADH-dependent metabolism of ethanol in the male rat, and this effect is completely reversed by testosterone (Cicero et al. 1980; Cicero et al. 1982a; Israel et al. 1977; Israel et al. 1979; Mezey and Potter 1985; Rachamin et al. 1980). Because narcotics and alcohol share the ability to substantially depress serum testosterone levels (Cicero 1980a; Cicero 1980b; Cicero 1982a; Cicero 1982b; Cicero 1982c; Cicero 1983; Cicero 1984; Cicero 1985; Cicero 1987), a number of investigators have examined whether the chronic administration of alcohol or morphine led to testosterone-reversible increases in the metabolism of ethanol (Cicero et al. 1982a; Israel et al. 1977; Israel et al. 1979; Mezey and Potter 1985; Rachamin et al. 1980; Rachamin et al. 1984).

The results of these studies demonstrated that chronic morphine or alcohol administration, at doses sufficient to markedly depress serum testosterone levels (greater than 85 percent), produced large increases in liver ADH activity and the *in vivo* clearance of ethanol, which were equivalent to those observed in the castrated male rat. However, it has been shown (Cicero et al. 1982a; Israel et al. 1979; Rachamin et al. 1984) that, in contrast to the castrated male rat, testosterone replacement only partially reduced the effects of long-term ethanol or opiate administration on the induction of ADH and the *in vivo* metabolism of alcohol. Thus, it appears that drug-induced changes in serum testosterone levels can only partially account for the development of metabolic tolerance to alcohol. However, further studies of this issue seem to be warranted, as the hormonal changes associated with castration and ethanol or morphine administration are not simply confined to changes in testosterone; many other direct and indirect effects on other hormones occur as a result of treatment with these two drugs and castration. Consequently, systematic studies should be carried out to determine whether any of these well-documented changes in hormonal status contribute to the effects of the chronic intake of alcohol or morphine on the development of metabolic tolerance to alcohol.

As should be obvious from the foregoing studies, there is very little information available about the role of steroids in mediating the chronic effects of commonly abused substances, particularly in the development of tolerance and physical dependence. However, there are some suggestive data available and, given the fact that steroids exert powerful effects on the organization and function of the CNS, drug-induced changes in steroid levels may very well participate in the long-term effects of substances of abuse on the brain. In this connection, it has been observed by many investigators that all commonly abused depressant drugs such as alcohol, barbiturates, and morphine have profound effects on the reproductive endocrine axis resulting in persisting reductions in serum testosterone levels (Cicero 1980a; Cicero 1980b; Cicero 1982a; Cicero 1982b; Cicero 1982c; Cicero 1983; Cicero 1984; Cicero 1985; Cicero 1987). This shared property of these substances has led many investigators to suggest that long-term reductions in serum testosterone levels would lead to changes in testosterone-dependent organs including the brain, which may be similar to the well-documented changes associated with castration. Whether these changes simply represent a mechanism mediating some of the adverse consequences of long-term drug abuse or are involved in the processes associated with tolerance and physical dependence remains to be determined. With the availability of an appropriate animal model to examine these issues, progress in evaluating this issue should be readily attainable.

CONCLUSION

Review of the literature suggests that the abuse liability of anabolic steroids has been studied in very little detail. It must be concluded at this time that the use of steroids by humans does not meet the criteria necessary to establish that steroids have significant abuse liability as defined in pharmacological terms. It should be noted, however, that very few investigators have carried out studies designed to directly answer this question. Consequently, it would be unwise to definitively conclude that steroids lack abuse liability. Rather, the only appropriate interpretation of the status of research in this area is that there is insufficient information at hand to draw any meaningful conclusions. Obviously, given the now widespread use and misuse of steroids, much more detailed studies are required to determine whether they have significant abuse liability analogous to that observed with more commonly abused substances such as opiates, stimulants, depressants, and alcohol.

Whether or not it can be concluded at this time that steroids have significant abuse liability, there seems to be little question that steroids are misused by an increasing number of individuals for a variety of anticipated effects, including most prominently an enhancement of physique and athletic performance. Aside from the fact that the evidence concerning the efficacy of steroids in this regard is not compelling, it must be recognized that users believe that these compounds produce such effects, and the misuse of steroids is, consequently, becoming an important problem in society that cannot be ignored. It is hoped that this chapter has not only placed into context the distinction between the abuse liability and misuse of steroids but will also serve as a stimulus to investigators to carry out more extensive studies to examine more fully the incidence and motivating factors responsible for the use of steroids, their efficacy in producing the anticipated effects, the distinction between expectancy and the immediate reinforcing properties of steroids, and, finally, whether these compounds have abuse liability in the true sense of this term. The latter would be particularly important to having these compounds scheduled under the Controlled Substances Act by the Drug Enforcement Agency, as has been suggested (Taylor 1987).

Aside from the important problems related to the misuse or abuse liability of steroids, there is now a growing body of data that suggests that steroids may be involved in mediating the acute effects of substances of abuse on at least certain parameters and could be involved in those processes associated with tolerance and physical dependence. Although this is a very new area of research, it is a very promising approach that is worthy of much further investigation. Three particularly fruitful areas of research are: (1) whether intrinsic changes in sex steroids modulate the acute or chronic effects of abused substances; (2) whether drug-induced alterations in the steroid milieu in humans and animals are involved in mediating the acute and, particularly, chronic effects of substances of abuse; and (3) whether the acute effects of commonly abused drugs or their self-administration are modified by long-term steroid misuse in chronic users.

FOOTNOTES

1. This chapter was not presented at the National Institute on Drug Abuse Technical Review Meeting on anabolic steroid abuse held on March 6-7, 1989.

REFERENCES

Ariel, G. The effect of anabolic steroid upon skeletal muscle contractile force. *J Sports Med* 13:187, 1973.

Ariel, G. Residual effect of an anabolic steroid upon isotonic muscular force. *J Sports Med* 14:103, 1974.

Ariel, G., and Saville, W. Anabolic steroids: The physiological effects of placebos. *Med Sci Sports* 4:124, 1972.

Arnold, A.P., and Breedlove, S.M. Organizational and activational effects of sex steroid on brain and behavior: A reanalysis. *Horm Behav* 19:469-498, 1985.

Bancroft, J. The relationship between hormones and sexual behavior in humans. In: Hutchinson, J.B., ed. *Biological Determinants of Sexual Behavior.* New York: Wiley, 1978. pp. 493-520.

Beach, F.A., and Omdoff, R.K. Variation in the responsiveness of female rats to ovarian hormones as a function of preceding hormonal deprivation. *Horm Behav* 5:201-205, 1974.

Belfer, M.L., and Shader, R.I. Premenstrual factors as determinants of alcoholism in women. In: Greenblatt, M., and Schuckit, M.A., eds. *Alcohol Problems in Women and Children.* New York: Grúne and Stratton, 1976. pp. 97-102.

Belfer, M.L.; Shader, R.I.; Carroll, B.J.; and Hermatz, J.S. Alcoholism in women. *Arch Gen Psychiatry* 25:540-544, 1971.

Brady, J.V. The reinforcing properties of drugs and assessment of abuse liability. In: Harris, L.S., *ed. Problems of Drug Dependence, 1987. Proceedings of the 49th Annual Scientific Meeting, The Committee on Problems of Drug Dependence, Inc.* National Institute on Drug Abuse Research Monograph 81. DHHS Pub. No. (ADM)88-1564. Washington, DC: Supt. of Docs., U.S. Govt. Print. Off., 1988. pp. 440-452.

Brady, J.V., and Lucas, S.E. Testing for drugs for physical dependence and abuse liability. In: Brady, J.V., and Lukas, S.E., eds. *Testing Drugs for Physical Dependence Potential and Abuse Liability.* National Institute on Drug Abuse Research Monograph 52. DHHS Pub. No. (ADM)84-1332. Washington, DC: Supt. of Docs., U.S. Govt. Print. Off., 1984.

Brawer, J.R.; Schipper, H.; and Naftolin, F. Ovary-dependent degeneration in the hypothalamic arcuate nucleus. *Endocrinology* 107:274-279, 1980.

Breedlove, M., and Arnold, A. Sexually dimorphic motor nucleus in rat spinal cord: Response to adult hormone manipulation, absence in androgen insensitive rats. *Brain Res* 225:297-307, 1981.

Chung, S.K; Pfaff, D.W.; and Cohen, R.S. Estrogen-induced alterations in synaptic morphology in the midbrain central gray. *Exp Brain Res* 69:522-530, 1988.

Cicero, T.J. Common mechanisms underlying the effects of ethanol and narcotics on neuroendocrine function. In: Mello, N.K., ed. *Advances in Substance Abuse, Behavioral and Biological Research.* Vol. I. Greenwich, CT: JAI Press, Inc., 1980a. pp. 201-254.

Cicero, T.J. Alcohol self-administration, tolerance and withdrawal in humans and animals: Theoretical and methodological issues. In: Rigter, H., and Crabbe, J.C., eds. *Alcohol Tolerance and Dependence.* Amsterdam: Elsevier/North Holland Biomedical Press, 1980b. pp. 1-51.

Cicero, T.J. Sex differences in the effects of alcohol and other psychoactive drugs on endocrine function: Clinical and experimental evidence. In: Kalant, O.J., ed. *Alcohol and Drug Problems in Women. New* York: Plenum Press, 1980c. pp. 545-593.

Cicero, T.J. Neuroendocrinological effects of alcohol. In: Creger, W.P., *cd. Annual Review of Medicine.* Palo Alto: Annual Reviews, Inc., 1982a. pp. 123-142.

Cicero, T.J. Involvement of hormones in the development of tolerance to and physical dependence on ethanol. In: Collu, R., ed. *Brain Peptides and Hormones.* New York: Raven Press, 1982b. pp. 379-390.

Cicero, T.J. Pathogenesis of alcohol-induced endocrine abnormalities. *Adv Alc Substance Abuse* 1:87-112, 1982c.

Cicero, T.J. Endocrine mechanisms in tolerance to and physical dependence on alcohol. In: Begleiter, H., ed. Biological *Pathogenesis of Alcoholism, Biology of Alcoholism.* New York: Plenum Press, 1983. pp. 285-*357.*

Cicero, T.J. Opiate-mediated control of luteinizing hormone in the male: Physiological implications. In: Delitala, G., ed. *Opioid Modulation of Endocrine Function.* New York: Raven Press, 1984. pp. 211-222.

Cicero, T.J. Opiate-mediated control of luteinizing hormone in the male: Role in the development of narcotic tolerance and physical dependence. In: Sharp, C.W., ed. *Mechanisms of Tolerance and Dependence.* National Institute on Drug Abuse Research Monograph 54. DHHS Pub. No. (ADM)84-1330. Washington, DC: Supt. of Docs., U.S. Govt. Print, Off., 1985. pp. 184-208.

Cicero, T.J. Basic endocrine pharmacology of opioid agonists and antagonists. In: Wakeling and Furr, eds. *Pharmacology and Clinical Uses of Inhibitors of Hormone Secretion and Action.* London: Bailliere Tindall, 1987. pp. 518-537.

Cicero, T.J.; Bernard, J.D.; and Newman, K.S. Effects of castration and chronic morphine administration on liver alcohol dehydrogenase and the metabolism of ethanol in the male Sprague-Dawley rat. *J Pharmacol Exp Ther* 215:317-324, 1980.

Cicero, T.J.; Greenwald, J.; Neck, B.; and O'Connor, L. Castration-induced changes in the response of the hypothalamic-pituitary axis to alcohol in the male rat. *J Pharmacol Exp Ther* 252:456-461, 1990.

Cicero, T.J.; Meyer, E.R.; and Schmoeker, P.F. Development of tolerance to morphine's effects on luteinizing hormone secretion as a function of castration in the male rat. *J Pharmacol Exp Ther* 223:784-489, 1982a.

Cicero, T.J.; Newman, K.S.; Schmoeker, P.F.; and Meyer, E.R. Role of testosterone in ethanol- and morphine-induced increases in the alcohol dehydrogenase-dependent metabolism of ethanol in the male rat. *J Pharmacol Exp Ther* 222:20-28, 1982b.

Collins, V.J.; Boling, J.L.; Dempsey, E.W.; and Young, W.C. Quantitative studies of experimentally induced sexual receptivity in the spayed guinea-pig. *Endocrinology* 23:188-196, 1938.

Commins, D., and Yahr, P. Acetylcholinesterase activity in the sexually dimorphic area of the gerbil brain: Sex differences and influences of adult gonadal steroids. *J Comp Neurol* 224:123-131, 1984a.

Commins, D., and Yahr, P. Adult testosterone levels influence the morphology of a sexually dimorphic area in the mongolian gerbil brain. *J Comp Neurol* 224:132-140, 1984b.

Crist, D.M.; Stackpole, P.J.; and Peake, G.T. Effects of androgenic-anabolic steroids on neuromuscular power and body composition. *J Appl Physiol* 54:366-370, 1983.

Damassa, D., and Davidson, J.M. Effects of ovariectomy and constant light on responsiveness to estrogen in the rat. *Horm Behav* 4:269-279, 1973.

Davidson, J.M. Hormones and reproductive behavior. In: Levine, S., ed. *Hormones and Behavior. New* York: Academic Press, 1972. pp. 63-103.

Dees, W.L., and Kozlowski, G.P. Differential effects of ethanol on luteinizing hormone, follicle stimulating hormone and prolactin secretion in the female rat. *Alcohol* 1:429-433. 1984.

Dee-s, W.L.; Rettori, V.; Kozlowski, G.P.; and McCann, S.M. Ethanol and the pulsatile release of luteinizing hormone, follicle stimulating hormone and prolactin in ovariectomized rats. *Alcohol* 2:641-646, 1985.

Doering, C.H.; Brodie, H.K.; Kraemer, H.; Becker, H.; and Hamburg, D.A. Plasma testosterone levels in psychologic measures in men over a two month period. In: Frideman, R.C.; Richard, R.M.; and Vande Wiele, R.O.L., eds. *Sex Differences in Behavior.* New York: Wiley, 1974. pp. 413-431.

Eaton, G.; Goy, R.W.; and Resko, J.A. Brain uptake and metabolism of oestradiol benzoate and estrous behavior in ovariectomized guinea pigs. *Horm Behav* 6:81-97, 1975.

Fahey, T.D., and Brown, C.H. The effects of an anabolic steroid on the strength, body composition, and endurance of college males when accompanied by a weight training program. *Med Sci Sports* 5:272-276, 1973.

Feder, H.H.; Landau, I.T.; Marrone, B.L.; and Walker, W.A. Interactions between oestrogen and progesterone in neural tissues that mediate sexual behavior of guinea pigs. *Psychoneuroendocrinology* 2:337-347, 1977.

Fischman, M.W., and Mello, N.K. Testing for abuse liability of drugs in humans. In: Fischman, M.W., and Mello, N.K., eds. *Testing for Abuse Liability of Drugs in Humans.* National Institute on Drug Abuse Research Monograph 92. DHHS Pub. No. (ADM)89-1613. Washington, DC: Supt. of Docs., U.S. Govt. Print. Off., 1989.

Fowler, W.M.; Gardner, G.W.; and Egstrom, G.H. Effect of an anabolic steroid on physical performance of young men. *J Appl Physiol* 20:1038-1040, 1965.

Freed, D.L.J.; Banks, A.J.; Longson, D.; and Burley, P.M. Anabolic steroids in athletics: Crossover double-blind trial on weightlifters. *Br Med J* 2:471-473, 1975.

Fuller, J.R., and LaFountain, M.J. Performance-enhancing drugs in sport: A different form of drug abuse,. *Adolescence* 22:969-976, 1987.

Garcia-Segura, L.M.; Baetens, D.; and Naftolin, F. Synaptic remodelling in arcuate nucleus after injection of estradiol valerate in adult female rats. *Brain Res* 366:131-136, 1986.

Garcia-Segura, L.M.; Olmos, G.; Tranque, P.; and Naftolin, F. Rapid effects of gonadal steroids upon hypothalamic neuronal membrane ultrastructure. *J Steroid Biochem* 27:615-623, 1987.

Gerall, A.A., and Dunlap, J.L. The effect of experience and hormones on the initial receptivity in female and male rats. *Physiol Behav* 10:851-854, 1973.

Golding, L.A.; Freydinger, J.E.; and Fishel, S.S. Weight, size and strength: Unchanged with steroids. *Phys Sports Med* 2:39-43, 1974.

Gurney, M. Hormonal control of cell form and number in the zebra finch song system. *J Neurosci* 1:658-673, 1981.

Gurney, M. Behavioral correlates of sexual differentiation in the zebra finch song system. *Brain Res* 231:153-172, 1982.

Gurney, M., and Konishi, M. Hormone induced sexual differentiation of brain and behavior in zebra finches. *Science* 208:1380-1382, 1980.

Haupt, H.A., and Rovere, G.E. Anabolic steroids: A review of the literature. *Am J Sports Med* 12:469, 1984.

Hervey, G.R.; Hutchinson, I.; Knibbs, A.V.; Burkinshaw, L.; Jones, P.R.M.; Norgan, N.G.; and Lewell, M.J. Anabolic effects of methandienone in men undergoing athletic training. *Lancet* 2:699, 1976.

Hervey, G.R.; Knibbs, A.V.; Burkinshaw, L.; Morgan, D.B.; Jones, P.R.M.; Chettle, D.R.; and Vartsky, D. Effects of methandienone on the performance and body composition of men undergoing athletic training. *Clin Sci* 60:457-461, 1981.

Holma, P. Effect of an anabolic steroid on central and peripheral blood flow in well-trained male athletes. *Ann Clin Res* 9:215, 1977.

Hutchinson, J. Hypothalamic regulation of male sexual responsiveness to androgen. In: Hutchinson, J., ed. *Biological Determinants of Sexual Behavior.* New York: Wiley, 1978. pp. 277-318.

Israel, Y.; Khanna, J.M.; Kalant, H.; Stewart, D.H.; MacDonald, J.A.; Rachamin, G.; Wahid, S.; and Orrego, H. The spontaneously hypertensive rat as a model for studies on metabolic tolerance to ethanol. *Alcohol Clin Exp Res* 1:39-42, 1977.

Israel, Y.; Khanna, J.M.; Orrego, H.; Rachamin, G.; Wahid, S.; Britton, R.; MacDonald, A.; and Kalant, H. Studies on metabolic tolerance to alcohol, hepatomegaly and alcoholic liver disease. *Drug Alcohol Depend* 4:109-129, 1979.

Johnson, L.C.; Fisher, G.; Silvester, L.J.; and Hofheins, C.C. Anabolic steroid: Effects on strength, body weight, oxygen uptake and spermatogenesis upon mature males. *Med Sci Sports* 4:43-45, 1972.

Johnson, L.C., and O'Shea, J.P. Anabolic steroids: Effects on strength development. *Science* 165:957-959, 1969.

Johnson, L.C.; Roundy, E.D.; Allsen, P.E.; Fisher, A.G.; and Silvester, L.J. Effect of anabolic steroid treatment on endurance. *Med Sci Sports* 7:287-289, 1975.

Johnson, M.D.; Jay, M.S.; Shoup, B.; and Rickert, V.I. Anabolic steroid use by male adolescents. *Pediatrics* 83(6):921-924, 1989.

LaBella, F.S.; Kim, R.S.S.; and Templeton, J. Opiate receptor binding activity of 17-alpha estrogen steroids. *Life Sci* 23:1797-1804, 1978.

Lamb, D.R. Anabolic steroids in athletics: How well do they work and how dangerous are they? *Am J Sports Med* 12:31-38, 1984.

Loughton, S.J., and Ruhling, R.O. Human strength and endurance responses to anabolic steroid and training. *J Sports Med* 17:285-296, 1977.

Matsumoto, A., and Arai, Y. Synaptogenic effect of estrogen on the hypothalamic arcurate nucleus of the adult female rat. *Cell Tissue Res* 198:427-433, 1979.

Matsumoto, A., and Arai, Y. Neuronal plasticity in the deafferented hypothalamic arcuate nucleus of adult female rats and its enhancement by treatment with estrogen. *J Comp Neurol* 197:197-205, 1981.

Mayer-Bahlburg, H.F.; Nat, R.; Boon, D.A.; Sharma, M.; and Edwards, J.A. Aggressiveness and testosterone measures in man. *Psychosom Med* 36:269-274, 1974.

Meisel, R.L., and Pfaff, D.W. Progesterone effects on sexual behavior and neuronal ultrastructure in female rats. *Brain Res* 463:153-157, 1988.

Mello, N.K. Effects of alcohol abuse on reproductive function in women. In: Galanter, M., ed. *Recent Developments in Alcoholism.* Vol. 6. New York: Plenum Publishing Corporation, 1988. pp. 253-276.

Mello, N.K., and Mendelson, J.H. Operate acquisition of marihuana by women. *J Pharm Exp Ther* 235:162-171, 1985.

Mello, N.K.; Mendelson, J.H.; Bree, M.P.; Ellingboe, J.E.; and Skupney, A.S. Alcohol effects on luteinizing hormone and testosterone in male macaque monkeys. *J Pharmacol Exp Ther* 233:588-596, 1985.

Mello, N.K.; Mendelson, J.H.; Bree, M.P.; and Skupny, A.S.T. Alcohol effects on luteinizing hormone-releasing hormone stimulated luteinizing hormone and follicle-stimulating hormone in ovariectomized female rhesus monkeys. *J Pharmacol Exp Ther* 239:693-700, 1986a.

Mello, N.K.; Mendelson, J.H.; Bree, M.P.; and Skupny, A.S.T. Alcohol effects on luteinizing hormone-releasing hormone stimulated luteinizing hormone and follicle-stimulating hormone in the female rhesus monkey. *J Pharmacol Exp Ther* 326:590-595, 1986b.

Mendelson, J.H., and Mello, N.K. Alcohol, aggression and androgens. *Res Publ Assoc Res Nerv Ment Dis* 52:225-247, 1974.

Mendelson, J.H., and Mello, N.K. Behavioral and biochemical interrelations in alcoholism. *Ann Rev Med* 27:321-333, 1976.

Mendelson, J.H., and Mello, N.K. Biologic concomitants of alcoholism. *N Engl J Med* 301:912-921, 1979.

Mendelson, J.H.; Mello, N.K.; Teoh, S.K.; and Ellingboe, J. Alcohol effects on luteinizing hormone releasing hormone stimulated anterior pituitary and gonadal hormones in women. *J Pharmacol Exp Ther* 250:902-909, 1989.

Mezey, E., and Potter, J.J. Effect of castration on the turnover of rat liver alcohol dehydrogenase. *Biochem Pharmacol* 34:369-372, 1985.

Nottebohm, F. Testosterone triggers growth of brain vocal control nuclei in adult female *canaries. Brain Res* 189:429-436, 1980.

O'Shea, J.P. The effects of an anabolic steroid on dynamic strength levels of weightlifters. *NutrRep Int* 4:363-370, 1971.

O'Shea, J.P. A biochemical evaluation of the effects of stanaolol on adrenal, liver and muscle function in humans. *Nutr Rep Int* 10:381-388, 1974.

O'Shea, J.P., and Winkler, W. Biochemical and physical effects of an anabolic steroid in competitive swimmers and weightlifters. *Nutr Rep Int* 2:351-362, 1970.

Parsons, B.; Maclusky, N.J.; Krieger, M.S.; McEwen, B.S.; and Pfaff, D.W. The effects of long-term estrogen exposure on the induction of sexual behavior and measurements of brain estrogen and progestin receptors in the female rat. *Horm Behav* 13:301-313, 1979.

Phoenix, C.; Goy, R.; Get-all, A.; and Young, W. Organizing action of prenatally administered testosterone propionate on the tissues mediating mating behavior in the female guinea pig. *Endocrinology* 65:369-382, 1959.

Podolsky, E. Women alcoholics and premenstrual tension. *J Am Med Womens Assoc* 18:816-818, 1963.

Pope, H.G., and Katz, D.L. Affective and psychotic symptoms associated with anabolic steroid use. *Am J Psychiatry* 145:487-490, 1988,

Price, M.T.; Olney, J.W.; and Cicero, T.J. Proliferation of lamellar whorls in arcuate neurons of the hypothalamus of castrated and morphine-treated male rats. *Cell Tiss Res* 171:277-284, 1976.

Rachamin, G.; Britton, R.S.; MacDonald, J.A.; and Israel, Y. The inhibitory effect of testosterone on the development of metabolic tolerance to ethanol. *Alcohol* 1:283-291, 1984.

Rachamin, G.; MacDonald, A.; Wahid, S.; Clapp, J.; Khanna, J.; and Israel, Y. Modulation of alcohol dehydrogenase and ethanol metabolism by sex hormones in the spontaneously hypertensive rat. *Biochem J* 186:483-490, 1980.

Ramirez, V.D., and Dluzen, D. Is progesterone a pre-hormone in the CNS? *J Steroid Biochem* 27:589-598, 1987.

Robel P.; Bourreau, E.; Corpechot, C.; et al. Neuro-steroids: 38-hydroxy-Δ5-derivatives in rat and monkey brain. *J Steroid Biochem* 27:649-655, 1987.

Samuels, L.T.; Henschel, A.F.; and Keys, A. Influence of methyl testosterone on muscular work and creatine metabolism in normal young men. *J Clin Endocrinol Metab* 2:649-654, 1942.

Scheff, S.W.; Morse, J.K.; and Dekosky, S.T. Neurotrophic effects of steroids on lesion-induced growth in the hippocampus. I. The asteroidal condition. *Brain Res* 457:246-250, 1988.

Simmonds, M.A.; Turner, J.P.; and Harrison, N.L. Interactions of steroids with the GABA-A receptor complex. *Neuropharmacology* 23:877-878, 1984.

Steger, R.W.; Esquifino, A.I.; Femandez-Ruiz, J.J.; and Bartke, A. Prolonged neuroendocrine effects of a brief exposure of adult male rats to diethylstilbestrol. *Neuroendocrinology* 49:191-196, 1989.

Stromme, S.B.; Meen, H.D.; and Aakvaag, A. Effects of androgen-anabolic steroid on strength development and plasma testosterone levels in normal males. *Med Sci Sports* 6:203-208, 1974.

Sturup, G.K. Treatment of sexual offenders in Herstedvester, Denmark. *Acta Psychiatr Stand [Suppl]* 204:5-62, 1968.

Su, T.P.; London, E.D.; and Jaffe, J.H. Steroid binding at σ receptors suggests a link between endocrine, nervous, and immune systems. *Science* 240:219-221, 1988.

Taylor, W.N. Synthetic anabolic-androgenic steroids: A plea for controlled substance status. *Phys Sports Med* 15(5):140-150, 1987.

Towle, A.C.; and Sze, P.Y. Steroid binding to synaptic plasma membrane: Differential binding of glucocorticoids and gonadal steroids. *J Steroid Biochem* 18:135-143, 1983.

Ward, P. The effects of anabolic steroid on strength and lean body mass. *Med Sci Sports* 5:277-282, 1973.

Walker, W.A., and Feder, H.H. Inhibitory and facilitory effects of various anti-oestrogens on the induction of sexual behavior by estradiol benzoate in guinea pigs. *Brain Res* 134:455-465, 1977.

Whalen, R.E., and Nakayarna, K. Induction of oestrous behavior: Facilitation by repeated hormone treatments. *J Endocrinol* 33:525-526, 1965.

Wilson, J.D. Androgen abuse by athletes. *Endocrine Rev* 9:181-199, 1988.

Wilson, J.D., and Griffin, J.E. The use and misuse of androgens. *Metabolism* 29:1278-1295, 1980.

Win-May, M., and Mya-Tu, M. The effect of anabolic steroids on physical fitness. *J Sports Med Fitness* 15:266-271, 1975.

Winslow, J.T.; Ellingboe, J.; and Miczek, K.A. Effects of alcohol on aggressive behavior in squirrel monkeys: Influence of testosterone and social context. *Psychopharmacology* 95:356-363, 1988.

Winslow, J.T., and Miczek, K.A. Androgen dependency of alcohol effects on aggressive behavior: A seasonal rhythm in high-ranking squirrel monkeys. *Psychopharmacology* 95:92-98, 1988.

Young, W.C.; Goy, R.W.; and Phoenix, C.H. Hormones and sexual behavior. *Science* 143:212-218, 1964.

Yu, H.A., and Srinivasan, R. Effect of testosterone and 5-alpha dihydrotestosterone in the regeneration of the hypoglossal nerve in rats. *Exp Neural* 71:431-435, 1981.

ACKNOWLEDGMENTS

The authors' research described in this chapter was supported in part by U.S. Public Health Service grants DA 03833, AA 07144, and AA 03935. Theodore J. Cicero is a recipient of Research Scientist Award DA 00095.

AUTHORS

Theodore J. Cicero, Ph.D.
Professor of Neuropharmacology in Psychiatry

Lynn H. O'Connor, Ph.D.
Research Assistant Professor of Neuroendocrinology

Department of Psychiatry
Washington University School of Medicine
4940 Audubon Avenue
St. Louis, MO 63110

History of Anabolic-Androgenic Steroids[1]

Charles D. Kochakian

INTRODUCTION

It has been known for centuries that castration of the male results in the loss of not only fertility but also the secondary male sex characteristics. Castration was practiced by farmers to domesticate animals for work or to improve meat production, by churches to preserve the trained soprano voices of choir boys, by the Ottoman Empire and China to produce eunuchs as guards of harems and as servants, and by religious cults as late as the early 20th century, e.g., Skoptzs of Russia (Hoskins 1941).

MALE HORMONE

Transplantation of Testis in Capons: Blood-Borne Factor

The general consensus was that changes after castration were mediated through the nervous system. The first inkling as to the real regulation of these changes was provided by Berthold (1849), professor of medicine at Gottingen. In a simple and excellently designed experiment with only six roosters, he demonstrated that the well-known regression of the comb, wattles, and behavior that occurred after castration (figure 1) was prevented by the return of a testis to the abdominal cavity.[2] The transplant developed a new blood supply and maintained the castrated roosters in the normal manner. Berthold correctly deduced that since the transplanted testis no longer had its nerve connections, it produced something that was secreted into the blood and was transported to the target tissues to regulate their growth and maintenance. The importance of this study was not the successful transplantation of the testis but the interpretation of the results.[3] Hunter had earlier (Forbes 1947) successfully transplanted testis and other tissues incidental to his studies on teeth. He seemed to be interested in compatibility of tissues.

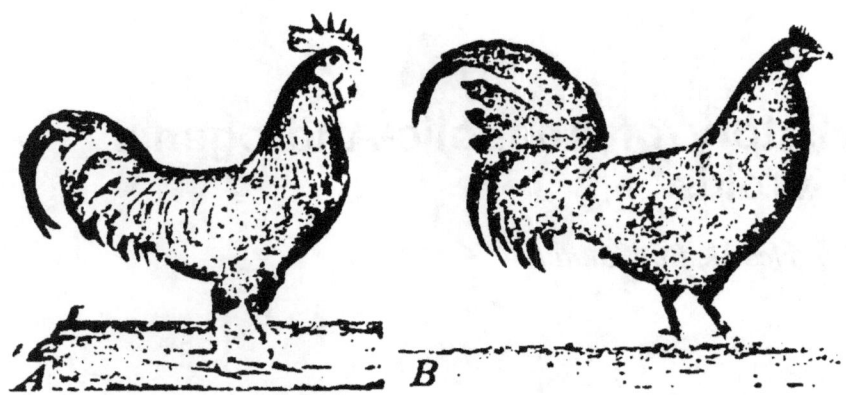

A. Normal brown leghorn cock. B. Brown leghorn capon. (After Domm

FIGURE 1. *Effect of castration on the comb and wattles of the brown leghorn rooster*

SOURCE: Moore 1939, copyright 1939, Williams and Wilkins Publishing Co.

In the subsequent 60 years, Berthold's results were questioned. Attempts by others to repeat the transplantation experiments were unsuccessful, except for Lode, who in 1891 did confirm Berthold's experiment; however, his results were ignored. After another 20 years, Pezard (1911) successfully repeated the effects of castration in roosters and, in 1912, fragmented the removed testes and deposited the fragments in the abdominal cavity of the castrated rooster (capon) (Pezard 1912). The combs and wattles of the capons were maintained. Shortly thereafter, an increasing interest in the development of the male reproductive tract resulted in many studies in laboratory rodents with attempts to produce extracts of the testis that would reverse the effects of castration (Moore 1939).

Testis Extract

Pezard (1911) also reported that an aqueous extract of pig testes maintained the comb and wattles of the capon.[4] F.C. Koch, professor of biochemistry at the University of Chicago, stimulated by the studies in the biology department by Lilly on the freemartin (Moore 1939) and by C.R. Moore on the development of the reproductive tract in male laboratory rodents, assigned McGee, for his doctoral dissertation, the extraction of bull testes. In 1927, McGee reported that an alcohol extract of bull testes stimulated the growth of the capon comb. Gallagher and Koch extended this seminal observation (Gallagher and Koch 1930; Gallagher and Koch 1934a). They improved the extraction procedure to produce a highly purified and active

30

preparation and developed the response of the capon comb into a quantitative assay method, which, with minor modifications, was adopted by most laboratories as the standard assay for "male hormone" activity (Gallagher and Koch 1930; Gallagher and Koch 1934a). At about the same time, regeneration of the accessory sex organs of the castrated rat (Moore and Gallagher 1930; Moore 1939) and the seminal vesicles of the castrated mouse (Voss 1930) were also suggested as methods of assay.

In the meantime, Pezard and Caridroit (1926) transplanted two fragments of the comb of a normal rooster to its back through an incision in its skin and found that they were maintained. One week after another rooster was castrated, two fragments of the comb were transplanted to its back. Both the comb *in situ* and the transplanted fragments exhibited the usual postcastration regression. He deduced, as had Berthold, that the active principal was in the blood and that it acted directly on the comb. On the basis of this observation, Funk and Harrow, in 1929, assumed that the active substance should be cleared by the kidney and appear in the urine. A crude cocentrate of alcohol-treated male urine stimulated the growth of the capon comb (Funk and Harrow 1929). Acidification of the urine, suggested by earlier studies on extraction of estrogens from female urine, followed by chloroform extraction, provided an oily active concentrate (Funk et al. 1930). Further purification and an increase in yield was effected by stronger acidification prior to chloroform extraction, followed by hydrolysis of the extract with sodium hydroxide solution, which removed many impurities and also estrogens (Funk et al. 1930). Other investigators (Freud et al. 1930; Loewe and Voss 1930) almost simultaneously developed similar extraction procedures. Thus, relatively simple methods for the production of highly active concentrates of what was designated "the male hormone" became available.

ANDROGENS

Isolation and Characterization of Androsterone

Butenandt in Windaus' laboratory at Gcttingen succeeded in isolating 15 mg of a pure substance from an extract of 25,000 L of male (policemen's) urine prepared by the Schering Corporation of Berlin by a modification of the Funk and Harrow procedure (Butenandt 1931; Butenandt and Tscherning 1934a). Butenandt had unsuccessfully attempted to isolate the active substance in bull testes before exploring the urine extract. Analysis of the urinary product indicated a hydroxyl and a ketone attached to a polycyclic nucleus like that of cholesterol; the compound was named androsterone (andro=male, ster=sterol, one=ketone) (Butenandt and Tscherning 1934a).

The structure of cholesterol had been and was being intensively studied in the laboratories of Windaus. The final elucidation of the ring structure of this compound was in the process of being accomplished (Fieser and Fieser

1959). Ruzicka, in the meantime, had become intrigued by the possible polycyclic structure of the compound and a possible relationship to the terpenes, which he had been successfully studying for the perfume industry. He reasoned that chromic acid oxidation of cholesterol should yield the polycyclic nucleus with a keto group at the site of the removed side chain. Therefore, he diverted the efforts of his young collaborators to this task (Ruzicka 1973; Ruzicka et al. 1934). Apparently Windaus had not considered that the polycyclic ring structure of cholesterol could survive the oxidative procedure and did not attempt to isolate the potential keto product. This is surprising, since he did isolate the intact side chain as the expected ketone. Ruzicka saturated the double bond of cholesterol prior to oxidation and treated the neutral fraction of the oxidized mixture for semicarbazone formation. He obtained the anticipated insoluble ketone derivative, albeit in small yield. The free compound possessed the comb-growth-producing property, but only at about one-seventh that of androsterone. It was assumed to be a stereoisomer of androsterone. Ruzicka's group then immediately proceeded, by known selective reductive and oxidative methods, to convert cholesterol to androsterone and its three possible isomers (figure 2) (Ruzicka et al. 1934). Thus, the chemical structure of androsterone and its relationship to the sterols was established.

Synthesis, Isolation, and Characterization of Testosterone

Studies on bull testes and on male urine were being conducted in parallel in a number of laboratories (Freud et al. 1930; Tausk 1984). Therefore, when androsterone was synthesized, its biological and chemical properties were compared with those of the testis extract. Two major differences became evident. The testis extract was more active in the stimulation of growth of the seminal vesicles and prostate of the castrated rat and mouse (Freud et al. 1930) and was labile to hot alkali (Gallagher and Koch 1934b). The alkaline lability, based on the recent studies with progesterone, suggested the presence of an unsaturated ketone in the testis product (Fieser and Fieser 1959; Tausk 1984). Both Ruzicka and Wettstein (1935a) and Butenandt and Kudszus (1935) recognized this possibility and immediately reported the synthesis of androstenedione from cholesterol. The compound possessed the chemical lability of the testis extract and showed a substantial increase in biological activity, but it was not as biologically active as the testis extract. Both investigators quickly converted the ketone at position 17 to a hydroxyl (Butenandt and Hanisch 1935; Ruzicka and Wettstein 1935b) (figure 3). This compound proved to have both the chemical and biological properties of the partially purified bull testis extract? In May 1935, David of Laqueur's group (David 1935) in Amsterdam reported the isolation of a crystalline compound from bull testes (10 mg from 100 kg), which had the chemical and biological properties of the newly synthesized compound, and named it testosterone (testo=testis, ster=sterol, one=ketone). Shortly thereafter, the Amsterdam group reported that the chemical structure of their compound was identical with that of the recently synthesized compound

32

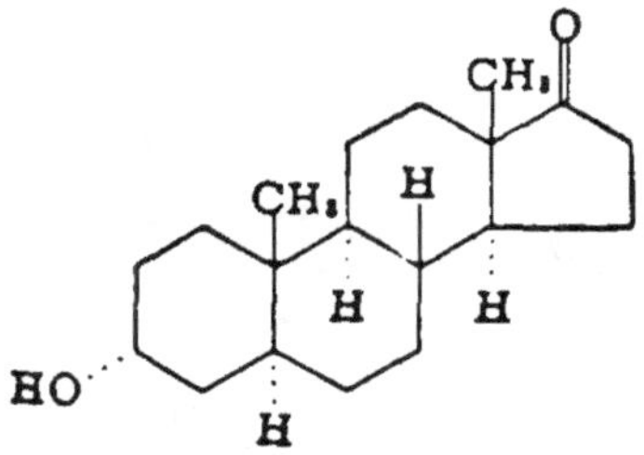

(1) Androsterone
183° +95° Al
I. U. 100γ

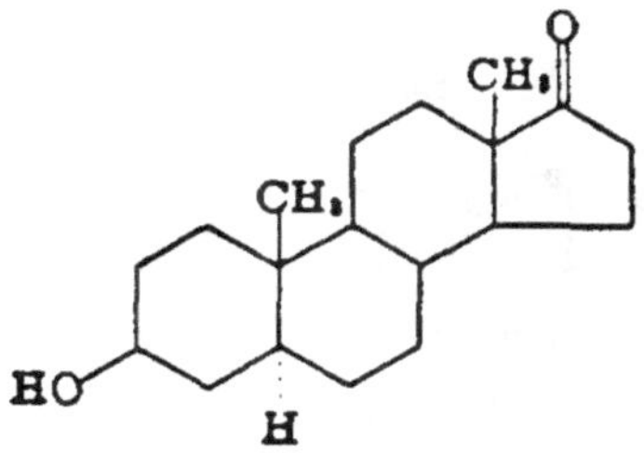

(2) Epiandrosterone
174° +87.5° Al
I. U. 700γ

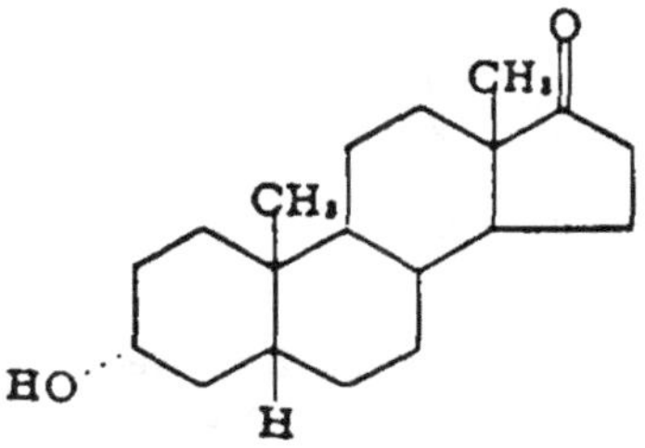

(3) 5β-Androsterone
151° +105° Al
Inactive

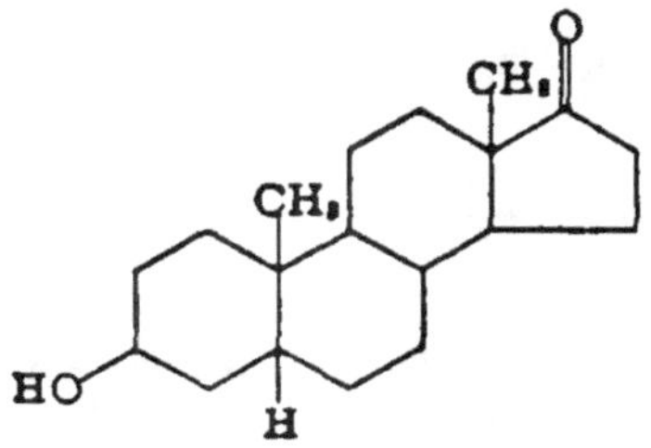

(4) 5β-Androstane-3β-ol-17-one
152° +88° Al
Inactive

FIGURE 2. *Androsterone and homers*

SOURCE: Fieser and Fieser 1959, copyright 1959, Reinhold Publishing Co.

(David et al. 1935). The slight delay in the report of the chemical structure was due to difficulty in the identification of the α,β-unsaturated keto character of the compound (Tausk 1984).

Family of Related C19 Steroids

It was becoming apparent that the body produced more than one compound with male hormonelike activity. Butenandt and Dannenbaum (1934) had already isolated a second compound from the male urine extract, an artifact (chlordehydroandrosterone) of dehydroandrosterone formed during the hydrochloric acid hydrolysis of the urine. Furthermore, they indicated that there probably were several more related compounds present in the urine, a conjecture which was amply confirmed over the subsequent years (Dorfman and

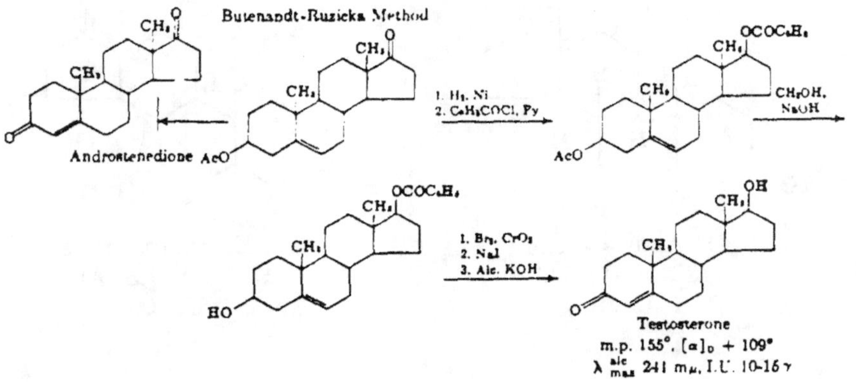

FIGURE 3. *Synthesis of androstenedione and testosterone from cholesterol via dehydrepiandrosterone*

SOURCE: Fieser and Fieser 1959, copyright 1959, Reinhold Publishing Co.

Ungar 1965). Thus, there was a family of compounds, and they were soon given the generic name of *androgens* (andro=male, gen=to produce).

Testosterone has the potential to be converted by tissue enzymes to 27 compounds (Kochakian 1959), three sets of nine steroids each: (1) Δ^4- and Δ^5-androstenes, (2) 5 α-androstanes, and (3) 5 β-androstanes with a difference of only 2 H+ between adjacent compounds (figure 4). The polycyclic nucleus of each compound had nine potential sites for α- or β--hydroxylation and also potential hydroxylation of the two angular methyls at C18 and C19. Thus the tissues have the possibility of producing at least another 540 compounds. Moreover, the unsaturated steroids may be converted to estrogens. In addition, a keto group may be formed at each of the nine positions on the ring nucleus, e.g., adrenosterone, and unsaturation may be introduced in the 3 and 16 positions by dehydration. Desaturation, however, at the 4 or 5 positions of the androstanes apparently does not occur. The metabolizing enzymes and the potential steroids, therefore, form a symphony that is kept in balance by delicate and skillful directorship to maintain a harmonious condition in the body. Many of these compounds are already recognized (Kochakian 1959; Kochakian and Arimasa 1976); others may be expected to become evident as the study of the metabolism of these steroids is extended to normal and abnormal conditions in both vertebrate and invertebrate animals and in humans.

The demonstration that testosterone could be prepared from cholesterol permitted organic chemists to synthesize all of the possible oxidized and reduced modifications (figure 4) and other modifications in search of a

34

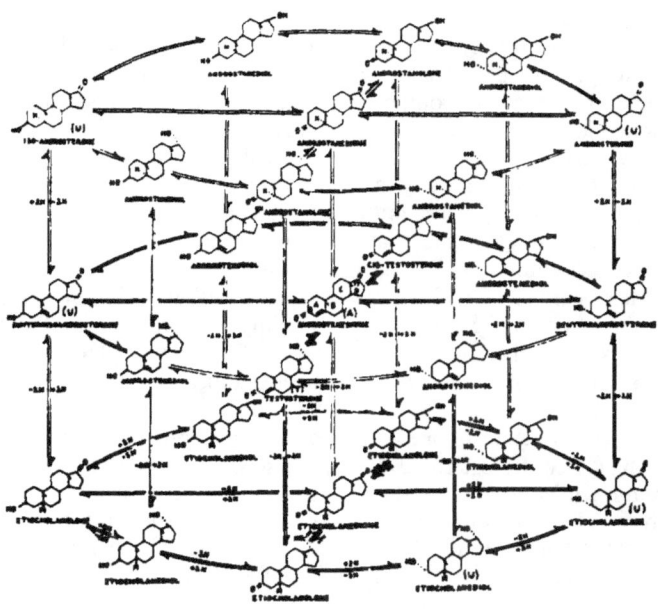

FIGURE 4. *The chemical interrelationship of metabolites of testosterone*

NOTE: The steric positions of the 17-hydroxyls are opposite to the accepted positions. This diagram was prepared in 1944 before the exact steric positions of the 17-hydroxyls had been established. Also, it is now apparent that the reverse reaction of **5α-** and **5β-**steroids to the **Δ⁴** or **Δ⁵** steroids does not occur.

SOURCE: Kochakian 1959, copyright 1959, Williams and Wilkins Publishing Co.

more biologically active compound for oral as well as parenteral administration. These two objectives were quickly achieved. The substitution of a methyl for the **17α** hydrogen yielded a highly effective oral compound, **17α** methyltestosterone, which was immediately accepted for clinical use. The later substitution of an ethyl instead of the methyl provided an even more effective steroid. Testosterone in the early studies appeared to be completely ineffective by oral administration. Later studies in mice (Kochakian 1952) and in man (Johnsen et al. 1974) demonstrated that testosterone was active by mouth if administered in sufficient quantity. An inefficient process.

It was observed early (Kochakian 1938) that the addition of fatty acids or impurities from extracts enhanced the biological activity of a parenterally administered oil solution of testosterone. These studies suggested that esters of testosterone would prove efficacious. The acetates of testosterone and related compounds already were available; they had been prepared to establish the presence of hydroxyl in the molecule. On bioassay, the acetate of testosterone proved to be more efficacious and also to provide a more prolonged activity. The propionate was even more effective (Kochakian 1938) and became the standard compound for parenteral administration. The further prolongation of activity with the propionate prompted the synthesis of several other esters with even greater extension of activity, which correlated with the length of the carboxylic acid of the ester. The prolongation has been extended as long as 4 months after the single injection of testosterone-trans-4n-butylcyclohexyl-carboxylate (Weinbauer et al. 1986). The introduction and recognition of 5α-dihydrotestosterone, 19-nortestosterone, and 5α-19-nortestosterone as effective agents was followed by the preparation of esters of the steroids. The rate of availability (absorption) of the esters to the tissues is an important factor in their effectiveness. Unfortunately, this property of these compounds has not been studied.

One of the esters (testosterone undecanoate) also proved to be orally more effective than free testosterone. It was absorbed through the lymphatic system and avoided rapid metabolism to less active forms by the enzymes of the liver. The minimum effective quantity still was much greater than that of a parenterally administered ester, e.g., 4x40 mg per day by mouth was less effective than 50 mg per week of testosterone isobutyrate by injection to transsexual women (Heresova et al. 1986).

ANABOLIC ACTIVITY AND NITROGEN BALANCE IN DOG AND MAN

The demonstration of male hormonelike activity in male urine provided not only a ready source of this substance for the isolation of androsterone but also stimulated many biological studies. Murlin, the discoverer of glucagon, was prompted to investigate whether this material also was responsible for the difference in basal metabolic rate (BMR) between males and females. He assigned two medical students in 1931 to conduct a pilot study as their class project. They found that a Funk and Harrow-type extract of medical student urine increased the BMR of a castrated dog. In the fall of 1933, I was appointed as a graduate assistant to confirm and extend this exciting observation (Kochakian 1984). In spite of repeated experiments at several dose levels, I was unable to confirm the increase in BMR. Thereupon, Murlin suggested the investigation of protein metabolism. This suggestion probably was prompted by his earlier studies on nitrogen balance during pregnancy in dogs (Murlin 1911). The urine extract produced an immediate and strongly positive nitrogen balance in two castrated dogs (figure 5). The results were reported in 1935 (Kochakian 1935; Kochakian and Murlin

36

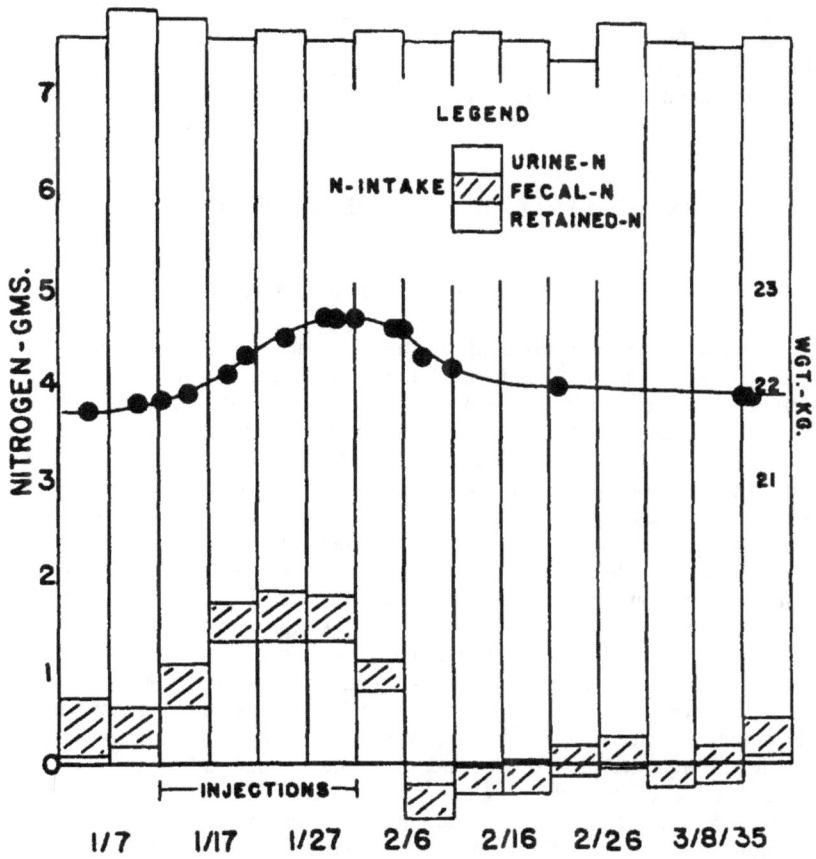

FIGURE 5. *Effect of "male hormone" urine extract on nitrogen metabolism and body weight of the castrated dog*

SOURCE: Kochakian and Murlin 1935, copyright 1935, American Institute of Nutrition.

1935) at the same time that androsterone, then androstenedione, and testosterone were being characterized and synthesized. The experiments were immediately repeated with androstenedione (Kochakian and Murlin 1936), which I synthesized, and testosterone and testosterone acetate (Kochakian 1937), which had become commercially available, to give results identical with those of the urinary extract. Shortly thereafter, Kenyon et al. (1938) reported identical results in eunuchoid men with the commercially available testosterone propionate. Kenyon, of the University of Chicago, was an unusual clinician with a keen interest in basic research. He not only became very interested in the research activity in the biology and biochemistry departments, but also recognized the potential application to clinical deficiencies. He developed a close friendship with Moore, Koch, and Gallagher, which produced many fruitful discussions. I was fortunate to make his acquaintance through our membership and participation in the Josiah Macy, Jr. Foundation Conferences on Bone and Wound Healing (later designated as the Metabolic Aspects of Convalescence).

PARTIAL DISSOCIATION OF ANABOLIC FROM ANDROGENIC ACTIVITY

Renotrophic Activity of Androgens in Mice and Rats

The potential therapeutic value of the anabolic activity of testosterone and its commercial availability stimulated many investigations in diverse anabolic-deficient conditions (Reifenstein 1942; Landau 1976), including intensive studies in women with breast cancer. A strong impetus was given to these investigations by the Josiah Macy, Jr. Foundation Conferences under the organization of Frank Fremont-Smith and the leadership of Fuller Albright. Clinical use of testosterone, however, always presented the objectionable accompanying vitilization, especially in women and children. A possible answer to this problem appeared imminent. As one aspect of my program to elucidate the nature and mechanism of the anabolic action, I decided to compare the effect of a number of steroids on their relative ability to stimulate growth in the sensitive mouse kidney (anabolic) (figure 6) (Selye 1939; Pfeiffer et al. 1940) with that in the seminal vesicles and prostate (androgenic). The synthesis of the many modifications of testosterone provided a ready source of steroids for my proposed study. These steroids were made available through the generous cooperation and support of Ernst Oppenheimer, director of research at CIBA Pharmaceutical Products, Summit, NJ. In 1942 I reported (table 1) (Kochakian 1942) that 5α-androstane-3α, 17β-diol (figure 7) possessed the same renotrophic (anabolic) as, but lesser androgenic activity than, testosterone at physiological doses (figure 8). The dichotomy disappeared with excessive doses, which produced comparable maximum responses in both organs (Kochakian 1946; Kochakian 1977). A similar relationship was noted in the rat (table 2) (Kochakian 1977).

The partial separation of the two biological activities by reduction in the A-ring of testosterone suggested the testing of steroids with an oxygen substituent in only the 3- or 17-position. These compounds proved to be too insoluble to be absorbed in sufficient quantity by parenteral administration (implanted pellets) to provide a growth response in either of the organs. I decided, then, to test them by oral administration. Not all of the mono-oxygenated steroids could be assayed, because of their limited quantities. The available steroids, however, produced an exciting result. The lack of an oxygen substituent at the 3-position gave a compound, 17α-methyl-5α-androstan-17β-ol, which possessed a similar renotrophic but a much lesser

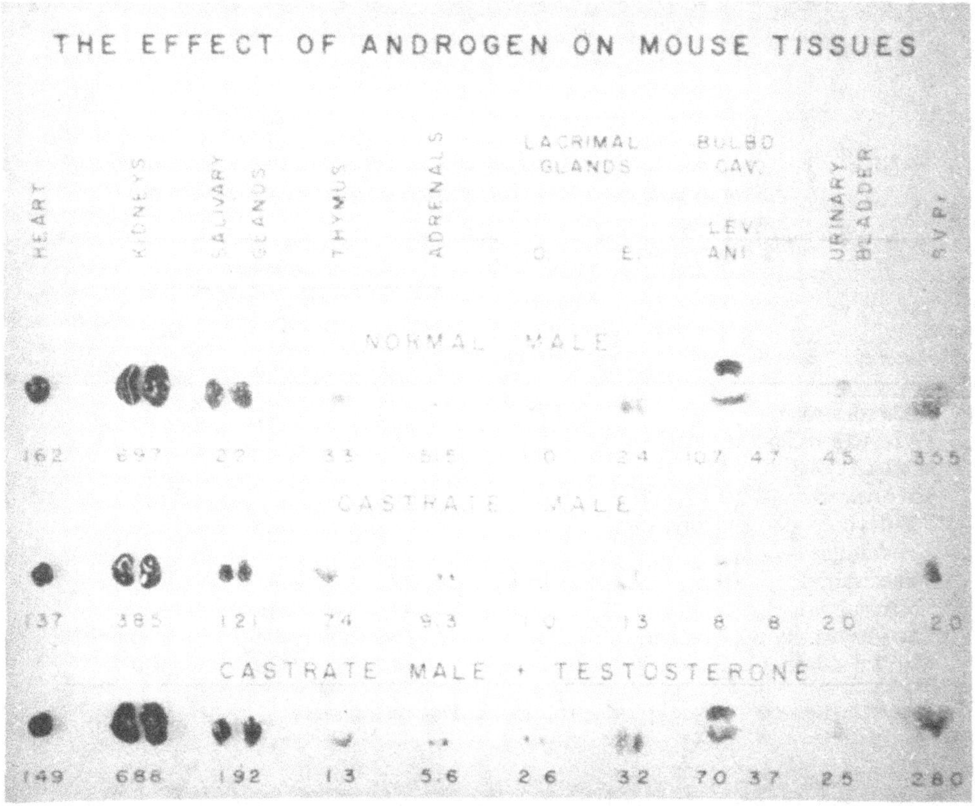

FIGURE 6. *The effect of castration and testosterone propionate on the weight of several organs of the mouse*

NOTE: The body weight and the seminal vesicles, prostate, kidney, salivary glands, lachrymal glands, and the bulbocavernosus and "levator ani" muscles exhibit a log-dose response to active steroids. Thus, the castrated mouse is a potential model for multiple assay.

SOURCE: Kochakian 1975, copyright 1975, Pergamon Press.

(one-third) androgenic effect than 17α-methyltestosterone (Kochakian 1953) providing further confirmation of importance of the nature of the A-ring for androgenic activity.

Myotrophic Activity of Androgens in Guinea Pigs

Papanicolaou and Falk (1938) had reported that the temporal and the masseter muscles of the guinea pig were much larger in the male than in the female and that castration of the male resulted in female-size muscles. Administration of testosterone propionate restored the weight of the muscles in the castrated male and increased those of the female to those of the male. They assumed this to be a general effect on skeletal muscles. These observations were made incidental to their studies on the reproductive cycle of the female guinea pig, which led to the now well-known "Pap smear" for vaginal cancer. I reported a confirmation of these results with the

TABLE 1. *Comparison of effect of chemical structure on the renotrophic-androgenic activities of various steroids in the castrated mouse*

| Steroid | Steroid Absorbed mg/30 days | Increase | | |
		Kidney mg	Sem. Ves. and Pros. mg	K/Sv. Pr. mg/mg
Androsterone	13.0	65	20	3.3
17α-Methyl-5α-androstane-3α,17β-diol	2.6	261	157	1.7
5α-Androstane-3α,17β-diol	1.7	202	137	1.5
17β-Hydroxy-17-methyl -5α-androstan-3-one	0.2	193	148	1.3
Testosterone	0.14	125	144	0.9
Normal mice	—	162	216	0.7
5α-Androstane-3,17-dione	32.3	60	95	0.6
Androst-4-ene-3.17-dione	10.6	84	173	0.5

SOURCE: Kochakian 1944, copyright 1944, American Physiological Society.

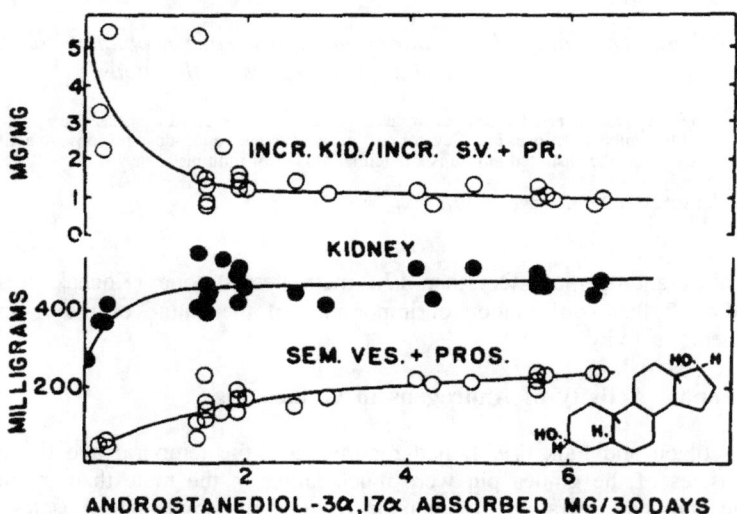

FIGURE 7. *A comparison of the renotrophic and androgenic activities in castrated mice at different doses of androstane-3α,17β-diol*

NOTE: The 17 hydroxyl was later proven to be in β and not the α position.

SOURCE: Kochakian 1946, copyright 1946, American Physiological Society

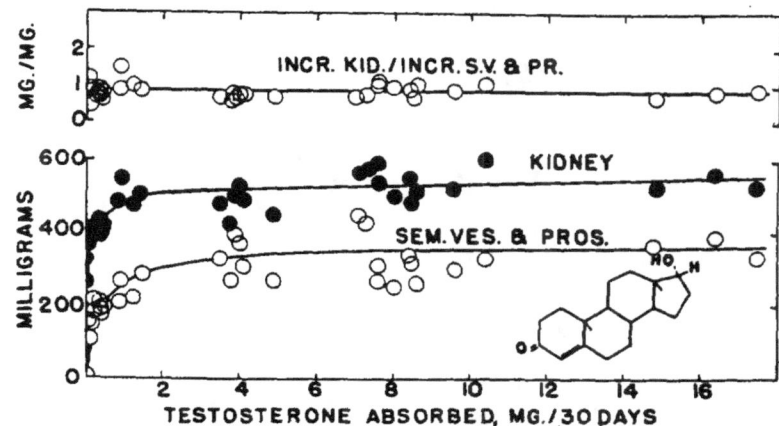

FIGURE 8. *A comparison of the renotrophic and androgenic activities in castrated mice at different doses of testosterone*

SOURCE: Kochakian 1946, coyright 1946, American Physiological Society.

TABLE 2. *Comparison of the renotrophic and androgenic action of various androgens at 1 mg/day for 21 days in the rat*

		Increase			
Treatment	Rats (No.)	Body Weight g	Kidney g	Sem. ves. and pros. g	K/Sv. Pr. g/g
Castrated	12	2	(2.00)	(0.21)	
Normal	6	0	—		
5α-Androstane-3α,17β-diol	2	25	0.94	3.30	0.29
17β- Hydroxy-5α-androstan-3-one	2	14	0.50	2.83	0.18
Testosterone propionate	8	21	0.22	4.27	0.05
Androst-4-ene-3,17-dione	2	10	0.15	1.70	0.09

NOTE: Rats on constant food intake for nitrogen balance studies; body weights approximately 300 g. The figures in parentheses are the absolute values.

SOURCE: Based on data in Kochakian 1977: Kochakian 1964.

temporal muscle (figure 9) (Kochakian et al. 1948). The increase in weight was due to hypertrophy (figure 10). A comparison of the effectiveness of several steroids revealed that 5α-andrastane-3α, 17β-diol produced a dichotomy between the growth of the muscle and the accessory sex organs similar

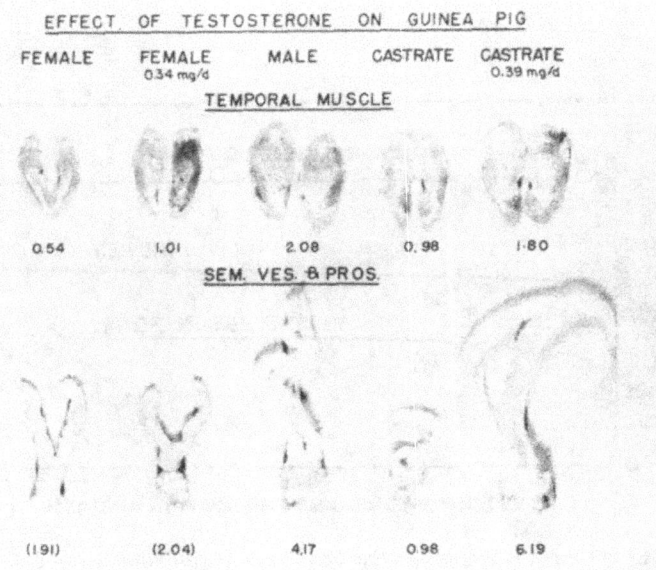

FIGURE 9. *Comparison of the size of the temporal muscle of the male and female guinea pig and the effect of castration and testosterone propionate*

SOURCE: Kochakian 1975, copyright 1975, Pergamon Press.

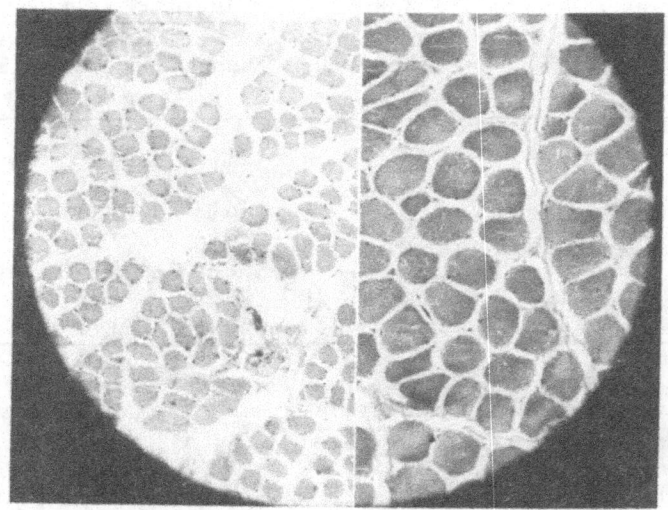

FIGURE 10. *A comparison of the diameter of the fibers in the temporal muscle of the normal and castrated guinea pig*

to that observed in a comparison of renotrophic and androgenic activity in the mouse and rat. The study was then extended to include 47 other muscles to determine the general nature of the response (Kochakian and Tillotson 1957; Kochakian 1975). The increase in size of the different muscles differed not only for the several steroids but also for the individual muscles (tables 3 and 4). The sensitivity of the muscles to the steroids was greatest in the head and neck region and gradually diminished from head to hindquarters (figure 11). The more responsive muscles exhibited a more favorable myotrophic than androgenic activity with 5α--androstane-3α, 17β-diol and the other 5α-androstanediols. Of further interest was the effect of 5α-dihydrotestosterone 5α-DHT). It was more active than testosterone in its androgenic effect and even more active in the myotrophic effect (tables 3 and 4). Furthermore, although testosterone and 5α-dihydrotestosterone produced no significant difference in the increase in weight of the uterus of the ovariectomized rat, they differ in their actions at the cellular level. Testosterone markedly increased the height of the luminal epithelium and stimulated glandular secretion, but 5α-dihydrotestosterone was ineffective in these actions. On the other hand, 5α-dihydrotestosterone stimulated a greater growth of the myometrium (Gonzalez-Diddi 1972).

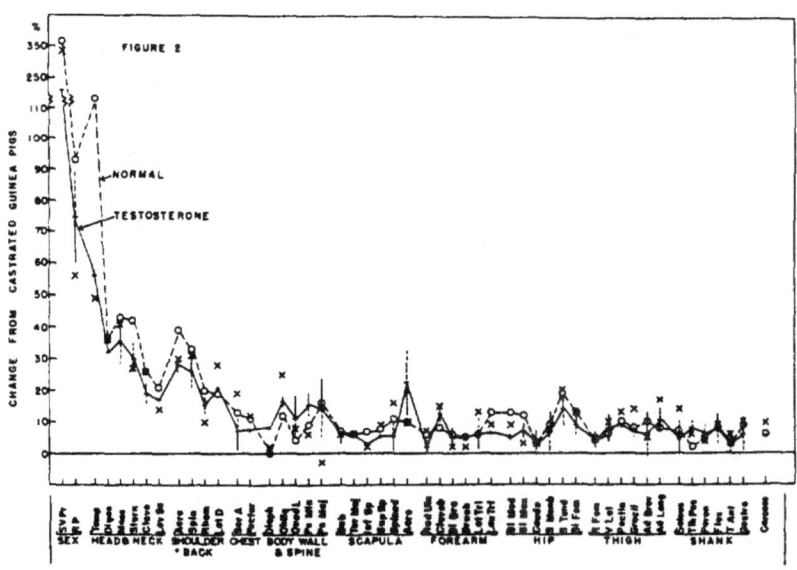

FIGURE 11. *Response of the individual muscles of the castrated guinea pig to testosterone stimulation*

SOURCE: Kochakian and Tillotson 1957, copyright 1957, The Endocrine Society.

TABLE 3. *Relative myotrophic and androgenic potencies of several C_{19} steroids*

Steroid	Sem. Ves. and Pros.	Digastric	Masseter	Clavo- trapezius	Temporal	Sterno- mastoid	Retractor Penis
Androstan-17β-ol,3-one	150	380	320	280	230	190	150
Testosterone	100	100	100	100	100	100	100
Methylandrosterone	100	140	120	80	90	100	80
Methylandrostan-17β-ol,3-one	50	60	70	280	70	90	30
Androstane-3α,17β-diol	50	60	50	40	30	20	100
Methyltestosterone	16	30	20	9	20	—	4
Methylandrostane-3α,17β-diol	17	10	10	—	10	3	20
Androstene-3,17-dione	16	20	10	20	10	8	8
Androstane-3,17-dione	15	10	4	20	10	3	4
Dehydroepiandrosterone	5	10	6	—	4	—	30
Epiandrosterone							

NOTE: The respective values are compared to those of testosterone set at 100.

SOURCE: Kochakian and Tillotson 1957, copyright 1957, The Endocrine Society.

TABLE 4. *Ratio of myotrophic to androgenic (seminal vesicles and prostates) activity of several C_{19} steroids*

Steroid	Digastric	Masseter	Clavo-trapezius	Temporal	Sterno-mastoid	Retractor Penis
Androstan-17β-ol,3-one	2.5	2.1	1.9	1.5	1.3	1.0
Androstane -3α,17β-diol	1.2	1.4	5.7	1.4	1.8	0.6
Methylandrostane -17β-ol,3-one	1.4	1.2	0.8	0.9	1.0	0.8
Methylandrostane -3α,17β-diol	1.8	1.2	0.6	1.3	—	0.3
Testosterone	1.0	1.0	1.0	1.0	1.0	1.0
Methyltestosterone	1.2	1.0	0.7	0.5	0.4	1.9
Androstane-3,17-dione	1.3	0.8	1.4	1.3	0.5	0.5
Epiandrosterone	2.6	1.2	—	0.8	—	5.8
Androstene3,17-dione	0.8	0.8	—	3.6	0.2	1.3
Dehydroepiandrosterone	0.7	0.3	1.5	0.7	0.2	0.3

NOTE: The respective values are compared to those of testosterone set at 1.0.

SOURCE: Kochakian and Tillotson 1957, copyright 1957, The Endocrine Society.

Nitrogen Balance in Rats

Although both the mouse kidney and several muscles of the guinea pig exhibited typical log-dose responses, they were not simple enough to be attractive as routine assay procedures. Nitrogen balance studies in the dog were too expensive and time consuming. The extension of the nitrogen balance studies to castrated rats as another phase in the delineation of the nature and mechanism of the anabolic action of steroids, showed a log-dose-response effect, but again the procedure was not sufficiently simple to provide a routine assay method (figure 12) (Kochakian 1950). However,

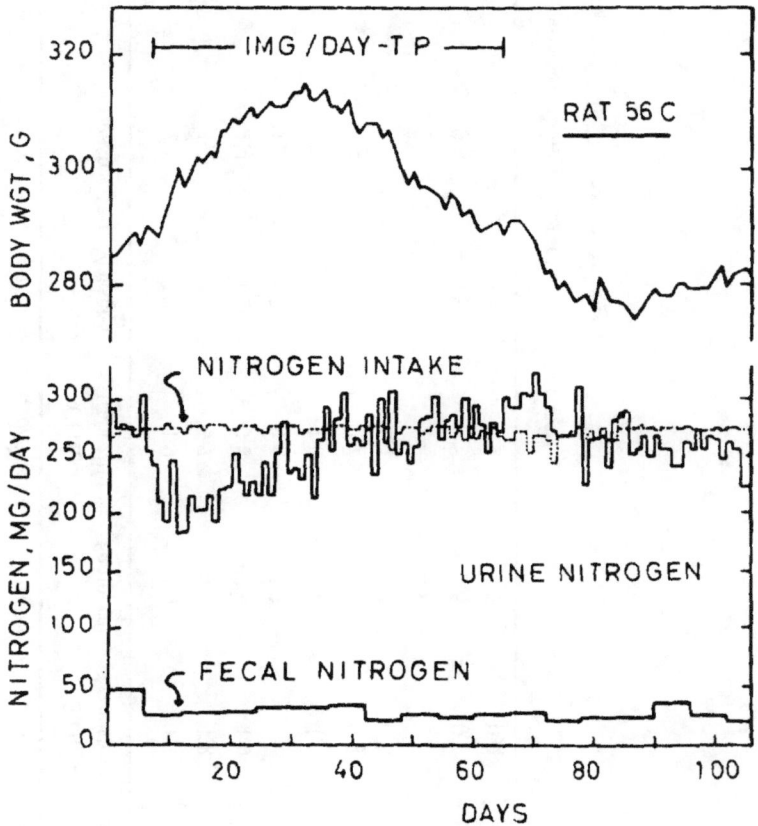

FIGURE 12. *The effect of testosterone propionate on the body weight and nitrogen balance of the adult castrated rat*

SOURCE: Kochakian 1950, copyright 1950, American Physiological Society.

the comparison of a number of natural steroids indicated testosterone propionate to be the most active steroid; androsterone showed only a trace of activity. Therefore, the anabolic activity in the urine extract could not have been due to the presence of androsterone. Furthermore, the urine extract was much more potent than androsterone in the stimulation of regeneration of the accessory sex organs of the castrated rat (Kochakian 1938).

Levator Ani Assay

The suggestion by Eisenberg and Gordan in 1950 that the observations of Wainman and Shipounoff (1941) on the dependency of the "levator ani" muscle of the rat to testosterone be used as representative of the anabolic action of androgens gained attention. Hershberger et al. (1953) reported a quantitative assay procedure in the castrated rat and found that 19-nortestosterone stimulated a greater response in this muscle than in the accessory sex organs. The "levator ani" muscle later proved to be the sex-linked dorsal bulbocavernosus muscle, but the assay, because of its inexpensiveness, simplicity, and use of the common laboratory animal, received wide use as a screening procedure. Overbeek et al. (1961) and Overbeek (1966) have made a careful study of the assay procedure and stipulate conditions to provide results that will permit a valid comparison of the biological activity of the steroids.

The synthesis of modifications of the natural compounds rapidly followed, approximately 2,000, to provide an interesting comparison of chemical structure with biological activity (Overbeek 1966; Vida 1969; Camerino and Sziacky 1975; Potts et al. 1976; Hilger and Hummel 1964). Many of the more active compounds (tables 5 and 6) have been further studied and confirmed by nitrogen balance experiments in castrated rats (table 6) by minor modifications of Kochakian's procedure (1984) and in monkeys and humans (tables 7 and 8) (Kochakian 1975; Potts et al. 1976).

The partial separation of the effect of the modified steroids on the "levator ani" muscle from that on the seminal vesicles or prostate of the castrated rat was achieved by modifications in the A-ring of both the orally and parenterally active steroids (tables 5 to 8). The efficacy of the parenterally active steroids was further enhanced by the esterification of the 17β-hydroxyl to provide an extended activity.

In several instances, the modification of the steroid not only effected a greater growth of the "levator ani" muscle than of the seminal vesicles or prostate, but also produced, in the weight of both of the organs, a greater increase than that produced by the unmodified steroid. In general, as in the case of the mouse and guinea pig experiments, the partial separation of the anabolic from the androgenic activity was due partly to a lesser stimulation of the growth of the accessory sex organs with a greater stimulation of the growth of the "levator ani" muscle. Esterification of the steroids further

TABLE 5. *Comparison of levator ani and ventral prostate potencies of various steroids*

| Steroid | Relative Potency | | Ratio |
	Levator Ani	Ventral Prostate	L.A./ Prostate
Testosterone Propionate	100	100	1
Testosterone	14	194	0.07
Methyl testosterone	159	168	0.9
Δ'-Testosterone	5	9	0.6
Δ'-1Methyltestosterone	9	9	1.0
4,5α-Dihydrotestosterone	74	50	1.5
2-Hydroxymethylene·17α-methyl-4, 5α-Dihydrotestosterone	7	5	1.4
Stanazol	13	3	4.3
1-Methyl-Δ'-4,5α-dihydrotestaterone Acetate	118	27	4.4
1-Methyl-Δ'-4,5α-dihydrotestasterone Enanthate	59	8	7.4
19-Nortestosterone	61	4	1.5
17α-Ethyl-19-nortestosterone	80	12	7
19-Nortestosterone β-Phenylpropionate	220	14	16
Wy3475	340	17	20

SOURCE: Edgren 1963, copyright 1963, Rhodes International Publishing Co.

enhanced the dissociation (table 5). Toth and Zaker (1982) postulated that 5α-reduction decreased the binding affinity of the reduced steroid to the androgen receptor in the accessory sex organs.

The failure of the "levator ani" assay to reveal a steroid with an increased effect on the skeletal muscle and minimal or no effect on the accessory sex organs of the rat could indicate that the selection of this muscle as representative of the anabolic action of testosterone was a poor choice (Kochakian 1975). The translation to clinical usage of the apparent favorable differential action has been a disappointment. Dianabol (17β-hydroxy-17α-methylandrost-1,4-diene-3-one), however, appeared to be a promising prospect. At very low doses, it initiated protein anabolism without any apparent sexual effects (Liddle and Burke 1960; Kochakian 1975).

Early doubt was cast on the selection of the "levator ani" muscle (Nimni and Geiger 1957) and was supported by the revelation that the muscle in reality was the sex-linked dorsal bulbocavernosus muscle (Hayes 1968). Furthermore, its response to castration and testosterone administration is like that of the accessory sex organs rather than like the skeletal muscles of the rat (Kochakian 1975) or those of the guinea pig (Kochakian and Tillotson

48

TABLE 6. *Summary of nitrogen-retaining, myotrophic, and androgenic activities of several orally active steroids relative to methyltestosterone*

Steroid	Anabolic Activity		Androgenic Activity	Activity Ratio	
	Nitrogen Retention	Levator Ani		Nitrogen Retention	Levator Ani
Methyltestosterone	1.0	1.0	1.0	1.0	1.0
Methandrostenolone	1.2 / 10		0.35	3.4	
		2.1 / 2.3	0.6		3.5
		0.9	0.45		2.0
Oxymetholone	1.75 / 3		0.2	8.75	
		1.5	0.3		5.0
Norethandrolone	3.9 / 2		0.19	20	
		2 / 5.6	(0-19)	—	(10.5)
		0.7	0.2		3.5
		1.0	0.34		3.1
Methylandrostano-lisoxazole	9.7		0.24	4.0	
		2	0.24		8.3
Stanozolol	10.0		0.33	3.0	
		2	0.33		6
		3.2	0.3		10.6

SOURCE: Arnold et al. 1963, copyright 1963, The Endocrine Society.

1951). A more representative tissue, such as a true skeletal muscle, possibly would reveal a steroid that would have a sufficient differential from its androgenic effect to make it a useful agent for the stimulation of anabolic activity with a minimal androgenic effect. Although testosterone and many of its natural metabolites have been assayed for the separation of their effect on 47 different muscles from their effect on the accessory sex organs of the guinea pig (Kochakian and Tillotson 1957), none of the large number of the synthetically modified steroids has been submitted to a similar examination.

At present the dissociation of anabolic from androgenic activity seems to be an impossible dream; nevertheless, encouragement may be derived from the fact that several natural and synthetic steroids already have been recognized to have a differential between androgenic and several of the other biological properties of testosterone sufficient to permit beneficial clinical applications (Kochakian, in press). Furthermore, the separation of the anti-inflammatory

TABLE 7. *Comparison of steroid protein activity index (SPAI)* of some newer oral steroids in convalescent adults*

Steroid	Number of Assays	Dosage mg/day	Average SPAI
Testosterone Propionate	12	10-25	+6
19-Nortestosterone	14	25-75	+9
Norethandrolone	10	30-60	+8
Oxandrolone	27	10-20	+20
4-Hydroxy-17α-methyltestosterone	14	15-45	+11
Methandrostenolone	16	5-30	+16
Stanozolol	10	6-12	+29
17β-Hydroxy-17α-methylandrost-4-ene-(3.20)-pyrazol	9	15-25	+30
Norbolethone	6	7.5-10	+34

*SPAI=steroid protein anabolic index, the formula of which is: $\dfrac{NBSP}{NISP} - \dfrac{NBCP}{NICP} \times 100.$

NBSP=nitrogen balance in steroid period; NISP=nitrogen intake in steroid period; NBCP=nitrogen balance in control period; NBIP=nitrogen intake in control period.

SOURCE: Albanese 1965, copyright 1965, Fort Orange Press.

TABLE 8. *Comparison of the nitrogen-retaining activity of orally administered steroids in man*

	Relative Activity
17α-Methyltestosterone	1
17α-Ethyl-19-nortestosterone	2
9α-Fluoro-11P-hydroxy-17α-methyltestosterone	3
2-Hydroxy-methylene-4,5-dihydro-17α-Methyltestosterone	3
Oxandrolone	6
Δ'-17α-Methyltestosterone	10

SOURCE: Liddle and Burke 1960, copyright 1960, Helvetica Medica Acta.

activity from the water balance property of cortisone has been effected by the alteration of the chemical structure to prednisone and particularly to dexamethasone.

Therapeutic and Other Applications

Many of the modified steroids are more active than testosterone (tables 5 to 8). The more active compounds have been used therapeutically in a variety of conditions (Camerino and Sziacky 1975; Kopera 1976; Kopera 1985) in man, in animal husbandry (meat production), in sports (Ryan 1976; Wright 1980; Haupt and Rovere 1984; Wilson 1988) and in horse and dog racing, with controversial results.

ANABOLIC-ANDROGENIC STEROIDS

These steroids became known as "anabolic steroids," but none of them exhibited a complete separation of anabolic from androgenic activity. They are now being more correctly recognized as "anabolic-androgenic steroids" (Kochakian 1976).

Although the new designation is more descriptive of the two better known effects of these compounds, it is not all-inclusive. Testosterone, directly or indirectly through its metabolites, influences the development and function of practically every organ in the body (Kochakian 1975). The tissues influenced by testosterone can be classified into at least four categories:

1. Complete Influence. The accessory sex organs and the bulbocavemosus muscles are decreased after castration to vestigial organs by the loss of cells and atrophy of the residual cells and are increased by testosterone administration to at least double their size in castrated and normal animals.

2. Supplementary Influence. The kidney, liver, heart, skeletal muscles, bone, bone marrow, salivary and orbital glands, urinary bladder, skin, sebaceous glands, and body hair are partially regressed after castration without an apparent loss in the number of cells and are restored to normal or greater size by testosterone administration.

3. Reverse Influence. Castration results in an increase in the size of the thymus, spleen, adrenals, and lymph glands. Testosterone administration decreases the thymus to a vestigial organ but only partially decreases the size of the adrenals, spleen, and lymph glands. Testosterone also causes a loss of scalp hair (male baldness).

4. Structural and Functional Changes in Specific Cells. The dendritic length and size of motoneurons in the lumbar region of the male rat are reduced by castration and restored by testosterone administration (Kurz et al. 1986; Breedlove 1984; Breedlove 1985). These units are involved in the mediation of the effect of steroids on the bulbocavernosus muscles ("levator ani muscle"). The ability of specific cells in the brain

to accumulate and metabolize testosterone is less in the castrated male and the female rat and is enhanced by testosterone administration.

These changes and the resulting metabolites of testosterone are correlated with behavior (Balthazart and Schumacher 1985). LH and FSH secretion by the anterior pituitary is enhanced after castration and decreased by testosterone administration. The degrees of responses of the tissues in category (1) are characteristic and the same for all species, but those in the other categories vary greatly among the different animal species and, in some instances, even among strains of the same species (Kochakian 1975). Furthermore, parallel changes are not produced in these tissues by the many anabolic-androgenic steroids. Some of the less studied, responsive tissues, e.g., epethelial cells of the gastrointestinal tract, have not been included in the classification.

What was conceived originally to be a male sex hormone has proven to be also a general supplementary metabolic agent. Perhaps Parkes (1966) was more prophetic than he realized when he reacted to the name for the crystalline substance isolated from bulls' testes as the "dreadful name, testosterone."

FOOTNOTES

1. Most of the material in this chapter was taken with permission from a lecture presented at a seminar of the Reynolds Historical Society of the University of Alabama at Birmingham on November 6, 1986 and published in *Ala J Med Sci* 25:96-102, 1988. The lecture was recorded on videotape and is available from the Reynolds Historical Library. The lecture was also presented at the "Panel on Steroid Abuse," sponsored by the National Institute on Drug Abuse on March 6, 1989, and is published in an abbreviated version in *Trends Biochem Sci* 11:399-400, 1966.

2. The effectiveness of the transplant attached to the intestine suggests that, in contrast to the rat, the secreted hormones of the rooster testis as it passes through the liver is not converted to less active or inactive metabolites. A pellet of testosterone propionate implanted in the spleen of castrated rats does not stimulate the regeneration of the accessory sex organs (Biskind and Mark 1939). In a comparable study with ovariectomized rats, estrogen stimulated estrus, but progesterone implanted in the mesentery of rabbits did not produce the typical endometrial changes in the uterus (Kochakian et al. 1944).

3. Berthold's experiments and interpretation of the results clearly anticipated the fundamentals of endocrinology, which were enunciated 56 years later by Starling (1905), who named the blood-borne factors "hormones" (excite or arouse).

4. In 1889, considerable excitement and stimulation were generated by the claims of Brown-Sequard (1889), a respected French scientist, that crude extracts of testis reversed the effects of old age not only in experimental animals but also in man, including himself. The claims, on the basis of our present knowledge, seem untenable. Yet it is remarkable that the dramatic effects on energy and other physical functions occurred presumably by suggestion. These reports stimulated many other similar studies with not only crude extracts but also transplants, with equally spectacular reports (Hoskins 1941; Moore 1939).

5. The enormous royalties from the patented synthetic procedures permitted Ruzicka (1973) to pursue his hobby of collecting 17th-century Dutch and Flemish masters, which he gave to the Zurich Museum of Paintings.

REFERENCES

Albanese, A.A. Newer methodology in the clinical investigation of anabolic steroids. *J New Drugs* 5:208-224, 1965.

Arnold, A.; Potts, G.O.; and Beyler, A.L. Evaluation of the protein anabolic properties of certain orally active anabolic agents based on nitrogen balance studies in rats. *Endocrinology* 72:408-417, 1963.

Balthazart, J., and Schumacher, M. Role of testosterone metabolism in the activities of sexual behavior in birds. In: Giles, R., and Balthazart, J., eds. *Current Comparative Approaches. Neurobiology*. Berlin: Springer-Verlag, 1985. pp. 121-140.

Berthold, A.A. Transplantation des Hoden. *Arch Anat Physiol Wiss Med* 16:42-46, 1849.

Biskind, G.R., and Mark, J. The inactivation of testosterone propionate and estrone in rats. *Bull Johns Hopkins Hospital* 65:212-217, 1939.

Breedlove, M.S. Steroid influences on the development and function of a neuromuscular system. In: DeVries, G.J.; DeBruin, J.P.C.; Vylings, H.B.M.; and Corner, M.A., eds. *Sex Differences in the Brain. Progress in Brain Research*. Vol. 61. Amsterdam: Elsevier Science Publishers, 1984. pp. 147-167.

Breedlove, M.S. Hormonal control of the anatomical specificity of motoneuron-to-muscular innervation in rats. *Science* 227:1357-1359, 1985.

Brown-Sequard, E.C. The effects produced in man by subcutaneous injections of a liquid obtained from the testicles of animals. *Lancet* 2:105-107, 1889.

Butenandt, A. Ueber die chemische Untersuchung der Sexualhormon. *Z Angew Chem* 44:905-908, 1931.

Butenandt, A., and Dannenbaum, H. Ueber Androsteron, un Kristallisietes mannliches Sexualhormone III. Isolierung eines neuen, physiological unwirksamen Sterinderivatives aus Mannerharn, seine Verknupfung mit Dehydro-Androsteron und Androsterons ein Beitrag zur Konstitution des Androsterons. *Z Physiol Chem* 229:192-208, 1934.

Butanandt, A., and Hanisch, G. Uber die Umwandlung des Dehydroandros-
terons in Androstenol-(17)-on(3) (Testosteron); un Weg zur Darstellung
des Testosterons aus cholesterins (Vorlauf Mitteilung). *Ber Dtsch Chem
Ges* 68:1859-1862, 1935.

Butenandt, A., and Kudszus, H. Uber Androstendion, einen hochwirksamen
mannlichen Pragungstoff. *Z Physiol Chem* 237:75-88, 1935.

Butenandt, A., and Tscherning, K. Uber Androsteron, ein Krystallisiertes
Mannliches Sexualhormon I. Isoliereng und Reindarstellung aus Manner-
ham. *Z Physiol Chem* 229:167-184, 1934a.

Butenandt, A., and Tscherning, K. Ueber Androsteron ein Krystallisiertes
Sexualhormon II. Seine Chemische Characterisierung. *Z Physiol Chem*
229:185-191, 1934b.

Camerino, B., and Sziacky, R. Structure and effect of anabolic steroids.
In: Laron, Z., ed. *International Encyclopedia of Pharmacology and
Therapeutics.* Vol. I. London: Pergamon Press, 1975. pp. 233-275.

David, K. Uber des Testosteron, des Kristallisierte Mannliche Hormon aus
Steerentestes. *Acta Brev Neerland Physiol Pharmacol Microbial* 5:85-86;
108, 1935.

David, K.; Dingemanse, E.; Freud, J.; and Laqueur, E. Uber Kristallin-
isches Mannliches Hormon aus Hoden (Testosteron) wirksamer als **aus**
Ham oder Cholesterin Bereitetes, Androsteron. *Z Physiol Chem* 233:281-
293, 1935.

Dorfman, R.I., and Ungar, R. *Metabolism of Steroid Hormones.* New
York: Academic Press, 1965.

Edgren, K.A. A comparative study of the anabolic and androgenic effects
of various steroids. *Acta Endocrinol* 87(44):1-24, 1963.

Eisenberg, E., and Gordan, G.S. The levator ani muscle as an index of
myotrophic activity of steroidal hormones. *J Pharmacol Exp Ther* 99:38-
44, 1950.

Fieser, L.F., and Fieser, M. *Steroids. New* York: Reinhold, 1959.

Forbes, T.R. Testis transplantation performed by John Hunter. *Endocrinology* 4:329-330, 1947.

Fox, M.; Minot, A.S.; and Liddle, G.W. Oxandrolone: A potent anabolic
steroid of novel chemical configuration. *J Clin Endocrinol* 22:921-924,
1962.

Freud, J.; deJongh, S.E.; Laqueur, E.; and Munch, A.P. Uber Mannliches
(Sexual) Hormon. *Klin Wchschr* 9:772-774, 1930.

Funk, C., and Harrow, B. The male hormone. *Proc Soc Exp Biol Med*
26:325-326; 569-570, 1929.

Funk, C., and Harrow, B. The male hormone. IV. *Biochem J* 24:1678-
1680, 1930.

Funk, C.; Harrow, B.; and Lejwa, A. The male hormone. *Am J Physiol*
92:440-449, 1930.

Gallagher, T.F., and Koch, F.C. The quantitative assay for the testicular
hormone by the comb growth reaction. *J Pharmacol Exp Ther* 40:327-
339, 1930.

Gallagher, T.F., and Koch, F.C. The testicular hormone. *J Biol Chem* 84:495-500, 1934a.

Gallagher, T.F., and Koch, F.C. Biochemical studies on the male hormone as obtained from urine. *Endocrinology* 18:107-112, 1934b.

Gonzalez-Diddi, M.; Komisaruk, B.; and Beyer, C. Differential effects of testosterone and dihydrotestosterone on the diverse tissues of the ovariectomized rat. *Endocrinology* 91:1129-1132, 1972.

Gurney, C.W. The hematological effects of androgens. In: Kochakian, C.D., ed. *Anabolic-Androgenic Steroids.* Berlin: Springer-Verlag, 1976. pp. 482-498.

Haupt, H.A., and Rovere, G.D. Anabolic steroids: A review of the literature. *Am J Sports Med* 12469-484, 1984.

Hayes, K.J. The so-called "levator ani" of the rat. *Acta Endocrinol* 48:337-347, 1968.

Heresova, J.; Pobisova, Z.; Hampl, R.; and Starka, L. Androgen administration to transsexual women. *Exp Clin Endocrinol* 88:219-223, 1986.

Hershberger, L.D.; Shipley, E.G.; and Meyer, R.K. Myotrophic activity of 19-nortestosterone and other steroids determined by modified levator ani method. *Proc Soc Exp Biol Med* 83:175-180, 1953.

Hilger, A.G., and Hummel, D.J. *Endocrine Bioassay Data: Androgenic and Myogenic.* Bethesda, MD: the National Cancer Institute, 1964. pp. 15-243.

Hoskins, R.G. *Endocrinology, the Glands and Their Functions.* New York: W.W. Norton, 1941. 388 pp.

Johnsen, S.G.; Bennett, E.P.; and Jensen, V.G. Therapeutic effectiveness of oral testosterone. *Lancet* 2:1473-1474, 1974.

Kenyon, A.T.; Sandiford, I.; Bryan, A.H.; Knowlton, K.; and Koch, F.C. The effect of testosterone propionate on nitrogen, electrolyte, water and energy metabolism in eunuchoidism. *Endocrinology* 23:135-153, 1938.

Kochakian, C.D. Effect of male hormone on protein metabolism of castrate dogs. *Proc Soc Exp Biol Med* 32:1064-1065, 1935.

Kochakian, C.D. Testosterone and testosterone acetate and the protein and energy metabolism of castrate dogs. *Endocrinology* 21:750-755, 1937.

Kochakian, C.D. The comparative efficacy of various androgens as determined by the rat assay method. *Endocrinology* 22:181-192, 1938.

Kochakian, C.D. In: Reifenstein, E.C. *Josiah Macy, Jr. Foundation Conference on Bone and Wound Healing.* Vol. 2, 1942. pp. 25-32.

Kochakian, C.D. A comparison of the renotrophic with the androgenic activity of various steroids. *Am J Physiol* 142:315-325, 1944.

Kochakian, C.D. The effect of dose and nutritive state on the renotrophic and androgenic activities of various steroids. *Am J Physiol* 145:549-556, 1946.

Kochakian, C.D. Comparison of protein anabolic property of various androgens in the castrated rat. *Am J Physiol* 160:53-61, 1950.

Kochakian, C.D. Renotrophic-androgenic properties of orally administered androgens. *Proc Soc Exp Biol Med* 80:386-388, 1952.

Kochakian, C.D. Mechanisms of androgen actions. *Lab Inves* 8:538-559, 1959.

Kochakian, C.D. Protein anabolic property of androgens. *Ala J Med Sci* 1:24-37, 1964.

Kochakian, C.D. Definition of androgens and protein anabolic steroids. In: Laron, Z., ed. *International Encyclopedia of Pharmacology and Therapeutics.* Vol. 1 (No. 2). London: Pergamon Press, 1975. pp. 149-177.

Kochakian, C.D. *Anabolic-Androgenic Steroids.* Berlin: Springer-Verlag, 1976.

Kochakian, C.D. Regulation of kidney growth by androgens. In: Briggs, M.H., and Christie, G.A., eds. *Advances in Steroid Biochemistry and Pharmacology.* Vol. 6. London: Academic Press, 1977. pp. 1-34.

Kochakian, C.D. *How It Was: Anabolic* Actions *of Steroids and Remembrances.* School of Medicine, University of Alabama at Birmingham, 1984. 116 pp.

Kochakian, C.D. Metabolites of testosterone: Significance in the vital economy. *Steroids 1990,* in press.

Kochakian, C.D., and Arimasa, N. The metabolism in vitro of anabolic-androgenic steroids by mammalian tissues. In: Kochakian, C.D., ed. *Anabolic-Androgenic Steroids.* Berlin: Springer-Verlag, 1976. pp. 287-359.

Kochakian, C.D.; Haskins, A.L., Jr.; and Bruce, R.A. The site of metabolism of progesterone in the rabbit. *Am J Physiol* 142:326-327, 1944.

Kochakian, C.D.; Humm, J.H.; and Bartlett, M.N. Effect of steroids on body weight, temporal muscle and organs of the guinea pig. *Am J Physiol* 155:242-250, 1948.

Kochakian, C.D., and Murlin, J.R. The effect of male hormone on the protein and energy metabolism of castrate dogs. *J Nutrition* 10:437-459, 1935.

Kochakian, C.D., and Murlin, J.R. The relationship of synthetic male hormone, androstendion, to the protein and energy metabolism of castrate dogs and the protein metabolism of a normal dog. *Am J Physiol* 117:642-657, 1936.

Kochakian, C.D., and Tillotson, C. Influence of several C19-steroids on the growth of individual muscles of the guinea pig. *Endocrinology* 60:607-618, 1957.

Kopera, H. Miscellaneous uses of anabolic steroids. In: Kochakian, C.D., ed. *Anabolic-Androgenic Steroiods.* Berlin: Springer-Verlag, 1976. pp. 535-625.

Kopera, H. The history of anabolic steroids and a review of clinical experiences with anabolic steroids. *Acta Endocrinologica* 110(Suppl. 271):11-18, 1985.

Kutz, E.M.; Sengelaub, D.R.; and Arnold, A.P. Androgens regulate dendritic length of mammalian motoneurons in adulthood. *Science* 232:395-398, 1986.

Landau, R.L. The metabolic effects of anabolic steroids in man. In: Kochakian, C.D., ed. *Anabolic-Androgenic Steroids.* Berlin: Springer-Verlag, 1976. pp. 45-72.

Liddle, G.W., and Burke, H.A., Jr. Anabolic steroids in clinical medicine. *Helv Med Acta* 27:505-513, 1960.

Lode, A. Zur Transplantation der Hoden bei Hahnen. *Wien Klin Wchscher* 4847, 1891.

Lode, A. Zur Transplantation der Hoden bei Hahnen. *Wien Klin Wchscher* 8:341-346, 1895.

Loewe, S., and Voss, H.E. Der Stand der Erfassung des Mannlichen Sexualhormons (Androkinins). *Klin Wchschr* 9:481-487, 1930.

McGee, L.C. The effect of the injection of a lipoid fraction of bull testicle in capons. *Proc Inst Med (Chicago)* 6:252, 1927.

Moore, C.R. Biology of the testes. In: Allen, E.; Danforth, C.H.; and Doisy, E.A., eds. *Sex and Internal Secretions.* Baltimore: Williams & Wilkins, 1939. pp. 354-451.

Moore, C.R., and Gallagher, T.F. Threshold relationship of testis hormone indicators in mammals. The rat unit. *J Pharmacol Exp Ther* 40:341-349, 1930.

Murlin, J.R. Metabolism of development III. Qualitative effects of pregnancy on the protein metabolism of the dog. *Am J Physiol* 28:422-454, 1911.

Nimni, M.E., and Geiger, E. Non-suitability of levator ani method as an index of anabolic effect of steroids. *Proc Soc Exp Biol Med* 94:606-610, 1957.

Overbeek, G.A. *Anabolic Steroids.* Berlin: Springer-Verlag, 1966. 80 pp.

Overbeek, G.A.; Delver, A.; and deVisser, J. Pharmacological comparisons of anabolic steroids (ethylestrenol, nandrolone esters). In: Everse, J.W.R., and van Keep, P.A., eds. Symposium on anabolic steroids. *Acta Endocrinol* 39(Suppl. 63):7-17, 1961.

Papanicolaou, G.N., and Falk, E.A. General muscular hypertrophy induced by androgenic hormone. *Science* 87:238-239, 1938.

Parkes, A.S. The rise of reproductive endocrinology, 1926-1940. *J Endocrinol* 34:xx-xxxii, 1966.

Pezard, A. Sur la determination des caracteres sexuels secondaire chez les gallinaces. *Compt Rend Acad des Sciences* 153:1027-1032, 1911.

Pezard, A. Sur la determination des caracteres sexuals secondaire chez les gallinaces. *Compt Rend Acad des Sciences* 154:1183-1186, 1912.

Pezard, A., and Caridroit, M. Le presence de l'hormone testiculaire dans le sang du coq normal, demonstration directe fondu sur la greffe autoplastique des cretillons. *Compt Rend Soc Biol* 95:296-298, 1926.

Pfeiffer, C.A.; Emmel, V.M.; and Gardner, W.U. Renal hypertrophy in mice receiving estrogen and androgen. *Yale J Biol Med* 12:493-501, 1940.

Potts, G.O.; Arnold, A.; and Beyler, A.L. Dissociation of the androgenic and other hormonal effects of steroids. In: Kochakian, C.D., ed. *Anabolic-Androgenic Steroids.* Berlin: Springer-Verlag, 1976. pp. 361-406.

Reifenstein, E.C. *The Protein Anabolic Activity of Steroid Compounds.* Josiah Macy, Jr. Foundation Conference on Bone and Wound Healing. Vol. 1 (Suppl). New York: Josiah Macy, Jr. Foundation, 1942.

Ruzicka, L. In the borderline between bio-organic chemistry and biochemistry. *Annu Rev Biochem* 41:1-20, 1973.

Ruzicka, L.; Goldberg, M.W.; Meyer, J.; Brunigger, H.; and Eichenberger, E. Zur Kenntnis der Sexualhormone II, Ueber die Synthese des Testikelhormons (Androsteron) und Steroisomers desselben durch Abbau hydrieter Sterine. *Helv Chim Acta* 17:1395-1406, 1934.

Ruzicka, L., and Wettstein, A. Sexualhormon V. Kunlsliche Herstellung des Mannlichen Sexualhormon, trans-Dehydroandrosteron und des Androsten-3, 17-dion. *Helv Chim Acta* 18:986-994, 1935a.

Ruzicka, L., and Wettstein, A. Uber die Krystallische Herstellung des Testikelhormons, Testosteron (Androsten-3-on-17-ol). *Helv Chim Acta* 18:1264-1275, 1935b.

Ryan, A.J. Athletics. In: Kochakian, C.D., ed. *Anabolic-Androgenic Steroids.* Berlin: Springer-Verlag, 1976. pp. 515-534.

Selye, H. The effect of testosterone on the kidney. *J Ural* 42:637-641, 1939.

Starling, E.H. The chemical correlation of the functions of the body. *Lancer* 1:339-341, 1905.

Tausk, M. Androgens and anabolic steroids. In: Parnham, M.J., and Bruinvels, J., eds. *Discoveries in Pharmacology,* Vol. 2. Amsterdam: Elsevier, 1984. pp. 305-320.

Toth, M., and Zaker, T. Relative binding activities of testosterone, nortestosterone, and their 5α-reduced derivatives to the androgen receptor and to other androgen binding proteins. A suggested role of 5α-reductive steroid metabolism in the dissociation of "myotrophic" and "androgenic" activities of 19-nortestosterone. *J Steroid Biochem* 17:653-660, 1982.

Vida, J.A. *Androgens and Anabolic Agents. Chemistry and Pharmacology.* New York: Academic Press, 1969. pp. xii, 332.

Voss, H.E. Die Vesiculardrusen (Samenblasen) des Kastraten Nach Hodentransplantation. *Pfluger's Arch ges, Physiologie des Menschen und der Tier* 226:138-147, 1930.

Wainman, P., and Shipounoff, G.C. The effects of castration and testosterone propionate on the striated perineal musculature in the rat. *Endocrinology* 29:975-978, 1941.

Weinbauer, G.F.; Marshall, G.R.; and Nieschlag, E. New injectable testosterone ester maintains serum testosterone of castrated monkeys in the normal range for four months. *Acta Endocrinol* 113:128-132, 1986.

Wilson, J.D. Androgen abuse of athletes. *Endocrine Rev* 9:181-199, 1988.

Wright, J.E. Steroids and athletics. *Exert Sports Sci Rev* 8:149-202, 1980.

AUTHOR

Charles D. Kochakian, Ph.D.
Professor Emeritus (Experimental Endocrinology)
  and former Director
Laboratory of Experimental Endocrinology
Medical Center
University of Alabama at Birmingham

Correspondence to:

3617 Oakdale Road
Birmingham, AL 35223

Anabolic-Androgenic Steroids

John A. Lombardo

INTRODUCTION

The use of anabolic-androgenic steroids (AS) by athletes to enhance their athletic performance has been reported since the 1950s (Wright 1978). Androgen use has spread to different groups of athletes, who use these drugs for various reasons. The common thread among all these groups, however, is the goal of enhancing muscular capacities and athletic performance and being successful (winning). Androgen use by weightlifters in order to enhance strength and thereby perform better in an event in which there is a direct correlation between strength and success is well known (Starr 1981). Bodybuilders, who are judged on muscle size, shape, definition, and symmetry, also see a direct correlation between the use of androgens and success in their activity. The throwers in track and field (hammer, shotput, discus, and javelin) are another group in which the use of androgens is frequently reported (Ljungqvist 1975; Todd 1987). Strength is a key factor in the ability to project a hammer, shot, discus, or javelin further than the competition. In collision sports such as football, in which the lean body mass and strength as well as the ability to efficiently repair "collision damage" are significant factors in the ability to succeed, players would benefit from the use of androgens in order to maximize their gains in these areas. This is especially true at Division I college and professional levels. At these levels, there is the greatest fame and financial reward; there are also more competitors for fewer positions.

In addition to these groups in which the use of androgens has been suspected and fairly well documented, other groups use androgens to allow frequent high-intensity work (Buckley et al. 1988; Anderson and McKeag 1985). Through these increases in the amount and intensity of training, performance is enhanced. These include the sprinters, middle- and long-distance runners in track, and swimmers who do not wish to gain lean body mass and in whom strength is not as great a factor. However, these athletes can be more successful if they can sustain training at a higher intensity level, over a longer period of time, or both.

Physical appearance has attained an important place in the present-day society. Self-esteem may be directly related to the size, shape, and attractiveness of one's body. To overcome genetic limitations or to speed the process of "bulking up," many individuals who are not involved in competitive athletics have become users of androgens. These "look-gooders" do not have a single competitive event or finite athletic career as their goal, but aim to overcome physical, psychological, emotional, and social limitations-especially low self-esteem. These are long-term problems being controlled or treated by physical conditioning with chemical enhancement; this method does not solve these problems, but compounds them.

The benefits that are desired by individuals who use androgens therefore include (1) alteration of body composition (increased lean mass and reduced fat); (2) increase in strength; (3) increase in endurance; (4) hastened recovery from exercise (ability to perform more frequent or higher intensity workouts); and (5) enhancement of athletic performance.

The question that needs to be answered is "Do androgens give the benefits desired by these individuals who take them?" There are two sources of information on this question. One is the scientific literature, both animal and human studies; the other is anecdotal evidence given by the athletes and users. It is important that scientists base their knowledge on accurate data. Scientifically, the literature is extremely confusing and contradictory.

ANIMAL STUDIES

The animal studies on the effects of androgens on weight and athletic performance are fairly consistent. Studies using male rats and monkeys have consistently shown no increase in body weight or improvement in performance (Young et al. 1977; Hickson et al. 1976; Richardson 1977). However, the activities generally studied were swimming and running on a treadmill. These do not compare favorably with progressive resistance training. Also, there is the difficulty of simulating the psychological drive of competition in the animal.

Interestingly, however, when castrated males (Kochakian and Endahl 1959; Heitzman 1976) and females (Exner et al. 1973; Heitzman 1976; Nesheim 1976; Hervey and Hutchinson 1973) are studied, significant increases in nitrogen retention and lean body mass in these animals have been found consistently.

HUMAN STUDIES

The literature on the effects of androgens on lean body mass, strength, and aerobic capacity in humans presents a great deal of contradiction and confusion.

A number of studies have shown an increase in aerobic capacity as measured by VO2 max (the maximum oxygen uptake as measured by a maximum exercise test) with the use of androgens (Albrecht and Albright 1969; Johnson and O'Shea 1969; Keul et al. 1976). However, there are also a number of studies using VO2 max as a criteria that have shown that there is no change in endurance with the use of androgens (Fahey and Brown 1973; Hervey et al. 1976; Johnson et al. 1972; Johnson et al. 1975). The theory being proposed when these studies were begun was that androgens would stimulate the bone marrow and therefore increase the oxygen-carrying capacity of the blood by increasing the red cell mass.

Two questions arise when looking at increases in endurance and androgens:

1. Is the VO2 max that was used in these studies an accurate indicator of success in endurance events?

2. Is it sensitive enough to record changes that would be significant in the results of an endurance event?

The answers to these questions are unknown.

A number of training studies have shown no significant increase in lean body mass with the use of androgens (Crist et al. 1983; Fahey and Brown 1973; Fowler et al. 1965; Golding et al. 1974; Stromme et al. 1974), although other studies have shown significant increases with the use of androgens (Hervey et al. 1976; Hervey et al. 1981; Stamford and Moffatt 1974; Ward 1973; Johnson et al. 1972; O'Shea 1971; Loughton and Ruhling 1977) (table 1).

Some more contradictory findings are discovered when the literature on the effects of androgen on strength training are reviewed. Some studies show a significant increase in strength with androgen use (Ward 1973; Stamford and Moffatt 1974; Hervey et al. 1981; O'Shea 1971), while others show there are no significant differences between control and androgen groups (Golding et al. 1974; Stromme et al. 1974; Hervey et al. 1976; Fahey and Brown 1973; Crist et al. 1983; Loughton and Ruhling 1977; Fowler et al. 1965) (table 1).

Hervey's two studies show a classic comparison. Hervey and colleagues (1976) found significant increases in fat-free mass but no significant increases in strength in a double-blind crossover study using physical education majors. However, Hervey and associates (1981) found significant increases in not only fat-free mass but also in strength when the study group was experienced weight trainers. Findings such as these lead the investigators to ask why there are so many differences in the studies reporting the ergogenic effects of androgens. Some of the reasons for these differences include the following.

62

TABLE 1. *Training and performance studies using AS*

Study	Golding	Stromme	Hervey et al. 1981	Hervey et al. 1976	Ward	Fahey/ Brown	Stamford/ Moffatt	Crist et al.	Loughton/ Ruhling	Fowler et al.	O'Shea
Duration (weeks)	12	8	6 x3	6 x3	5	9	8	3 x3	7	16	4
Intensity	Mod. ↓ Heavy	Mod. ↓ Heavy	Mod. ↓ Heavy	Mod. ↓ Heavy	Heavy	Light ↓ Mod.	Heavy	Mod. ↓ Heavy	Mod. ↓ Heavy	Light	Mod. ↓ Heavy
Frequency	4	3	-	-	3?	3	3	-	6	5	3
Drug/ Dosage	? 10 ?	Met. 75- 100	Met. 100	Met. 100	Met. 10	Nand. 1 kg/ week	Met. 10	Nand. test 100/week	Met. 10	Met. 20	Met. 10
Diet	Protein ↓	Protein ↓	-	-	-	-	Protein ↓	Protein ↓	Protein ↓	-	Protein ↓
Exp./ Inexp.	Exp.	Inexp.?	Exp.	Inexp.	Exp.	Inexp.	Exp.	Exp.	Exp.? Inexp.	Inexp.	Exp.
Weight/ LBM	- SF	- Ant.	+ UW SF Ant.	+ UW SF Ant.	+ UW	- UW	+ Ant.	- UW	+ BWT	- SF Ant.	+ SF
Strength	-	-	+	-	+	-	+	-	-	-	+

KEY: Mod.=moderate; Frequency=frequency of workouts (days); Met.=methandrostenolone; Nand.=Nandrolone; Exp.=experienced weight trainer, Inexp.=inexperienced weight trainer; LBM=lean body mass; SF=skin folds; Ant.=anthropometric; UW=underwater weighing; BWT=body weight.

1. *The weighr training experience of the subjects.* Many of the studies utilize inexperienced weight trainers who will make significant early gains when beginning a strength training program. These large gains in strength will not be significantly increased by the androgens in this early part of the program. Experienced weight trainers, on the other hand, have plateaued, and their gains in strength are smaller with continuation of their regular training. In these individuals, drug-assisted gains that might be small in comparison to the larger gains by the novice lifter will be significant compared to the smaller gains that could be attained in a 6-week training study (Wright 1978; Yesalis et al. 1989).

2. *The intensity of training.* Many studies utilize low-intensity, short duration, and low-frequency workouts, which are not comparable in terms of physiologic and biochemical effects to the high-intensity, long duration, and high-frequency workouts performed by many athletes who use androgens. These are not fair comparisons when assessing the efficacy of androgens on high-intensity weight training programs (Wright 1978; Yesalis et al. 1989).

3. *Dietary controls.* Many of the studies did not control dietary intake. There was no mention of the amount of calories or the percentage of carbohydrates, protein, and fat in the diet of the subjects. These factors are extremely important when one is looking at a study measuring lean body mass and strength as indicators of efficacy (Wright 1978; Yesalis et al. 1989).

4. *Dosage of the drug.* The athletes are using dosages 10 to 20 times therapeutic levels. No studies have approached these doses. Ethically, these studies could not be done, since the long-term effects of these doses are not known. The question of benefits of the high-dose and multiple drug regimens commonly used by the athletes remains unanswered (Wright 1978; Yesalis et al. 1989).

5. *Specificity of testing.* Some of the studies used isometric or isokinetic testing with isotonic training. The sensitivity and specificity of these measurements have been questioned (Wright 1978; Yesalis et al. 1989).

Table 2 has a review of these factors and others that affect the results of studies (Yesalis et al. 1989).

WOMEN AND CHILDREN

There have been no studies performed on two groups of individuals in which the use of androgens has reportedly increased. These are young males and women. Studies in these two groups pose an ethical problem. However, in view of the animal studies on castrated males (Kochakian

TABLE 2. *Reasons for lack of consensus on AS effects on health and performance variables in human subjects*

Subjects	The number of subjects, their experience in weight training, and their physical condition at the start of the study varied.
Diet	Most not controlled or recorded.
Training Programs	Volumes and intensities varied.
Testing Programs	Strength often not measured in the training mode. Body compositions often assessed from skinfold estimates. Health effects often mismeasured (not organ specific) or not measured.
Drugs	Variable, and few have reported on athletes self-administering multiple drugs.
Study	Some crossover, some single blind, some double blind, some not blind, some no controls.
Drugs Mechanisms Action	Unknown and varying degrees of anabolic, anticatabolic, and motivational effects depending upon the circumstances.
Dosages	Variable, only two studies administered dosages approximating those currently used by competing athletes.
Length of Study	Variable and generally short; very few have reported on prolonged training and AS self-administration.
Placebo Effect	Well documented for most drugs; yet most data suggest that athletes can readily detect AS administration making it virtually impossible to conduct blind studies.
Data Interpretation	Variable, dependent upon the background and experience (scientific, clinical, athletic, administrative), general perspective, and goals of interpreters.
Legal and Ethical Issues	Preclude design and execution of well-controlled studies using doses and patterns of administration of drugs with unknown long-term effects in healthy volunteers in a manner comparable to those of many current AS users.

SOURCE: Yesalis et al., in press.

and Endahl 1959; Heitzman 1976) and females (Exner et al. 1973; Heitzman 1976; Nesheim 1976; Hervey and Hutchinson 1973) and the effects of andmgens, a positive ergogenic effect can be expected.

SUMMATION

After a critical review of the literature and in view of the overwhelmingly consistent anecdotal evidence, I wholeheartedly agree with the statement of the American College of Sports Medicine Position Stand (1984) on the Use of Anabolic-Androgenic Steroids in Sports when it states that:

> Anabolic/androgenic steroids, in the presence of an adequate diet, can contribute to increases in body weight often in the lean mass compartment . . . The gains in muscular strength achieved through high intensity exercise and proper diet can be increased by the use of anabolic/androgenic steroids in some individuals.

It is extremely difficult to make any statement about endurance other than stating that, using VO2 max as an indicator of endurance, there is not significant evidence to show that anabolic-androgenic steroids improve endurance.

MECHANISM OF ACTION

A number of mechanisms have been proposed for the actions of androgens on muscular strength and lean body mass. These include (1) increase in protein synthesis; (2) inhibition of the catabolic effect of glucocorticoids; (3) effects on central nervous system and neuromuscular junction; and (4) placebo effect.

Rogozkin (1976; Rogozkin 1979) has shown that exercise increases the rate of transcription as measured by increased RNA polymerase activity. He has also shown that androgens further increase the rate of transcription over that found with exercise alone.

The interaction between the catabolic glucocorticoids and the anabolic androgens is not completely understood. However, there are some connections that are known. Goldberg (1969) has shown that glucocorticoids are catabolic, causing protein degradation and muscle atrophy. Konagaya and associates (1986) have shown that glucocorticoid blockade decreases muscle atrophy. Doerr and Pirke (1976) have shown that cortisol causes a decrease in the nocturnal rise in testosterone. Snochowski and coworkers (1981) have shown that there are separate receptors for androgens and glucocorticoids, but they did not find competitive binding for these receptors. Mayer and Rosen (1975) have shown that testosterone can displace dexamethasone from glucocorticoid receptors. Many studies have shown that physical and psychological stress can decrease testosterone and increase cortisol levels.

66

This has been shown by Aakvag and colleagues (1978) in Army recruits undergoing severe physical and psychological stress. Wheeler and associates (1984), Guglielmini and coworkers (1984), Villaneuva and colleagues (1986), Urhausen and Kindermann (1987), and Mather and associates (1986) have shown that in strenuous exercise for more than 3 hours, there is an increase in cortisol and a decrease in testosterone, while with exercise for less than 3 hours, there is an increase in testosterone. This is all with submaximal work. No work has been done in the area of chronic exercise of 2 to 3 hours on successive days, although this is the training regimen of many athletes at this time. Based on this evidence, one can speculate that one of the actions of the androgens is inhibition of the catabolic effect of glucocorticoids in athletes undergoing strenuous physical training. This inhibition may occur by maintaining a steady-state level of androgen by exogenous supplementation. More research is needed in this area.

There are known to be androgen receptors in both the brain and alpha-motor neurons, the size and number of which can be influenced by the use of androgens (Sar and Stumpf 1977; Stumpf and Sar 1976). There has been an implication that androgens can facilitate the release of acetylcholine at the neuromuscular junction and elevate monoamine levels in the central nervous system (Vyskocil and Gutmann 1977). Electroencephalographic recordings have shown changes in individuals given anabolic steroids (Itil et al. 1974; Itil 1976). Aggression has been associated with increases in testosterone in both animals (Simon et al. 1985) and humans (Persky et al. 1971; Kreuz and Rose 1972; Ehrenkranz et al. 1974; Scaramella and Brown 1978). Brooks (1980) has suggested that this increase in aggressive behavior is a mechanism for the action of androgens. Perhaps the increases in aggression and energy that the athlete feels may be a result of the neurologic changes previously discussed.

The placebo effect has been suggested as the mechanism of action of androgens by Ryan (1981). This has been shown to be effective in one study (Ariel and Saville 1972).

The mechanism of action of androgens is most likely not any one of these but a combination of them.

ATHLETIC PERFORMANCE

Do androgens enhance athletic performance? To answer this important question, it is necessary to understand the multifactorial nature of athletic performance. Rarely, if ever, is there a solitary factor that contributes to success; success is a result of optimal development of many factors (Lombardo 1987) (table 3). The following is a list of the factors contributing to athletic performance.

1. *Level of conditioning.* Conditioning includes not only strength **but** also flexibility and endurance (both cardiovascular and muscle endurance). The importance of these various aspects of conditioning differs among sports.

2. *Skill.* Development of skill is a learned behavior based on genetic predisposition and repetition (practice). Some sports successes may require not only development of gross motor skills but also fine and complex motor skill development. This is an extremely important factor in success in most sports.

3. *Diet.* One of the most neglected areas, until recently, is nutrition. An athlete's diet provides the fuel that the athlete needs to perform. A high-performance athlete, like a high-performance car, needs premium fuel. The fund of knowledge in this area is rapidly expanding and the role of diet is increasing as the field of nutrition develops.

4. *Psyche.* Many phrases, such as "getting up for a game," "raising the intensity level," and "concentrating," have long been a part of sports. As the field of psychology applies its knowledge and energy to the world of sports, new phrases such as "focus," "visualization," and "relaxation" have been added to sports jargon. This is another rapidly developing area that is a major factor in athletic performance.

5. *Opponent.* Often the individual or team against whom one is competing makes a difference. Due to style of play or strengths and weaknesses of an opponent (commonly referred to as "matchups"), performance and success is affected.

6. *Arena.* The home field advantage is a real phenomenon that occurs in the world of sports. It may be the influence of the spectators, the familiarity with environment, maintenance of daily routine, or a combination of these and others, which gives the home team an edge.

7. *Sleep.* Proper rest is important in the performance of any task, especially when complex motor skills are involved. Because of pre-event anxiety, a new environment, or the circuslike atmosphere surrounding certain events, athletes may have difficulty sleeping.

8. *Drugs.* Drugs can have two effects. If the athlete is abusing illicit drugs, such as cocaine or marijuana, or legal drugs, such as alcohol, his or her athletic performance can be adversely affected. The ergogenic drugs are used to enhance performance. Some of these drugs and procedures will positively affect the performance of the athlete and potentially make a difference in the outcome of an event.

9. *Genes.* The most important factor and one over which the athlete has absolutely no control is genetic makeup. Many of the characteristics that are key to success in sports are a result of these genetic expressions. These have been referred to as "natural ability," "raw talent," or "God-given ability."

In events in which centimeters or milliseconds are the difference between success and failure, how much does manipulation of one factor contribute? When 20 to 30 pounds of lean mass can make the difference between a professional contract worth over $100,000 a year and the adulation and fame of such a career and the $40,000 to $50,000 a year and routine of many jobs, how many athletes will use androgens to reach their goal?

CONCLUSION

The individual who takes androgens desires an increase in strength, lean body mass, or decreases in recovery time between workouts to enhance athletic performance or to "look good." The scientific studies that have been reported in this area are fraught with problems. However, it can be concluded that androgens are associated with increases in strength and lean body mass, especially in experienced weight trainers, when performing high-intensity work in the presence of an adequate diet. This can be concluded through the available scientific evidence and the overwhelmingly consistent anecdotal reports of the athletes. Recovery time is based solely on anecdotal evidence, since it has not yet been studied.

REFERENCES

Aakaag, A.; Bentdol, O.; Quigstod, K.; Walstod, P.; Renningen, H.; and Fonnum, F. Testosterone and testosterone binding globulin (TeBg) in young men during prolonged stress. *Int J Androl* 1:22-31, 1978.

Albrecht, H., and Albrecht, E. Ergometric, rheographic, reflexographic, and electrographic tests at altitude and effects of drugs on human physical performance. *Fed Proc* 28:1262-1267, 1969.

American College of Sports Medicine position stand on the use of anabolic-androgenic steroids in sports. *Med Sci Sports Exer* 19:13-18, 1984.

Anderson, W., and McKeag, D. The substance use and abuse habits of college student-athletes. Research paper #2, National Collegiate Athletic Association, Mission, KS, 1985.

Ariel, G., and Saville, W. Anabolic steroids: The physiological effects of placebos. *Med Sci Sports* 4:124-126, 1972.

Brooks, R.V. Anabolic steroids and athletes. *Phys Sportsmed* 8(3):161-163, 1980.

Buckley, W.; Yesalis, C.; Friedl, K.; Anderson, W.; Streit, A.; and Wright, J. Estimated prevalence of anabolic steroid use among male high school seniors. *JAMA* 260(23):3441-3445, 1988.

Crist, D.M.; Stackpole, P.J.; and Peake, G.T. Effects of androgenic-anabolic steroids on neuromuscular power and body composition. *J Appl Physiol* 54:366-370, 1983.

Doerr, P., and Pirke, K.M. Cortisol-induced suppression of plasma testosterone in normal adult males. *J Clin Endocrinol Metab* 43:622-629, 1976.

Ehrenkranz, J.; Bliss, E.; and Sheard, M.H. Plasma testosterone: Correlation with aggressive behavior and social dominance in man. *Psychosomatic Med* 36(6):469-475, 1974.

Exner, G.U.; Staudte, H.W.; and Pette, D. Isometric training of rats— effects upon fast and slow muscle and modification by an anabolic hormone (nandrolone decanoate). I. Female rats. *Pflugers Arch* 345:1-14, 1973.

Fahey, T.D., and Brown, C.H. The effects of an anabolic steroid on the strength, body composition, and endurance of college males when accompanied by a weight training program. *Med Sci Sports* 5:272-276, 1973.

Fowler, W.M., Jr.; Gardner, G.W.; and Egstrom, G.H. Effect of an anabolic steroid on physical performance in young men. *J Appl Physiol* 20:1038-1040, 1965.

Guglielmini, C.; Paolini, A.R.; and Conconi, F. Variations of serum testosterone concentrations after physical exercises of different duration. *Int J Sports Med* 5:246-249, 1984.

Goldberg, A.L. Protein turnover in skeletal muscle. II. Effects of denervation and cortisone on protein catabolism in skeletal muscle. *J Biol Chem* 244:3223-3229, 1969.

Golding, L.A.; Freydinger, J.E.; and Fishel, S.S. The effect of an androgenic-anabolic steroid and a protein supplement on size, strength, weight, and body composition in athletes. *Phys Sportsmed* 2(6):39-45, 1974.

Heitzman, R.J. The effectiveness of anabolic agents in increasing rate of growth in farm animals; report on experiments in cattle. In: Lu, F.C., and Rendell, J., eds. *Anabolic Agents in Animal Production.* Stuttgart: George Thieme Publishers, 1976. pp. 89-98.

Hervey, G.R., and Hutchinson, I. The effects of testosterone on body weight and composition in the rat. *J Endocrinol* 57:xxiv-xxv, 1973.

Hervey, G.R.; Hutchinson, I.; Knibbs, A.V.; et al. Anabolic effects of methandienone in men undergoing athletic training. *Lancer* 2:699-702, 1976.

Hervey, G.R.; Knibbs, A.V.; Burkinshaw, L.; et al. Effects of methandienone on the performance and body composition of men undergoing athletic training. *Clin Sci* 60:457-461, 1981.

Hickson, R.C.; Heusner, W.W.; VanHuss, W.D.; Jackson, D.E.; Anderson, D.A.; Jones, D.A.; and Psaledas, A.T. Effects of dianabol and high-intensity sprint training on body composition of rats. *Med Sci Sports* 8(3):191-196, 1976.

Itil, T. Neurophysiological effects of hormones in humans: Computer EEG profiles of sex and hypothalamic hormones. In: Schar, E.J., ed. *Hormones, Behaviour and Psychopathology.* New York: Raven Press, 1976.

Itil, T.; Ackpinar, C.; Harrmann, W.; and Patterson, C. "Psychotropic" action of sex hormones: Computerized EEG in establishing the immediate CNS effects of steroid hormones. *Curr Ther Res* 16:1147-1170, 1974.

Johnson, L.C.; Fisher, G.; Silvester, L.J.; and Hofheins, C.C. Anabolic steroid: Effects of strength, body weight, oxygen uptake and spermatogenesis upon mature males. *Med Sci Sports* 4:43-45, 1972.

Johnson, L.C., and O'Shea, J.P. Anabolic steroid: Effects on strength development. *Science* 164:957-959, 1969.

Johnson, L.C.; Roundy, E.S.; Allsen, P.E.; Fisher, A.G.; and Silvester, L.J. Effect of anabolic steroid treatment on endurance. *Med Sci Sports* 7:287-289, 1975.

Keul, J.; Deus, H.; and Kinderman, W. Anabole hormone: Schadigug, Leistungsfahigkeit und Stoffwechses. *Med Klin* 71:497-503, 1976.

Kochakian, C.D., and Endahl, B.R. Changes in body weight of normal and castrated rats by different doses of testosterone propionate. *Proc Soc Exp Biol Med* 100:520-522, 1959.

Konagaya, M.; Bernard, P.A.; and Max, S.R. Blockage of glucocorticoid receptor binding and inhibition of dexamethasone-induced muscle atrophy in the rat by RU38486, a potent glucocorticoid antagonist. *Endocrinology* 119(1):375-580, 1986.

Kreuz, L.E., and Rose, R.M. Assessment of aggressive behavior and plasma testosterone in a young criminal population. *Psychosom Med* 34(4):321-332, 1972.

Ljungqvist, A. The use of anabolic steroids in top Swedish athletes. *Br J Sports Med* 9(2):82, 1975.

Loughton, S., and Ruhling, R. Human strength and endurance responses to anabolic steroid and training. *J Sports Med* 17:285-296, 1977.

Mather, D.N.; Toriola, A.L.; and Dada, O.A. Serum cortisol and testosterone levels in conditioned male distance runners and nonathletes after maximal exercise. *J Sports Med* 26:245-250, 1986.

Mayer, M., and Rosen, F. Interaction of anabolic steroids with glucocorticoid receptor sites in rat muscle cytosol. *Am J Phys* 229(5):1381-1386, 1975.

Nesheim, M.C. Some observations on the effectiveness of anabolic agents in increasing the growth rate in poultry. In: Lu, F.C., and Rendel, J., eds. *Anabolic Agents in Animal Production.* Stuttgart: Georg Thieme Publishers, 1976. pp. 110-114.

O'Shea, J.P. The effects of an anabolic steroid on dynamic strength levels of weightlifters. *Nutr Rep In* 4:363-370, 1971.

Persky, H.; Smith, K.D.; and Basu, G.K. Relation of psychologic measures of aggression and hostility to testosterone production in man. *Psychosom Med* 33(3):265-277, 1971.

Richardson, J.H. A comparison of two drugs on strength increase in monkeys. *J Sports Med Phys Fitness* 17:251-254, 1977.

Rogozkin, V.A. The role of low molecular weight compounds in the regulation of skeletal muscle genome activity during exercise. *Med Sci Sports* 8:104, 1976.

Rogozkin, V.A. Anabolic steroid metabolism in skeletal muscle. *J Steroid Biochem* 11:923-926, 1979.

Ryan, A.J. Anabolic steroids are fool's gold. *Fed Proc* 40:2682-2688, 1981.

Sar, W., and Stumpf, W. Androgen concentration in motor neurons of cranial nerves and spinal cord. *Science* 197:77-79, 1977.

Scaramella, T.J., and Brown, W.R. Serum testosterone and aggressiveness in hockey players. *Psychosom Med* 40(3):262-265, 1978.

Simon, N.G.; Whalen, R.E.; and Tate, M.P. Induction of male typical aggression by androgens but not by estrogens in adult female mice. *Horm Behav* 19:204-212, 1985.

Snochowski, M.; Dahlberg, E.; Eriksson, E.; and Gustafsson, J.A. Androgen and glucocorticoid receptors in human skeletal muscle cytosol. *J Steroid Biochem* 14:765-771, 1981.

Stamford, B.A., and Moffatt, R. Anabolic steroid: Effectiveness as an ergogenic aid to experienced weight trainers. *J Sports Med Phys Fitness* 14:191-197, 1974.

Starr, B. Defying gravity: How to win at weightlifting. Wichita Falls, TX: Five Star Production, 1981. pp. 84-94.

Stromme, S.B.; Meen, H.D.; and Aakvaag, A. Effects of an androgenic-anabolic steroid on strength development and plasma testosterone levels in normal males. *Med Sci Sports* 6:203-208, 1974.

Stumpf, W., and Sar, W. Steroid hormone target sites in the brain: The differential distribution of estrogen, progestin, androgen and glucocorticosteroid. *J Steroid Biochem* 7:1163-1170, 1976.

Todd, T. Anabolic steroids: The gremlins of sport. *J Sport Hist* 14(1):87-107, 1987.

Urhausen, A., and Kindermann, W. Behaviour of testosterone, sex hormone binding globulin (SHBG), and cortisol before and after a triathlon competition. *Int J Sports Med* 8:305-308, 1987.

Villaneuva, A.L.; Schlosser, S.; Hopper, B.; Liu, J.H.; Hoffman, D.I.; and Rebar, R.W. Increased cortisol production in women runners. *J Clin Endo Meta* 63(1):113-136, 1986.

Vyskocil, E., and Gutmann, E. Electrophysiological and contractile properties of the levator ani muscle after castration and testosterone administration. *Pflugers Arch* 368:104-109, 1977.

Ward, P. The effect of an anabolic steroid on strength and lean body mass. *Med Sci Sports* 5:277-283, 1973.

Wheeler, G.D.; Wall, S.R.; Belcasto, A.N.; and Cumming, D.C. Reduced serume testosterone and prolactin levels in male distance runners. *JAMA* 252(4):514-516, 1984.

Wright, J. *Anabolic Steroids and Sports.* Natick, MA: Sports Science Consultants 3, 1978.

Wright, J. *Anabolic Steroids and Sports.* Natick, MA: Sports Science Consultants 3, 1978.

Yesalis, C.; Wright, J.; and Lombardo, J. Anabolic-androgenic steroids: A synthesis of existing data and recommendations for future research. *Clin Sports Med* 1(3):109-134, 1989.

Young, M.; Crookshank, H.R.; and Ponder, L. Effects of an anabolic steroid on selected parameters in male albino rats. *Res Q* 48:653-656, 1977.

AUTHOR

John A. Lombardo, M.D.
Professor and Chairman
Department of Family Medicine
The Ohio State University
1114 University Hospitals Clinic
456 West 10th Avenue
Columbus, OH 43210

Anabolic Steroids: An Ethnographic Approach

Paul J. Goldstein

INTRODUCTION

The intent of this chapter is to make two sorts of contributions. The first is conceptual—to provide a sociological framework and a substance abuse perspective from which the emergent social problem of anabolic steroid misuse may be viewed. The second contribution is to present some preliminary empirical findings from participant observation research that was done in health clubs and gyms in the New York City area. As part of this effort, interviews were conducted with bodybuilders, personal trainers (PTs), and gym staff.

The poor quality of available data on the use and effects of anabolic steroids and their frequent contradictory nature is consistently bemoaned. There is clearly a need to advance beyond anecdotes, rumors, and locker room gossip. Yet, it is important to realize that reports of such "gossip" provide an insight into the manner in which users perceive anabolic steroids, their motivations for use, and both their functional and dysfunctional experiences with these substances.

The approach employed herein is part of a methodological tradition common to the study of drug abuse. It focuses on understanding users' interpretations of the etiology and meaning of drug abuse within their own sociocultural environment. This tradition, with its roots in phenomenology, is usually called qualitative methodology, or ethnography. Its primary focus is on users' perceptions of meaning and the contexts of initiation and sustaining of drug-abusing behavior (McBride and Clayton 1985).

Data about the nature and scope of anabolic steroid use are difficult to collect, and becoming more so, owing to recent upgrading of penalties for both steroid possession and sale. The Anti-Drug Abuse Act of 1988 upgraded Federal penalties in this area. Some States had preceded the Federal Government in this regard, e.g., California; others have followed suit since

74

the Federal legislation; others are considering doing so. For example, Georgia has recently upgraded penalties for steroid trafficking to a third-degree felony status. This has reportedly made steroid users and traffickers in that State more reluctant to talk to researchers. According to one social scientist, who had been interviewing high school and college steroid users, mainly football players, many participants in competitive athletics will no longer discuss their steroid experiences with outsiders because they are afraid of being turned in (John R. Fuller, personal communication, January 1989).

The key informants, or "guides," who have been introducing me into various health clubs and gyms in New York City and Long Island all cautioned me against publicly declaring any special interest in steroids. I was told that everybody would just "clam up" if they learned that was my primary interest. I have been presenting myself simply as a sociologist interested in the workout and fitness world.

There are three principal areas in which information about steroid use and distribution must be generated: epidemiology, distribution, and consequences.

EPIDEMIOLOGY

Some sources provide a rough indication of the extent of steroid use. The Mayo Clinic estimated more than 1 million regular steroid users in America (Couzens 1988). It has been suggested that as many as 96 percent of professional football players may have taken steroids (Jacobson 1988; Schuckit 1988). It has also been suggested that between 80 and 99 percent of male bodybuilders have taken steroids (Schuckit 1988, Hecht 1984; Lee 1985). There has been talk of increasing steroid use among female bodybuilders, as the trend in that sport has moved away from the goal of obtaining a "dancer's physique" towards increasing muscularity (Lee 1985).

Buckley and colleagues (1988) found that 6.6 percent of a national sample of 12th-grade males reported using *or* having used anabolic steroids. Other scattered high school level epidemiological information includes an unscientific survey by Miami's South Plantation High School student newspaper in 1986. It sampled 200 of the school's 2,000 pupils. Sixty-five percent knew someone who was taking steroids (Miami Herald 1988). This sort of statistic is important because other research in the substance abuse field has shown that having drug-using peers is one of the best predictors of drug use. Eleven percent of high school football players in Arkansas were reported to be using anabolic steroids (Herrmann 1988). Thirty-eight percent of high school football players surveyed in Portland, OR, knew where to get steroids (Charlier 1988).

Many individuals who are informed about the high school scene stress the importance of the steroid issue. Fred Rozelle, Executive Secretary of the Florida High School Activities Association, stated that "We face a lot of problems, but we feel that the number one concern is steroids" (Phillips and Lohrer 1989, p. 4D). Don Leggett, a Food and Drug Administration (FDA) official, said, "Bulging muscles are in. Guys want to look good at the beach. High school kids think steroids may enhance their ability to get an athletic scholarship, play professional sports, or win the girl of their heart. Steroid use in this country has spread down to general people" (Penn 1988, p. A1). A Philadelphia physical therapist, who works with athletes, stated, "People think the cocaine issue is big. It's not as big as anabolic steroids. Among kids, it's epidemic" (Charlier 1988, p. A20).

Within the context of epidemiology, substance abuse researchers have tended to emphasize the concepts of a drug-using "career" or a "natural history" of drug use. Such careers, or natural histories, may be conceptualized as having three steps:

1. Initial stage of exploration.

2. Continuing stage, in which use is regular, and the identity of the user is established.

3. Cessation from use (usually preceded by growing ambivalence towards regular use and unsuccessful attempts at detachment).

Exploration Stage

Steroid use may be viewed as a search for a competitive edge in athletics. Many athletes have a win-at-any-cost mentality. Of course, this mentality is common to areas other than athletics. The rhetoric in these other areas is remarkably similar to the steroid rhetoric. For example, I recently received a brochure for a February 1989 conference on "Achieving Excellence." The conference included seminars in financial planning, organization, innovation, and leadership skills. One of the presenters was Nancy K. Austin, author of the 1985 publication *A Passion for Excellence: The Leadership Difference.* The brochure announced her presentation as follows:

> Nancy K. Austin highlights how "winners"—even those in
> mundane, decaying, battered or regulated environments—
> create and sustain their competitive edge. They don't just
> do a percent or two better than the rest, they do hundreds of
> percentage points better . . . This presentation will highlight
> those who have achieved extraordinary results under fire and
> how they succeeded while others faded away.

I suspect that if a pill or an injectable were available that was touted to guarantee such a competitive edge in business, or in grant writing, it would be used eagerly. Steroids function in this fashion with regard to athletics and body development. Of course, what happens is similar to the arms race. Those with early access to an innovation do have an edge. Soon, however, the 'have nots' catch up. In the case of steroids, the word now is that everybody is doing it and competitive steroid users no longer have an edge; they must use just to stay even with their rivals.

There can be no question that there has been an escalation of muscularity in those areas in which muscularity is important. Professional athletes are bigger and stronger now than they ever were. The old cinema muscle men, like Victor Mature, look fairly puny compared to modem titans like Arnold Schwarzenegger. Charles Atlas, in his famous advertisements of three decades ago, looks like a pretty ordinary guy today. Competitive body-builders claim that persons who won major titles 10, or even 5 years ago, would have little chance against today's competitors. One bodybuilder claimed that today "the only way you can make even the beginnings of an amateur is by taking steroids."

The use of performance enhancers in athletic competitions are neither new nor limited to steroids. Participants in 6-day bicycle races in 1879 were alleged to have prepared as follows: the French used a mixture made from a caffeine base; the Belgians ate sugar cubes dipped in ether; others drank alcohol cordials; and sprinters used nitroglycerine (STASH 1978). In 1886, a British cyclist died from using a drug containing ephedrine, a stimulant alleged to mask fatigue and remove physiological restraints intended to prevent overexertion (STASH 1978). In remarks to the January 1984 meeting of the FDA Endocrinologic and Metabolic Drugs Advisory Committee, Thomas Murray of the Hastings Center noted that performance enhancers were popular at the turn of the century. Vin Muriani, a widely used mixture of coca leaf extract and wine, was advertised as the wine for athletes. It was reportedly used by French cyclists and by a champion lacrosse team in Peru (Hecht 1984).

A variety of other substances or techniques are employed by athletes who try to give themselves an edge on the competition. These include special dietary regimens, vitamins, bicarbonate loading (for short events), caffeine loading (for long events), and such psychological techniques as hypnosis.

Some gyms sell a wide variety of products to their clientele. A blender will mix up an Aminofuel or Carbofuel drink for $2. For an extra $1 a banana will be added. Fruit punchlike concoctions that are billed as being rich in amino acids are sold for $2. In speaking with gym regulars, it becomes clear that some persons lack the sophistication to discriminate between such products and steroids.

For young high school athletes, getting big and strong enough to compete on the collegiate level may be vital for their future. Don Reynolds, chairman of the drug abuse committee of Florida High School Activities Association, stated, "I think there is a lot more steroid use than we think there is. High schools is where it's at. That's where the competition for college scholarships begins" (Phillips and Lohrer 1989, p. 4D). Parents may contribute to this pressure to obtain athletic scholarships.

Steroid use should also be viewed in the context of the search for substances that increase feelings and appearances of strength. Steroid research has been likened to the search for a "superman formula" (Schuckit 1988). Stories of great strength have intrigued our imaginations for centuries. We have television series like "The Bionic Man"; comic book superheroes like Superman and the Hulk; biblical supermen like Samson; legendary strongmen like Hercules; that staple of carnivals, the sideshow strong man; professional wrestlers; a long list of male movie stars, such as Victor Mature, Steve Reeves, and Arnold Schwarzenegger, whose muscular bodies were their main attraction for the ticket-buying public. Weight-lifting competitions are popular Olympic events. Bodybuilding contests attract large audiences and are frequently shown on cable television. Children watching Saturday morning cartoon shows aspire to the impossible-to-achieve muscularity of superheroes such as He-Man. Popeye's spinach eating produces the great strength that allows him to vanquish his comical opponents.

Clearly, there is something about muscular development and great strength that taps into something very basic to the male mentality. Sexual attractiveness is part of this. Young boys want to impress the girls with their muscles. One young man that I spoke to in a gym remarked that it is tough for high school kids when a muscular guy takes their girl away. Some boys feel that they cannot compete with a guy who has a great body. It is a real incentive for them to try to develop their own bodies as fast as possible. Steroids present the promise that such aspirations can be achieved through chemistry.

In health clubs and gyms, I have observed the frustration felt by those who are working out intensely, yet who are not achieving substantial results. This frustration is intense for persons who are working out next to someone who is enjoying good results, i.e., getting bigger and stronger much more rapidly than they are. Such frustrated persons become targets of pushers who offer a short cut to physical development. Pushers may compliment persons on their successful workout regimen but stress that, if the person continues to work out at such a pace, it may take 5 or 6 more years of struggle and pain before the person will look that certain way. Of course, there is a way to get there a lot sooner. That way is, of course, the use of anabolic steroids.

78

Successful bodybuilders, especially competitors, are usually approached in a different fashion. Pushers of steroids may begin their sales pitch to successful bodybuilders by saying such things as the following:

1. "You're looking good, but you look unfinished. You need something in order to get that finished look."

2. "You look good enough to enter a competition. But you don't look good enough to win. You'll need something else for that."

However, a former steroid user and PT who has worked with adolescents cautions against attributing most steroid use to competitive bodybuilders or other athletes.

> Forget that! I think the majority of people who use steroids don't have any idea of going into a contest. Let's not go in a direction that these steroids arc being used **by** bodybuilders who aspire to be Mr. Universe. That's baloney. Steroids are being used mostly by men and women and young kids just for their ego.

> . . . I see the kids using it today. It just blows my mind. They are using at a young age for one reason only, for their egos. Whcthcr to get dates, whether to be part of a gang . . . The peer pressure is enormous for strength. If you're not a rock singer, you damn well better be a muscle man.

> . . . once bodybuilding hits you, it doesn't matter. Once the idea of strength and size, and feeling good about yourself and being admired and looked at hits you, you could be from anywhcrc.

Users also describe a euphoric state produced by steroids. One user said, "The anabolics make you feel good mentally. They are a high."

Continuing Stage

For whatever reasons people begin steroid use, it appears that the addictive nature of the substance. the habituating effect of the workout routine itself, and the feelings of muscularity and strength that arise create a syndrome of continued and habitual use.

Addiction is a difficult concept to operationalize. Previous research with heroin users indicated that individuals who are typically classified as heroin addicts, in fact, have patterns of use that contain many peaks and valleys, and days of nonuse arc frequently intermixed with days of use (Johnson et al. 1985). In other words, operational definitions of addiction, especially those employing a medical model, may be of limited value in predicting actual behavior of substance users in their environments over time.

The classic behavioral definition of addiction was that advanced by Alfred Lindesmith (1947). Essentially, he argued that persons might begin using a drug for a variety of reasons, usually involving positive feelings produced by the drug. Individuals might continue to use the drug for this reason. However, real addiction sets in when the individual experiences negative feelings, such as pain or dysphoria in the absence of the drug, attributes these negative sensations to the lack of the drug, and begins to administer the drug to ward off the negative sensations rather than attempting to achieve a positive feeling.

A variety of knowledgeable sources, including Robert Voy, have argued that an addiction syndrome exists with regard to anabolic steroids (Jacobson 1988; Schuckit 1988). Craig Whitehead, who directed the drug rehabilitation unit of the Haight-Ashbury Clinic, stated, "The dependence many people develop on steroids is classic" (Cowart 1987a, p. 427).

The addiction syndrome that has been described to me by habitual steroid users harmonizes well with Lindesmith's definition. Users claim that steroids function to anesthetize the body. Steroids enable the user to work out intensely without feeling pain. However, when the user stops taking steroids, muscles and joints (especially) become very sore. Old injuries or strains that were not even noticed before begin to be very painful. The ex-user cannot work out anywhere near the level that he or she did while taking steroids. It is just too painful now. Indeed, common everyday physical tasks may become difficult and painful. Psychological feelings of depression set in. If the user returns to steroids, the pain disappears. The depression disappears. One's body feels good again. One can return to one's workout regimen.

A PT whom I interviewed described some manifestations of this addictive state of mind.

> I hear it all the time. I heard it just yesterday . . . three guys . . . I asked them how they're doing. They said, "Well, good. I just got back from skiing. I can't wait to get back on the stuff." That's all you hear. And another guy, "How you been?" "Good, doing all right, you know, maintaining, but in 2 weeks I got all my stuff together now, I'm going back on the stuff." These arc not competitive bodybuilders. These are just gym guys who are printers and going to school.

A steroid user described to me the manner in which steroids affect the psychology of users and function to perpetuate use.

If you never use [steroids], you use your natural inclination
to drive forward. Whatever may have been your driving
force, whether it was to show your father that you can succeed in life, or whether it was being insecure and needing to
have assurance from the world that you can be somebody
. . . If you have that burning up so hard in you, then you
can make it with that. But once you get on the steroids,
you'll lose that ability to call upon self. It then controls
you, and you actually lose the ability to ever do that again.
There's a part of you that goes and never comes back . . .
If you do it for one little 12-week cycle, and you can
manage to get off it, and you say, "this was not for me,"
God bless you. But if you're stuck on that stuff for a year,
you're hooked for life. You're no longer a virgin . . .
you're finished. You forget a lot of the innocence that you
had. Or a lot of the natural drive that is in there. 'Cause
this stuff gives you a new level of aggression and power
that you can't achieve on your own by thinking it out on
your own anymore. You just can't. You try! Like you're
lifting a dumbbell, and you give up. "I ain't going to do it.
I'm leaving." But you go to the gym when you're on that
stuff, and everything is going good, and your levels are real
built up high . . . You take that weight, 40 pounds heavier,
and you do it. Screaming! Crazy joy! Ecstasy! It is like
having an orgasm. It's better. You don't have any idea
what it's like . . . It's total orgasm. Oneness. It is like a
one cell creature reproducing itself. It's just incredible . . .
The fire. the escalation of joy and excitement, the conquer-
ing of it. And it's nowhere near as exciting when you're
off the stuff as when you're on it. You just feel so good
that you just want to buy 20 bottles more. That's the way
it is. It's crazy.

Some users say that feelings of power become so associated with steroid
use that persons begin to use steroids for social situations in which they
feel insecure. For example, adolescents may take steroids before going to a
party because they feel nervous, and the steroids give them a sense of being
able to handle the situation. In this case, the drugs address basic feelings
of inadequacy. One user stated, "You get to believe in the drugs so much,
that if you need a crutch, you will take a few extra pills."

Several factors appear inextricably linked in a steroid addiction syndrome.
For example, steroid users find it almost impossible to analytically separate
the drug from the workout itself. They say that one would just not exist
without the other. Without the drug, there would be no workout. Without
the workout, there would be no need for the drug. It should be noted that
persons who do not use steroids, yet who are also committed to working

out, frequently talk about the addictive nature of a workout regimen. But serious steroid use and habitual working out seem to dissolve into a unitary lifestyle. One user vividly described this reality.

> You get into the vicious cycle of doing more and more and more and doing new sophisticated stuff . . . Then once you're on the stuff, you feel differently. See you're on it and all of a sudden you're making the gains . . . And you're strong. And you have no pains like you had before. You're very euphoric. You kind of feel indestructible. And nothing matters. They can steal your car. You know, so what? If you caught the guy, you would kill him. But if you didn't, all right, the car's gone. As long as the gym is open . . . Don't steal your food. Don't steal your steroids. But you can take my car, my wife, take anything you want. That's really how you become. And you don't know it. You're in this fog.

The gym culture itself tends to perpetuate steroid use. The gym culture is very competitive. Bodybuilders are always comparing themselves to other gym regulars or to the proverbial "new guy" as to who is biggest and strongest. Persons who are getting bigger and stronger may feel puny and weak, because a gym buddy is progressing faster than they-lifting more weight or adding more lean muscle. Girls hanging around the gym gravitate towards the biggest, strongest guys. Friends exert pressure to get back on "the stuff." The grapevine is filled with gossip about who is selling what. Special "deals" may be offered. The peer pressure to continue steroid use is strong.

Cessation From Use

Steroid users that I have talked with tend to cease their use for one of two reasons. Most younger persons seem to "mature out" when they reach an age at which career, marriage, and all the trappings of conventional lifestyles become more highly valued than a macho image of great strength and size. Older, long-term steroid users tend to quit only when their health is seriously threatened. A long-term steroid user, who had been a highly successful competitive bodybuilder, claimed to have almost died from liver problems about 3 years ago.

> After I got sick, I had to come off it, or I never would have come off it. I would never have come off of steroids if I didn't get sick. Never! I'd still be using it today and trying to compete at 40. But I was forced. I almost died. So you choose between that and living. You find out living is not so bad.

DISTRIBUTION

Until recently, black market sale of steroids was estimated at more than $100 million per year (Couzens 1988; Penn 1988; Kahler 1989). However, this estimate was recently upgraded to between $300 and $400 million per year by Leslie Southwick, Deputy Assistant Attorney General (1990).

It has been estimated that more than half the steroids smuggled into the United States are counterfeit, frequently bearing the names of reputable manufacturers. Most supplies are alleged to come from Mexico (Penn 1988; Kahler 1989). These counterfeits are often produced in crude, unsanitary laboratories and are of dubious purity. Counterfeit steroids are also being manufactured in this country, in makeshift laboratories that are springing up around the United States. My own sources in gyms in the New York City area have suggested that as much as 80 percent of the steroids that they encounter are counterfeit.

One clandestine laboratory, Fountain Valley Research Laboratories, Inc., located 35 miles south of Los Angeles was shut down recently. It produced what were labeled as East German steroids. The labels read: *Eigentum Der DDR-Versenden Gesetzlich Verboten*—"Property of GDR, export prohibited." The steroids fetched $180 per bottle. "East German steroids are rated the best," said a California lawman. "Their athletes have the reputation of being better, bigger, and stronger" (Penn 1988, p. A20).

The Department of Justice has recently expressed an interest in the use and trafficking of steroids. Assistant Attorney General John Bolton stated the following.

> Not only are we concerned with the risks associated with the unprescribed use of legitimate steroids (by adolescents), risks such as upsetting the hormonal balance and stunting growth, but of equal or greater concern is the unauthorized use of illegitimate steroids which have no FDA approval and are made under less than sanitary conditions. We think it's a very dangerous problem . . . You will see a lot more prosecutions. Prosecution of steroid cases is a priority for the civil division. (Kahler 1989, p. 29)

Justice officials have reportedly obtained Federal convictions or guilty pleas against 60 steroid traffickers in the 2 1/2 years preceding October 1988. About 120 more persons face charges (Penn 1988). In December 1988, former British Olympic medalist David Jenkins was sentenced to 7 years in prison followed by 5 years probation and was fined $75,000 for his role in arranging for a Tijuana plant, Laboratorios Milano de Mexico, to produce anabolic steroids and smuggle them across the border for distribution in the United States (Kahler 1989).

There are indications that traditional drug traffickers are involved in steroid distribution. There are also indications that they are conducting their business in the traditional ways of drug traffickers The following account appeared in the *Wall Street Journal.*

> According to criminal charges filed in San Diego last year, when a man in Phoenix reneged on a steroid deal, his supplier sent an emissary named Leonard T. Swirda. Mr. Swirda took along an accomplice carrying a 12 inch club, a double edged knife and leather gloves weighted with metal, says the indictment, which accuses Mr. Swirda of beating and cutting the dealer. In a separate action, Mr. Swirda last May was indicted for cocaine trafficking in Spokane, Washington. (Penn 1988, p. A1, A20)

The underground world of steroid use and trafficking is prone to the same sorts of hustles and scams that we are more used to hearing about with regard to street drugs, such as cocaine or heroin. One common hustle concerns the difference in price between generic and name brand steroids. Brand names, of course, fetch a higher price. Inexperienced users are frequently sold generic steroids, but are charged brand name prices.

A former steroid user, speaking of the great prevalence of bogus steroids, recalled a product called Bolasterone.

> Bolasterone. It swept the country. They made millions. Millions, these California guys. All it was, was vegetable oil, a little bit of testosterone, and liquid aspirin. And they called it Bolasterone. And they hyped it up so much. It was selling for $250 to $275 a bottle. You would do anything to get this stuff. [They said] "Mr. Olympia used it! Secretly." I tell you, Madison Avenue could not have come up with a better campaign to sell this stuff . . . If you had a bottle of it, I me-an you could sell it for anything . . . [It was hyped] through the grapevine. Underground. The network is incredible. From gym to gym to gym . . . They'll say, "Did you see M.? He put on 15 pounds in a week." "What the hell is he using?" "Don't say anything. He's using Bolasterone!" "Wow. What the hell is it? Can you get it?" "Yeah, I can."

It is difficult to estimate actual costs to users because of a wide variability in patterns of use. Serious long-term uses may spend as much as $200 to $400 per week on steroids and the accompanying pharmacopoeia. Since such users may go on cycles of steroid use lasting 12 to 14 weeks, each cycle can cost in the thousands of dollars. Users are generally afraid of being caught short in the middle of a cycle, and like to have all the drugs that they will be using in hand before they start their cycle.

Cycles generally begin with a few pills of this kind, a few pills of that kind during the first week; gradually the number and strength of pills is increased; then injectibles are introduced into the cycle. As the weeks go by, the number of pills and shots increase until a plateau is reached; for example, about the ninth week of a 14-week cycle. Then users come back down the same way they went up.

Younger, or less experienced or committed users, will use considerably less. Some persons may be long-term users, but take only one injection per week. Adolescents may go on shorter cycles, perhaps only 6 weeks. Some adolescents will only use when they have the money to do so. These youngsters may take a very few pills or shots on an irregular basis.

As with most drug use, a primary way of supporting one's own steroid use is trafficking in the substance. Also, since many users do not use that much, they are able to support their steroid use by working, getting money from women, stealing from their parents, or engaging in petty theft. Competitive athletes may be supplied by coaches, promoters, or other interested parties.

Steroid use may also be supported by male friends. Older or wealthier homosexuals are frequently interested in the company of young, male bodybuilders. These homosexual liaisons may involve sexual activity or remain at the friendship level. Older bodybuilders report that this phenomenon was more common prior to the advent of AIDS than it is today.

Male bodybuilders may obtain employment for which their muscularity especially qualifies them. Some examples of these sorts of jobs include bouncers, male dancers in such clubs as Chippendales, and models.

PTs

One of the hallmarks of the sociological approach is a focus on social structure and social roles. David Matza summarized the sociological approach nicely in a discussion of delinquency.

> The distinguishing feature of sociological theory, in contrast
> to formulations stressing personality, lies in the prominence
> of the social situation. Sociology brings to the foreground
> the social circumstances that form the backdrop for personal-
> ity theory. (Matza 1964, p. 17)

In doing ethnographic research in health clubs and gyms, I was struck by a particular social role—the PT. PTs enjoy a high status in the "workout" world. They are the cognoscenti, the knowledgeable insiders, the gurus. They instruct their clients in a wide variety of areas including workout techniques, diet, nutritional supplements, and sometimes in the use of steroids. PTs typically work with a heterogeneous clientele that may include overweight housewives, professional football players, competitive bodybuilders, adolescents who want to look better, and simple gym habituees.

Most clients do not appear interested in ascertaining potential PTs' educational or professional credentials; they are more concerned with how PTs look. If a PT has a title, e.g., Mr. America, that seems to carry the most weight with potential clients. The title is proof of the PT's ability to condition a body; it is a real status thing to be able to say that Mr. America is one's PT. Additional status is held by PTs with ties to professional athletics. It enhances clients' status to be able to say that their PT trains football players. It is also fun to feel like an insider, e.g., to get some gossip about sports celebrities.

Individuals become PTs for a variety of reasons. The basic reason is, of course, money. PTs tend to be young men and women beginning a career in the fitness business, young athletically oriented persons who reject a 9-to-5 office existence, or older athletes who are retired from competition and who may have few marketable job skills. Health clubs pay very low wages. At one health club that I visited, the fitness director, who had 3 years experience. a bachelor's degree, and some credits towards a masters degree, mode $19,000 per year. There is a need to supplement salary by taking on private clients, who will pay about $25 per hour.

Bartering is not uncommon among PTs. For example, one young female PT that I spoke with has a client who is a psychiatrist. They exchange hours of physical training for hours of therapy.

PTs' income may be erratic. Clients go in and out of phases of life dedicated to working out. Clients are usually fairly wealthy and may do lots of traveling. They may go south during the winter, cutting substantially into a PT's income.

PTs may recruit and see clients at a number of different health clubs or gyms. They may spend some mornings at this gym; some afternoons at that gym; some evenings at yet another. They may also go to client's homes. Their network of contacts tends to be far reaching.

There appears to be a growing professionalization of the fitness field, exemplified by the growth of degree programs in physical education, biomechanics, exercise physiology, and so on. New young holders of professional certifications are in conflict with older fitness and bodybuilding trainers whose knowledge is experiential rather than learned from books.

Older PTs used their own bodies as their laboratories, experimenting with various workout routines, nutritional programs, and drugs, including steroids. The success of particular regimens was subjectively determined and also objectively determined in terms of looks, performance, and titles achieved.

I have observed conflict in health clubs between younger credentialed PTs and older noncredentialed PTs. They argue over which pieces of equipment to install and what sort of training regimens are appropriate to use. They are in competition for clients, scarce jobs, and the acceptance of their point of view as to how the subject matter in their field should be taught. The situation may be viewed, from the standpoint of occupational sociology, as a case of developing professionalism, which poses interesting sociology-of-knowledge issues, regarding experiential vs. academic knowledge.

The prevalence of PTs is difficult to estimate. Most trainers that I spoke with were reluctant to make any quantitative estimates. The best "guesstimates" that I was able to obtain were that there are about 1,000 PTs in New York's Nassau County going to persons homes, and about 1,500 working in clubs. The American College of Sports Medicine certifies trainers, but it appears that most trainers work without certification, and, hence, it would be difficult to ascertain how many PTs there actually are.

For comparative purposes, there arc approximately 1,200 Aerobics & Fitness Association of America (AFAA)-certified aerobics instructors teaching on Long Island, which includes Nassau and Suffolk counties, according to Peg Jordan, editor of *American Fitness* magazine. However, about 50 percent of all Long Island instructors have had no professional training at all. That percentage is better than the national average in which only an estimated 17,000 of 100,000 acrobic instructors are AFAA certified (Hancock 1989).

PTs play an interesting role with regard to steroid use and distribution. Some may be users themselves. PTs may be motivated to use steroids because they feel a need to look perfect. Their ability to secure and maintain clients may depend on how good they look, how good their clients perceive them as looking, and how they perceive themselves as looking.

More important, PTs, as bodybuilding gurus, have a strong influence on their clients. This influence may be exerted to encourage or discourage steroid use. Experienced PTs, because of their wide networks of contacts, may be pressured by clients to supply them with steroids. PTs may be financially motivated to supply steroids to clients that ask for them. In addition to the profit to be made from selling steroids, PTs are primarily concerned with maintaining clientele. If they do not supply steroids to a client that requests them, the client may find another PT that will supply steroids. The original PT then loses a client. One PT remarked that, for this reason. he will not train bodybuilders anymore.

It just got to be too nuts. What with you trying to please
everybody. Who wants this, who wants that, and you're
watching everybody self-destruct. I couldn't take it. When
you train bodybuilders, that one-to-one trainer will certainly
be looked upon as the guru of many things. And certainly
it affords the trainer an opportunity to make a lot of money.
But it isn't the one-to-one trainer who is the source of distribution of the stuff. Really. It occurs, and it happens, but
he isn't the main. He doesn't get into it to do that.

Older PTs, especially those who are or have been steroid users themselves,
express horror at the naivete with which many young persons approach the
use of steroids. Many PTs feel a responsibility to coach the young person
in the proper use of these substances to minimize the potential health consequences. A 57-year-old man who claimed to have taken one shot of deca-
durabolin per week, "forever," said that the kids today were worrying him.

[They are] . . . using so much stuff. I walk into the gym,
and they're all 17 years old, and they all look like pus
heads . . . They are all puffed out with water. And they
have very little muscle. Because they are just throwing crap
into their bodies. They have no idea . . . And who knows
what they are doing to their insides . . . They're stupid by
taking the steroids so wrong.

A PT remarked that everyone is different and that steroid users must be
medically monitored, both while on cycles and when between cycles.

Blood tests . . . white cell counts. We're looking to see
liver, kidney problems. We are looking to set pancreatic
and pituitary problems. We want to see their testrosterone
levels, estrogen levels. nitrogen levels. We want to see their
blood-sugar level, thyroid, adrenal, and if they have normal-
ized, they can go back on them. If it's 4 weeks, they can
go back on them. If it is 4 months, they have to keep
taking the test until they're normal. If not, no sense going
back on it again. The body won't react. They just keep
getting worse. You do need a healthy body to keep this
stuff working to the maximum.

Additional factors mentioned as important were levels of minerals, such as
calcium and magnesium. Steroids are calcium depleting.

With regard to steroids currently being used, I am told that the trend today
is towards veterinary steroids. One user described this trend in the following way.

88

Veterinary drugs are cheaper, they come in much larger quantities and they're much better . . . They're more anabolic. The androgenic ones tend to build fat, hold water . . . Race horses are the biggest users of anabolic steroids. They cannot breed a horse that's full of water and fat. Every tiny micro-ounce must be muscle, or he's not going to win a race. He cannot carry any extra weight. So if you have ever seen a race horse up close, it's built like the greatest bodybuilders of the world. They are tipped to the bone. And they are very muscular and thick. So that has certainly seeped its way down . . . in the last 20 years. And a lot of the drugs they are using now are the veterinary drugs. The Winstrol-V, [and others] . . . They come in these huge 50-cc bottles.

I don't think the veterinarians are selling them to bodybuilders. I think they're a lot more sensible than that. But it is filtering down through the veterinary market. I think maybe the distributors or the salesmen have found the market.

CONSEQUENCES

Some experienced steroid users place much of the responsibility for the current problem on pharmaceutical companies, and suggest that the nature and scope of health consequences are likely to increase in the future. A long-term steroid user stated the following:

Athletes that used them in the late forties, they . . . used it very sparingly, so anybody who developed a tumor here or there, it had to be very scarce. Then the fifties came, and some synthetics came in to being used. Then the sixties came, and a little more research got involved in it. Around the late sixties or early seventies, the drug companies realized there was a hell of a market here for the stuff. So they threw some dollars into research. Now the steroids are so sophisticated and are getting even more sophisticated. The old ones are not even available anymore. They got a whole new line . . . The more powerful ones weren't being used, certainly not as often as today. Now, in the eighties, and going into the nineties, they are using anabolics that . . . work so fast, they are so powerful . . . I don't think the body has caught up with the dosage or the science of it all . . . And not as many people were using it as they are today, because the sport [bodybuilding] was not as popular in the past as it is today . . . So 20 years from now, you're

going to see a whole bunch of people dying. But you are
going to have to wait 20 years.

There is a long list of health consequences that have been associated with
the use of anabolic steroids. Unfortunately, good clinical documentation
and elaboration, obtained through rigorously controlled experimental studies,
is lacking in most areas. However, the list of commonly discussed health
consequences of steroid use includes liver problems (tumors, peliosis hepatitis), kidney problems, hypertension, psychiatric problems (depression,
aggression), sexual problems in males (testicular atrophy, decreased sperm
production, gynecomastia), sexual problems in females (menstrual irregulari-
ties, shrinkage of breast tissue, hypertrophy of the clitoris, facial hair, deepened voice), acne, physical injuries, cholesterol difficulties, cardiovascular
problems, stunted growth in adolescents, male pattern baldness, fetal damage, gallstones, and so on. Since most of these topics are covered by other
chapters in this volume, I chose to focus my discussion of health consequences on only two areas that are of traditional interest to drug abuse
researchers: (1) interactions between steroids and other drugs, and
(2) needle sharing.

Steroids and Other Drugs

In the area of health consequences, the National Institute on Drug Abuse
(NIDA) should have a special interest in interaction effects between steroids
and other drugs of abuse. In this regard, experienced steroid-using bodybuilders hold a taken-for-granted prohibition against using cocaine while on
a steroid cycle. They claim that there is a great danger of heart attacks if
the two substances are mixed. One user stated that whenever he reads of a
young athlete dying suddenly of a heart attack, he immediately suspects an
interaction between steroids and cocaine.

Amphetamines may be used to help drive the workout regimen. Long-term
steroid users report that, as the years go by, steroids lose their ability to
provide the driving force for the workout routine. At this point, "speed"
may come to be used. Under the influence of speed, bodybuilders report
going "nuts," working out until totally exhausted, and then "falling out."

No one that I have spoken with reported any specific interactions between
alcohol and steroids. In fact, most of the bodybuilders who shared their
experiences with me were very moderate drinkers or abstainers. Interestingly, one person observed that, in his opinion, persons who have great tolerance to alcohol tend to have a great tolerance to steroids.

Those who get drunk on a beer really get a lot of side
effects real quick on steroids. Migraine headaches, bloody
noses, deep acne--tremendous scarring of the face. It is
funny . . .

90

Experienced steroid users also report using a wide variety of other drugs along with steroids. The primary purpose of these other drugs is to cope with the side effects of the steroids. For example, in order to prevent or retard the spread of acne, antibiotics are used. Nolvadex is medicine used in the treatment of breast cancer. It is an antiestrogen. Bodybuilders may use Nolvadex during steroid cycles to keep their estrogen levels down.

When coming off a steroid cycle, human chorionic gonadotropin (HCG) and Clomid are used. HCG is a polypeptide hormone produced by the human placenta. It is derived from the urine of pregnant women. The use of exogenous hormones (steroids) tends to depress the body's natural hormone production. Heavy steroid users wish to return to normal levels of testosterone as quickly as possible when they come off a steroid cycle. They claim the body is usually sluggish and just takes too long to return to normal hormonal activity. HCG is reportedly used to simulate an estrogen buildup in the male, which "shocks" the system into a more rapid recovery. Clomid, a female fertility drug, is alleged to perform the same trickery. Teslac and Halotestin are also reported to accomplish this result.

Long-term steroid users claim that there is a right way to do steroids, which involves full knowledge of pharmacological "chain reactions." The above discussion has just presented a few of the substances that are commonly employed by anabolic steroid users who were interviewed in the New York City area. Some of these users maintain amazing pharmacopeias.

There are two contrary health-consequence aspects of this multiple drug use. The first relates to the utility and dangers of this wide range of drugs being used by the most pharmacologically sophisticated steroid users. The other health-consequence aspect refers to the fact that many users are not sophisticated; they are not aware of potentially damaging side effects or the means for circumventing them. Many young men can barely afford the steroids that they are using. They see the purchase of these other substances as a low-priority item in an already strained budget. A sophisticated PT stated the following.

> These. kids, of course, don't know anything about this . . . I get the reaction from them like I have two heads. Some of them don't want to listen to it. They say, "I'm just taking my 'tes' or my Dianabol 'cause my friend is taking them." But anybody who is serious about going on them . . . and who is really interested in his health and going on a couple of cycles will have to absorb this.

Needle Sharing

Persons using injectable steroids are prone to all the health hazards common to needle users of any substance. This includes diseases associated with

91

bacterial infections caused by injections with nonsterile equipment. This practice may lead to localized infection problems, such as abscesses and cellulitis, or systemic problems such as endocarditis, hepatitis, and AIDS.

A competitive bodybuilder reported that a number of his colleagues had problems when they were first learning how to inject themselves.

> A lot of people don't know how to do it. They do it eventually because they feel they have to. Or they get a friend who learned from a friend, who learned from a sister who is a nurse. That's generally how it works. And you learn how to put it in a muscle. A lot of guys have come to me that they hit a vein and they are black or blue . . . You hit too much in the same site and you get tumors all the time. A lot of bodybuilders had to get those cut out . . . Actually you get huge fibroid lumps that develop from hitting the same sites.

Harold Connelly, an Olympic gold medalist in the hammer throw, testified to the following before a U.S. Senate Committee in 19'73.

> It was not unusual in 1968 to see athletes with their own medical kits, practically a doctor's, in which they would have syringes and all their various drugs . . . I know any number of athletes on the '68 Olympic team who had so much scar tissue and so many puncture holes on their backsides that it was difficult to find a fresh spot to give them a new shot. (Hecht 1984, p. 14)

All competitive athletes that I have spoken with denied using dirty needles or sharing needles. As one person stated, "The guy who's selling you the needles wants you to buy 100 needles. He don't want to sell you two needles."

However, in some inner-city gyms, I did get reports that heterosexual lovers, perhaps spouses, who are working out together, will sometimes share needles. It's part of the "we do everything else together so why not this" feeling. A young woman told me that such couples decide which muscles they will work on that day, inject into that muscle sharing the needle, and then go and do their workout.

A 1984 letter to the editor of *The New England Journal of Medicine* from six physicians at Nassau Hospital in New York described a case of AIDS in a bodybuilder using anabolic steroids. This was a 37-year-old white male who denied any history of homosexual activity. He did admit to injecting cocaine intravenously on one occasion approximately 6 months prior to hospital admission. During the 4 years before admission, the patient had injected anabolic steroids intramuscularly on a weekly basis. The needles were often shared with other bodybuilders at various gyms. The physicians state that their experience with this patient indicates that intramuscular injection of anabolic steroids through shared needles may serve as a mode for dissemination of the AIDS virus. "Because this practice appears to be common among many athletes . . . persons at risk must be warned" (Sklarek et al. 1984, p. 1701).

A recent issue of *Sports Illustrated* featured a story on Benji Ramirez, a 17-year-old boy from Ashtabula, OH, who was alleged to have died from steroid-related heart problems. While there appears to be some question as to both the cause of death in this case and the nature and extent of Ramirez's actual involvement with steroids, the story does contain the following account.

> Another of Ramirez's classmates . . . says that on two occasions last summer he purchased steroids from Ramirez and used them in his company. In both instances, Ramirez injected the classmate in the buttock and then injected himself (Telander and Noden 1989, p. 78).

It is not clear from this account whether the boys shared the needle. The possibility seems to be present here and in other cases in which naive youngsters with limited financial resources may be involved with injectable steroids.

NEEDS FOR FURTHER RESEARCH

It is customary, and frequently gratuitous, to end a research paper with a statement of the need for future research. However, in the area of anabolic steroids, that need is clear and immediate. The following sorts of data are needed.

1. Good epidemiological data are needed regarding incidence and prevalence of steroid use in different populations.

2. Data are needed on the frequency and volume of steroid use in different populations, including data on concomitant use of other substances with steroids.

3. Data are needed regarding the consequences of increasing criminal penalties for use or possession of steroids.

4. Data are needed on the health consequences and other effects of long-term use of steroids.

5. Data are needed on the natural history of steroid use in different populations, including patterns of use and cessation associated with different stages of life.

6. Given the general trend in society towards drug testing and the specific trend towards steroid testing in both amateur and professional athletics, data are needed on (a) what should be done when a steroid-problem area, e.g., high school football, is identified, and (b) what should be done when a specific steroid user is identified.

7. Data are needed on the patterns of steroid distribution, and how they are similar to or different from distribution patterns associated with other substances. Of special interest in this regard is the extent to which systemic violence may be beginning to be associated with black market steroid sales.

8. Data are needed on the cost of steroid use, and how users support their consumption.

9. Data are needed on the extent to which counterfeit steroids have penetrated the market, and the specific sorts of problems associated with these substances.

10. Data need to be generated on the extent of needle sharing among steroid users. Special attention should be paid to gay populations in this regard.

11. Data are needed on the effect of steroid use among persons with existing mental disorders.

12. The role of steroid use in sports injuries needs to be further explored.

REFERENCES

Buckley, W.E.; Yesalis, C.E.; Friedl, K.E.; Anderson, W.A.; Streit, A.; and Wright, J.E. Estimated prevalence of anabolic steroid use among male high school seniors. *JAMA* 260(23):3441-3445, 1988.

Chapman, ES. Steroid edge: Real or illusion. *Washington Post,* October 18, 1988. p. 8.

Charlier, M. For teens, steroids may be bigger issue than cocaine use. *Wall Streer Journal,* October 4, 1988. p. A20.

Couzens, G.S. A serious drug problem. *Newsday,* November 26, 1988. p. II, 5.

Cowart, V. Steroids in sports: After four decades, time to return these genies to the bottle? *JAMA* 257(4):421-427, 1987a.

Cowart, V. Physician-competitor's advice to colleagues: Steroid users respond to education, rehabilitation. *JAMA* 257(4):427-428, 1987b.

Hancock, L. Have body, will travel. *Long Island Monthly* 2(2):21-23, 1989.

Hecht, A. Anabolic steroids: Pumping trouble. *FDA Consumer,* September 1984. pp. 12-15.

Herrmann, M. Steroids: A vague threat. *Newsday,* October 30, 1988. pp. 36, 31.

Huapt, H.A., and Rovere, G.D. Anabolic steroids: A review of the literature. *Am J Sports Med* 12(6):469-484, 1984.

Jacobson, S. NFL is late in seeing the light. *Newsday,* November 6, 1988. pp. 9, 40.

Johnson, B.D.; Goldstein, P.J.; Preble, E.; Schmeidler, J.; Lipton, D.S.; Spunt, B.J.; and Miller, T. *Taking Care of Business: The Economics of Crime by Heroin Abusers.* Lexington: Lexington Books, 1985.

Kahler, K. Steroids 'mania' spawning perilous new drug traffic. *The Sunday Star Ledger* (Newark), January 8, 1989. pp. 1, 29.

Lee, B.L. Growth drug hitting black market. *The Journal,* Addiction Research Foundation 15(9):4, 1985.

Lindesmith, A.R. *Opiate Addiction.* Evanston: Principia Press, 1947.

Mann, F. Dark side of steroids plagues former boxer. *Miami Herald* December 27, 1988. pp. 1D, 4D.

Matza, D. *Delinquency and Drift.* New York: John Wiley, 1964.

McBride, D., and Clayton, R.C. Methodological issues in the etiology of drug abuse. *J Drug Issues* 15(4):509-529, 1985.

Miami Herald Study: 6% of teen boys use steroids. December 23, 1988. pp. 1A, 7A.

Penn, S. Muscling in. *Wall Street Journal,* October 4, 1988. pp. Al, A20.

Phillips, M., and Lohrer, R. High schools are considering steroid tests. *Miami Herald* January 14, 1989. pp. 1D, 4D.

Schuckit, M.A. Weight lifter's folly: The abuse of anabolic steroids. *Drug Abuse and Alc Newsletter* 17(8), October, 1988.

Scott, J. Use of steroids by youths widespread, study finds. *Los Angeles Times,* December 16, 1988. pp. 1, 45.

Sklarek, H.M.; Mantovani, R.P.; Erens, E.; Heisler, D.; Niederman, M.S.; and Fein, A.M. AIDS in a bodybuilder using anabolic steroids. *N Engl J Med* 311(26):1701, 1984.

Southwick, L. Testimony before U.S. House of Representatives Subcommittee on Crime, May 17, 1990.

STASH Staff. *Drugs in Sports.* Educational Offprint Series #219. Madison, WI: STASH, Inc., 1978.

Strauss, R.H. Controlling the supply of anabolic steroids. *Phys Sports Med* 15(5):41, 1987.

Telander, R., and Noden, M. The death of an athlete. *Sports Illustrated* 70(8):68-78, 1989.

Toufexis, A. Shortcut to the Rambo look. *Time Magazine,* January 30, 1989. p. 78.

Wieberg, S. All quiet on drug-test front—but why? *USA Today,* December 30, 1988. p. E1.

AUTHOR

Paul J. Goldstein, Ph.D
Deputy Director
Narcotic and Drug Research, Inc.
11 Beach Street
New York, NY 10013

Incidence of the Nonmedical Use of Anabolic-Androgenic Steroids

Charles E. Yesalis, William A. Anderson,
William E. Buckley, and James E. Wright

INTRODUCTION

The use of drugs to enhance physical performance predates the ancient Greek Olympiads (Strauss and Curry 1987). Throughout history, athletes have used a variety of drugs as ergogenic aids. These have included alcohol, cocaine, ether, and strychnine (Boje 1939; Wright 1978). Currently there are over 100 substances banned by the International Olympic Committee (IOC), including over 17 anabolic-androgenic steroids (AS) and related compounds (United States Olympic Committee 1989).

Only 4 years after testosterone was synthesized, Boje (1939) suggested that sex hormones, based on their physiologic actions, might enhance physical performance. It has been rumored, but not documented, that during World War II a number of German soldiers were given some type of androgen to increase aggressiveness in combat (Wade 1972).

Several prominent older athletes have indicated that various forms of testosterone were being used by a few bodybuilders in the United States in the late 1940s and early 1950s (Wright 1978). However, the most often referenced account of the initiation of systematic use of AS in sports credits the Soviet weightlifting team in the early 1950s. In 1954, at the world weightlifting championships in Vienna, Dr. John Ziegler, the U.S. team physician, reportedly was told by his Soviet counterpart that the Soviets were taking testosterone (Goldman 1984; Starr 1981; Todd 1987). Dr. Ziegler returned to the United States and experimented with testosterone on himself and a few weightlifters in the York Barbell Club. Dr. Ziegler was concerned, however, with the androgenic effects of testosterone and, in 1958, when the Ciba Pharmaceuticals Company released Dianabol (methandrostenolone), he began experimentation with this new drug. After several of the early AS users achieved championship status, the efficacy of these drugs apparently spread by word of mouth during the early 1960s to other strength-intensive

97

sports from field events to football (Starr 1981; Todd 1987). Thereafter, use of AS apparently diffused to endurance sports such as long-distance running and swimming; however, this has not been chronicled.

Until the mid-1970s all that was known regarding the incidence of the non-medical use of AS was based on rumors, anecdotes, and testimonials (Goldman 1984; Wade 1972; Wright 1978). High levels of use were attributed to such sports as professional football, weightlifting, powerlifting, bodybuilding, and throwing events in track; even use by high school athletes has been rumored as early as 1959 (Gilbert 1969; Morris, personal communication, 1989). Although rumors still abound, estimates of the incidence of AS use are now available, based on the results of drug testing associated with athletic competition and on the results of systematic surveys.

Drug Tests

Owing to the lack of satisfactory screening techniques, AS were not banned by the IOC until 1975, and it was not until the 1976 Montreal Games that testing for these drugs was initiated (Catlin 1987). Testosterone esters were not added to the banned list until 1982 because of the previous unavailability of testing techniques (Todd 1987). Exogenous testosterone can be detected only by examining the peak height of the testosterone:epitestosterone ratio (Catlin et al. 1987). Normally the ratio is approximately 1:1; a value of 6:1 or greater is considered positive.

In 1986, the National Collegiate Athletic Association (NCAA) began testing for AS at football bowl games and championship events (National Collegiate Athletic Association 1987). The results of these announced drug tests are shown in table 1. Generally, less than 2 percent of athletes tested positive for AS. In addition, less than 1 percent of athletes tested positive during announced drug testing in sporting events sponsored by the U.S. Olympic Committee (USOC) from 1984 to 1988 (Voy, personal communication, 1989). However, when the USOC conducted *unannounced* drug tests with no punitive actions at a number of "Olympic Sports" events in the United States in 1984 and 1985, approximately 50 percent of athletes tested positive for AS use (Voy, personal communication, 1989). There are two explanations for this rather large discrepancy: (1) athletes knew when they would be tested, and (2) the detection time for most AS is relatively short (i.e., a few days to several weeks). Thus, it seems that to escape detection, athletes have avoided certain long-lasting injectable steroids, e.g., nandrolone decanoate (Deca Durabolin), which may have a detection time of up to 6 months or longer, in favor of oral steroids and injectable esters of testosterone (Yesalis et al. 1988). Based on recent IOC pronouncements (deMerode 1988) it seems that some athletes have had themselves tested by laboratories in order to titrate the doses of particular AS to their own biochemistry; thus they know when to stop use prior to official testing during

98

TABLE 1. *Anabolic steroid use based on announced drug testing*

Year	Event	Results	Percent Positive
1976	Olympic Games (Montreal)	8 positives 275 analyses	2.9
1980	Olympic Games (Moscow)	0 positives 1,500 analyses	0
1983	Pan American Games (Caracas)	15 positives 825 analyses	1.8
1984	Olympic Games (Los Angeles) (10 "sanctioned" positives; 17 positives)*	17 positives 1,510 analyses	1.1
1986-1987	NCAA Championships and Bowl Games	26 positives 3,360 analyses	0.8
1987	U.S. Olympic Festival (Greensboro)	6 positives 628 analyses	0.9
1987-1988	NCAA Championships and Bowl Games	9 positives 2,385 analyses	0.4
1988	Olympic Games (Seoul) (10 "sanctioned" positives; 30 positives)	30 positives 1,500 analyses	2.0

*For the past two Summer Olympiads, the number of laboratory "positives" has exceeded the number of athletes sanctioned (Catlin et al. 1987). No satisfactory explanation is available.

competitions. Athletes usually discontinue oral AS 2 to 4 weeks and testosterone esters, which are injectable, 3 to 6 weeks before testing (DiPasquale 1987).[1]

The results of a recent study by Friedl et al. (1989) cast further doubt on the sensitivity of drug tests for testosterone esters. Two volunteers were administered 300 mg of testosterone cypionate per week for 6 weeks. This dose equals or exceeds that used by many strength athletes during the 1960s and early 1970s (Wright 1978) and exceeds the dose used by most of today's track and endurance athletes.

Two other volunteers were administered 100 mg of testosterone cypionate per week for 6 weeks. At the end of the sixth week, urine samples were screened and testosterone:epitestosterone ratios were determined. All four subjects had ratios at or below 4.2:1. Backup samples were tested and yielded the same results.

Little can be said at present about the effect of purported masking drugs such as probenecid or the use of designer steroids (substances with minor structural modifications that shift the gas chromatographic signature of currently existing steroids). Neither the extent of use nor the efficacy of either strategy in subverting the testing process has been scientifically documented (DiPasquale 1987).

Finally, the recent negotiations between the United States and the U.S.S.R. to establish year-round, unannounced random testing for AS bears witness to the impotence of infrequent, announced testing for these drugs (Cowart 1988; Janofsky 1988).

Surveys

A number of surveys are available that attempted to measure the incidence or prevalence of AS use among a designated population. These surveys of AS use are categorized here as (1) high school age (or younger) students, (2) college students, and (3) athletes not fitting in categories 1 or 2. The results of these surveys are summarized in tables 2 to 4.

HIGH SCHOOL

Corder et al. (1975) surveyed students in 10 Arizona high schools in 1971 and 1975 and found a prior AS-use rate of less than 1 percent. They did not report their findings by sex, but 4 percent of athletes in the 1975 survey reported previous use of AS. In a study of 8th, 10th, and 12th graders in 11 public school districts in Michigan, 3 percent, 2 percent, and 2 percent of students, respectively, reported previous AS use, while 1 percent of respondents in each of the grades acknowledged AS use in the prior month (Newman 1986). The lifetime AS-use rate among seniors was 5 percent for boys and 1 percent for girls. Of the respondents, 25 percent of males and 7 percent of females believed that an athlete's performance is safely improved by AS (Newman 1986).

Polen et al. (1986) surveyed 200 randomly selected students at a Florida high school with an enrollment of 2,000, and 18 percent of males (but no females) reported prior AS use. Of 190 varsity football players in 6 high schools in Oregon, only 1.1 percent admitted AS use (Bosworth et al. 1987).

TABLE 2. *Self-reported anabolic steroid use among high school students*

Investigator and Year	Site and Population	Subjects (Number)	Percent AS use	Percent Response
Corder et al. 1975	Arizona 10 schools	1,393	0.7	NR
	Arizona 10 schools	1,099 208 athletes	0.7 4	NR
Newman 1986	Michigan 11 districts grade 8 grade 10 grade 12	5,029 (—) (—) 1,426	3 3 2 2 (M=5, F=1)	NR
Polen et al. 1986	Florida 1 school	200	M=18, F=0	NR
Bosworth et al. 1987	Oregon 6 schools varsity foot-ball players	190	1.1	NR
Buckley et al. 1988	24 States 46 high schools 12th-grade males	3,403	6.6	50
Johnson et al. 1989	Arkansas 6 schools 11th grade	1,775	5.7 (M=11, F=.5)	99.5
Terney and McLain 1990	Illinois 1 school	2,075	4.4 (M=6.5, F=2.5)	98
Windsor and Dumitru 1989	Texas 5 schools	901	3.0 (M=5.0, F=1.4)	89

KEY: NR=Not Reported.

In the first nationwide study of AS use, Buckley et al. (1988) found that 6.6 percent of male high school seniors reported having used these drugs. There was no difference in the level of reported AS use between urban and rural areas, but there was a small but significant difference by size of enrollment, with larger high schools reporting higher levels of AS use. Almost 40 percent of the AS users repotted five or more cycles of use.[2] In addition, of the self-reported AS users, 38 percent initiated use before age 16, 44 percent used more than one steroid at a time, i.e., stacking, and

TABLE 3. *Self-reported anabolic steroid use among college students*

Investigator and Year	Site and Population	Subjects (Number)	Percent AS Use	Percent Response
Toohey and Corder 1981	6 universities intercollegiate swimmers	67 (M=17, F=50)	M=5.8, F=0	NR
Dezelsky et al. 1985	5 universities 1970, 1973, 1976, 1980, 1984	4,171	athletes=15 (1970) athletes=20 (1976 to 1984) nonathletes=1 (1984)	NR
Anderson and McKeag 1985	11 universities intercollegiate athletes	2,100	football=9 Division I athletes=5 men's basketball and track=4 women's swimming=1	72
Anderson and McKeag, in press	11 universities intercollegiate athletes	2,300	M=6.4, F=1 football=10 Division I and II athletes=5 Division II athletes=4 men's track and field=5 women's swimming, track and field, softball=1	78
Pope et al. 1988	3 universities	males=1,010 varsity athletes=147	2 9.4	30

KEY: NR=Not Reported.

38 percent used injectable AS. Over one-third of the AS users did not intend to participate in interscholastic sports. Approximately 21 percent of AS users reported that a health professional was their primary source for these drugs, while the remainder identified "black market" sources, e.g., contacts at gyms and academic institutions, mail order, visits to foreign countries, etc. Only 15 percent of the public and private high schools that

TABLE 4. *Self-reported anabolic steroid use among athletes*

Investigator and Year	Site and Population	Subjects (Number)	Percent AS Use	Percent Response
Ljungqvist 1985	elite Swedish track and field athletes	99	31 throwers=75 middle- and long distance runners=8	69
Frankle et al. 1984	weightlifters in 3 gymnasiums	250	44	NR
Newman 1987	elite women athletes in more than 15 sports	271	3	59
Yesalis et al. 1988	elite powerlifters	45 questionnaires 20 telephone	33.3 55	74

KEY: NR=Not Reported.

participated in this study had no reported AS use. However, in a recent survey by Swenson of 472 high school head football coaches in Michigan, only 12 percent admitted that they had at least one player who used AS prior to 1988 (Duda 1988).

Three more recent studies in Illinois, Texas, and Arkansas confirm Buckley et al. (1988) findings and show that 5 to 11 percent of high school males admit having used AS (Johnson et al. 1989; Temey and McLain 1990; Windsor and Dumitru 1989). These three studies also examined AS use among high school girls and found that approximately 1 to 2 percent reported use.

Johnson et al. (in press) surveyed 1,775 male and female 11th-grade students in 6 Arkansas high schools, and the results indicated that 11 percent of males and 0.5 percent of females had used AS. The most common reason for AS use was to increase strength (64 percent) and size (50 percent); however, 27 percent of users wanted to improve their physical appearance.

McLain (1989) surveyed over 2,100 students in a high school (grades 9 to 12) in Illinois and found a total incidence of use of 4.1 percent (6.5 percent for males and 2.5 percent for females). Incidence of AS use did not vary significantly by grade. Of reported AS users, 83 percent participated in sports, and the use rate among all athletes surveyed was 9.4 percent. In addition, 35 percent of AS users said they obtained the drugs from a physician, while the remainder cited black market sources.

103

In a study of 901 male and female students in 5 Texas high schools, an overall use rate of 3 percent was reported (5 percent for males and 1.4 percent for females) (Windsor and Dumitru 1989). The AS-use rate among athletes was greater for males (6.7 percent vs. 1.8 percent) but, surprisingly, less for females (0.7 percent vs. 2.5 percent). AS use by grade was not reported. This was the first study to examine use by socioeconomic status (SES), with high-SES males exhibiting the highest AS-use rates. Once again, the large majority of users obtained their drugs from black market sources (85 percent), while only 7 percent obtained them from a physician.

COLLEGE

Of 67 intercollegiate swimmers (male and female) from 6 universities surveyed, only 1 athlete (a male) reported prior use of AS (Toohey and Corder 1981). In a study of nonmedical drug-use behavior of students at five public universities from 1970 to 1984 by Dezclsky et al. (1985), only 1 percent of nonathlete students reported using AS in 1984. However, the percent of intercollegiate athletes who reported AS use rose from 15 percent in 1970 to 20 percent in 1984. Separate AS-use rates for men and women were not reported.

Anderson and McKeag (1985) surveyed over 2,100 NCAA men and women athletes at 11 universities regarding alcohol and drug use. Heaviest AS use was among football players (9 percent). Other men's sports not typically considered to be associated with AS use but that did include AS users were baseball (3 pcrccnt). basketball (4 percent), track and field (4 percent), and tennis (4 percent). For women, only one sport reported AS use-women's swimming (1 percent). Altogether, 5 percent of Division I athletes, 4 percent of Division II athletes. and 2 percent of Division III athletes reported AS use.

Athletes who used AS obtained them from several different sources: non-team physicians (25 percent), teammate (22 percent), friend or relative (22 percent), other source (22 percent), coach (5 percent), team physician (5 percent), and pro scout or agent (2 percent).

Anderson and McKeag (in press) replicated their study of NCAA athletes during the 1988 to 1989 academic year. Data were collected from 2,300 men and women athletes at 11 universities nationwide. Of the original 11 universities. 8 participated in the replication study. In general, AS use had increased over the past 4 years. For Division I male and female athletes, reported AS use remained at 5 percent. However, for Division II and Division III athletes, AS use rose to 5 percent and 4 percent, respectively, of all the athletes surveyed.

Heaviest reported AS users were again football players (10 percent of all football players surveyed). Anabolic steroid USC also rose for track and field athletes (5 percent) but declined for baseball (2 percent), basketball (2 percent), and tennis (2 percent). Unlike the 1984 to 1985 study in which only one women's sport reported AS use, in the replication study, three women's sports reported a small amount of AS use. Track and field, basketball, and swimming all reported 1 percent of the women athletes in those sports using AS.

The sources for obtaining AS also changed over the past 4 years. The two largest sources for obtaining AS in the 1988 to 1989 study were teammates (49 percent) and friends or relatives (29 percent). Additional sources were: nonteam physicians (10 percent), other sources (6 percent), pro scout or agent (4 percent), and coach or trainer (2 percent).

For those athletes using AS, 25 percent began use before college, 25 percent initiated use during the first year of college, and 50 percent began after the first year of college. When asked whether members of their coaching staff knew that they were using AS, 23 percent of AS users said their coaches knew, 15 percent were uncertain, and 62 percent did not think their coaches were aware of their AS use.

Of the 1,010 respondents in a survey of college men at 3 eastern universities, 2 percent acknowledged AS use, while 9.4 percent of the 147 varsity athletes in the sample reported use of these drugs (Pope et al. 1988). More than 40 percent of AS users reported personal appearance as their primary reason for use.

OTHER ATHLETES

Ljungqvist (1975) surveyed elite Swedish male track-and-field athletes and found 31 percent had used AS. None of the middle- or long-distance runners admitted AS use compared to 75 percent of the throwers.

Weight trainers in three gymnasiums in the Chicago area were questioned 6 years ago, and 44 percent reported prior AS use (Frankle et al. 1984); however, no details of study methods, including sample selection, were provided. Of a subsample of 50 AS users interviewed in depth, only 44 percent were competing in athletics. AS-use rates by sex were not reported. The majority of respondents obtained their drugs illegally, but 20 percent claimed to have received them by prescription.

Elite women athletes in over 15 sports reported a lifetime AS-use rate of 3 percent, but only 1 percent acknowledged using these drugs in the past year (Newman 1987). The lifetime-use rate was slightly higher for those over the age of 26 (4 percent) and members of professional teams (5 percent). Of the respondents, 11 percent believed that their performance could be safely enhanced by AS.

Yesalis et al, (1988) surveyed elite powerlifters at a major contest using both a questionnaire at a major contest and followup telephone interviews. One-third of the questionnaire respondents admitted prior AS use; however, 55 percent of those interviewed later by telephone conceded use. The acknowledged AS users (via questionnaire) reported a lifetime average of eight cycles each. The primary sources of AS for this group were black market (73 percent) and physician or pharmacist (20 percent).

The extent to which the respondents in the surveys reviewed here honestly reported their AS use is not known. It is possible that they intentionally underreported or overreported their AS use. Intentional overreporters could be characterized as "braggarts," who overemphasize drug use to present themselves in a more worldly manner. This is unlikely to be a major source of bias, however, since virtually all surveys dealing with AS use are written and anonymous. Reasons for unintentional reporting errors include the reading levels of the respondents, the reporting timeframes for drug use, and the complexity of the scales for reporting frequencies and amounts of drug use.

The respondents may have underreported their drug use to meet more socially acceptable standards of behavior. The use of AS is in violation of not only the rules of all sport federations, but also of the traditional ethics of fair play in sports and would likely meet with the disapproval of family, friends, and fans. Indeed, even though these surveys guaranteed personal anonymity, the potential for underreporting could have existed because of concern for the reputation of their sport, school, or athletic conference. The difficulty of convincing athletes to be open about steroid use has been described as "getting only a glimpse of a large, underground subculture" (Pope and Katz 1988, p. 489). The underreporting of drug use is also undoubtedly due partly, if not largely, to the lack of trust and communication between members of the athletic and the scientific and medical communities. This, in turn, is a function of poor understanding on the part of researchers and physicians of the motivation of athletes and vice versa. The medical community lost much credibility as a result of repeated denials that steroids enhance performance (American College of Sports Medicine 1977). Until recently, statements from physicians and scientists dogmatically reported that any weight gained while taking steroids was mainly the result of fluid retention and that any strength gain was largely psychological (a placebo effect).

The studies reviewed here had a mean response rate of 73 percent. Thus, we have no information on individuals who chose not to volunteer, but, again, it could be hypothesized that those who did not participate were more likely to be AS users.

On the other hand, the research on the use of self-report methods has shown them to be valid for documenting recreational drug use, especially for adolescents (McClary and Lubin 1985; Smart and Blair 1978). When the recreational drug-use rates from self-report studies have been compared with external methods of documenting drug use (reports by others, blood, urine samples, etc.), the self-report-use rates have been similar or only slightly lower than rates derived by the other methods (Ausel et al. 1976; Bonito et al. 1976; Deaux and Callaghan 1984; Petzel et al. 1973; Stacy et al. 1985).

On the whole, it is reasonable to infer that the level of AS use as determined by the survey method likely reflects a lower bound and that the level of underreporting may vary by age, sport, level of competition, and sex. Adolescents may be more open regarding their AS use than older athletes whose scholarships or livelihood depend on their participation and success in sport. Because of the virilizing qualities of AS (Wright 1980; Haupt and Rovere 1984) women might be more secretive about their AS use than men.

CONCLUSIONS

1. The nonmedical use of AS is reported from early adolescence to adulthood. It is believed that, of high school seniors, at least 7 percent of males on average and 1 percent of females have used AS. Less information is available on the AS-use levels in adult populations.

2. Significant variation in the incidence of AS use has been reported among high schools and colleges.

3. AS use has been reported by both urban- and rural-dwelling adolescents attending schools of all sizes.

4. The level of AS use among all groups has likely increased significantly over the past two decades.

5. The level of AS use by women appears to be significantly less than that for men.

6. Although higher AS-use rates are reported by elite and competitive athletes, a significant number of recreational athletes appear to be using AS, probably to improve their appearance.

7. The results of surveys based on self-reports likely represent a lower bound of the level of AS use.

8. The results of announced drug tests at athletic events are a poor indicator of the overall level of AS use.

9. Although the black market serves as the primary source of AS, between one-fifth and one-third of users identify medical professionals as their source for the drugs.

FOR THE FUTURE

The medical community has identified the nonmedical use of anabolic steroids as a potentially significant health problem (American Academy of Pediatrics 1988; American College of Sports Medicine 1977; American College of Sports Medicine 1984; American Medical Association 1988). However, development of an effective response to this problem requires that a clearer picture of the magnitude of the problem-the extent of use, characteristics of users, and the real health implications-be obtained. Although much more information is available now than 5 years ago, further research is strongly indicated in the following areas:

1. The incidence and prevalence of AS use by males and females and among competitive and recreational athletes of all ages needs to be more accurately measured;

2. the dose and frequency of use of AS among high-risk groups needs to be established;

3. adolescent and adult AS users need to be profiled, and a better understanding of the processes involved in initiating and continuing AS use needs to be achieved; and, finally,

4. the association of AS use with other illicit drugs or alcohol use needs to be examined.

FOOTNOTES

1. Athletes view steroids primarily as training drugs. Because the effects on physiologic capacities and performance linger for a signficant time after steroids are discontinued, athletes can use them during training and stop before being tested at the time of competition. Thus, it appears likely, based on anecdotal information, that steroid users who abstain for a time continue to have enhanced capacities relative to nonusers.

2. A cycle is an episode of AS use that is usually 6 to 12 weeks or more in length.

REFERENCES

American Academy of Pediatrics. Policy statement: Anabolic steroids and the adolescent athlete. Elk Grove Village, IL: the Academy, 1988.

American College of Sports Medicine. Position statement on the use and abuse of anabolic-androgenic steroids in sports. *Med Sci Sports Exerc* 9(4):11-13, 1977.

American College of Sports Medicine. Position stand on the use of anabolic-androgenic steroids in sports. *Sports Med Bull* 19:13-18, 1984.

American Medical Association, Council on Scientific Affairs. Drug abuse in athletes: Anabolic steroids and human growth hormone. *JAMA* 259(11):1703-1705, 1988.

Anderson, W., and McKeag, D. The substance use and abuse habits of college student-athletes. Research Paper #2. Mission, KS: National Collegiate Athletic Association, 1985.

Anderson, W., and McKeag, D. Replication of the national study of substance use and abuse habits of college student athletes. Mission, KS: National Collegiate Athletic Association, in press.

Ausel, S.; Mandell, W.; and Mathias, L. Reliability and validity of self-reported illegal activities and drug use collected from narcotics addicts. *Int J Addict* 11:325-336, 1976.

Boje, O. Doping. *Bull Health Org League Nations* 8:439-469, 1939.

Bonito, A.; Nucro, D.; and Schaffer, J. The veridicality of addicts' self-reports in social research. *Int J Addict* 11:719-724, 1976.

Bosworth, E.; Bents, R.; Trevisan, L.; and Goldberg, L. Anabolic steroids and high school athletes. *Med Sci Sports Exerc* 20(2) Supplement:S3:17, 1987.

Buckley, W.; Yesalis, C.; Friedl, K.; Anderson, W.; Streit, A.; and Wright, J. Estimated prevalence of anabolic steroid use among male high school seniors. *JAMA* 260(23):3441-3445, 1988.

Catlin, D. Detection of drug use by athletes. In: Strauss, R.H., ed. *Drugs and Performance in Sports.* Philadelphia: W.B. Saunders Company, 1987. pp. 103-120.

Catlin, D.; Krammerer, R.; Hatton, C.; Sekera, M.; and Merdink, J. Analytical chemistry at the games of the XXIIIrd Olympiad in Los Angeles. *Clin Chem* 33(2):319-327, 1987.

Corder, B.W.; Dezelsky, T.L.; Toohey, J.V.; and DiVito, C.L. Trends in drug use behavior at ten Central Arizona high schools. *Ariz J Health Phys Ed Recreation Dance* 18:10-11, 1975.

Cowart, V. Accord on drug testing, sanctions sought before 1992 Olympics in Europe. *JAMA* 260(23):3397-3398, 1988.

Deaux, E., and Callaghan, J. Estimating statewide health risk behavior: A comparison of telephone and key informant survey approaches. *Eval Rev* 8:467-492, 1984.

deMerode, A. International Medical Commission Code of Ethics for IOC Accredited Laboratories, Lucerne, Switzerland, April 1988.

Dezelsky, T.; Toohey, J.; and Shaw, R. Non-medical drug use behavior at five United States universities: A 15-year study. *Bull Narc* 27(2-3):49-53, 1985.

DiPasquale, M.G. *Drug Use and Detection in Amateur Sports.* Warkworth, ON: MGD Press, 1984. Updates 1-4, 1986-1987.

Duda, M. Gauging steroid use in high school kids. *Physiol Sports Med* 16(8):16-17, 1988.

Frankle, M.; Cicero, G.; and Payne, J. Use of androgenic anabolic steroids by athletes. Letter. *JAMA* 252(4):482, 1984.

Friedl, K.; Jones, R.; Hannan, C.; and Plymate, S. The administration of pharmacological doses of testosterone or 19-nortestosterone to normal men is not associated with increased insulin secretion or impaired glucose tolerance. *J Clin Endocrinol Metab* 68:971-975, 1989.

Gilbert, B. Drugs in sport: Part 2, something extra on the ball. *Sports Illustrated,* June 30, 1969. pp. 30-42.

Goldman, B. *Death in the Locker Room.* South Bend, IN: Icarus Press, 1984. pp. 93-94.

Haupt, H., and Rovere, G. Anabolic steroids: A review of the literature. *Am J Sports Med* 12(6):469-484, 1984.

Janofsky, M. East Germany wants to join U.S.-Soviet plan for drug tests. *New York Times,* December 9, 1988.

Johnson, M.; Jay, M.; Shoup, B.; and Rickert, V. Anabolic steroid use in adolescent males. *Pediatrics* 83(6):921-924, 1989.

Ljungqvist, A. The use of anabolic steroids in top Swedish athletes. *Br J Sports Med* 9(2):82, 1975.

McClary, S., and Lubin, B. Effects of type of examiner, sex, and year in school on self-report of drug use by high school students. *J Drug Educ* 15:49-55, 1985.

Morris, R.E., Executive Director, National High School Athletic Coaches Association, Ocala, FL, personal communication, 1989.

National Collegiate Athletic Association. 1987-88 NCAA Drug Testing Program. Mission, KS: the Association, 1987. p. 4.

Newman, M. *Michigan Consortium of Schools Student Survey.* Minneapolis, MN: Hazelden Research Services, 1986.

Newman, M. *Elite Women Athletes Survey Results.* Minneapolis, MN: Hazelden Research Services, 1987.

Petzel. T.; Johnson, J.; and McKillip, J. Response bias in drug surveys. *J Consult Chin Psychol* 40:437-439, 1973.

Polen, L.; Shnider, L.; Sirotowitz, A.; and West, J. Teenage drug epidemics: Build up on steroids. *Sword and Shield* (South Plantation High School newspaper, Broward County, FL), October 1986,

Pope, H., and Katz, D. Affective and psychotic systems associated with anabolic steroid use. *Am J Psychiatry* 145(4):487-490, 1988.

Pope, H.; Katz. D.; and Champoux, R. Anabolic-androgenic steroid use among 1,010 college men. *Physiol Sports Med* 16(7):75-81, 1988.

Smart, R., and Blair, N. Test-retest reliability and validity information for a high school drug use questionnaire. *Drug Alcohol Depend* 3:265-271, 1978.

Stacy, A.; Widaman, K.; and Hays, R. Validity of self-reports of alcohol and other drug use. A multitrait-multimethod assessment. *J Pers Soc Psychol* 49:219-232, 1985.

Starr, B. *Defying Gravity: How to Win at Weightlifting.* Wichita Falls, TX: Five Starr Productions, 1981. pp. 84-86.

Strauss, R.N., and Curry, T.J. Magic, science and drugs. In: Strauss, R.H., ed. *Drugs and Performance in Sports.* Philadelphia: W.B. Saunders Company, 1987. pp. 3-9.

Temey, R., and McLain, L. The use of anabolic steroids in high school students. *Am J Dis Child* 144:99-103, 1990.

Todd, T. Anabolic steroids: The gremlins of sport. *J Sport Hist* 14(1):87-107, 1987.

Toohey, J., and Corder, B. Intercollegiate sports participation and nonmedical drug use. *Bull Narc* 23(3):23-26, 1981.

United States Olympic Committee. *Guide to Banned Medications.* Colorado Springs, CO: February 14, 1989. pp. 4-5.

Voy, R.O., Director, Division of Sports Medicine and Science, U.S. Olympic Committee, Colorado Springs, CO, personal communication, 1989.

Wade, N. Anabolic steroids: Doctors denounce them, but athletes aren't listening. *Science* 176:1399-1403, 1972.

Windsor, R.; and Dumitru, D. Anabolic steroid use by adolescents: Survey. *Med Sci Sports Exerc* 21:494-497. 1989.

Wright, J.E. *Anabolic Steroids and Sports.* Natick, MA: Sports Science Consultants, 1978. p. 3.

Wright, J. Anabolic steroids and athletics. In: Hutton, R., and Miller, D., eds. *Exercise and Sport Sciences Reviews.* Vol. 8. New York: Macmillan Publishing Company, 1980. pp. 149-202.

Yesalis, C.E.; Herrick, R.T.; Buckley, W.E.; Friedl, K.E.; Brannon, D.; and Wright, J.E. Self-reported use of anabolic-androgenic steroids by elite power lifters. *Physiol Sports Med* 16(12):91-100, 1988.

AUTHORS

Charles E. Yesalis, Sc.D.
Professor of Health Policy and Administration
  and Exercisc and Sport Science
College of Health and Human Development
The Pennsylvania State University
115 Henderson Building
University Park, PA 16802

William A. Anderson, Ph.D.
Associate Professor of Medical Education
Michigan State University
East Lansing. MI

William E. Buckley, Ph.D.
Assistant Professor of Health Education
The Pennsylvania State University
19 White
University Park, PA 16802

James E. Wright, Ph.D.
Sports Science Consultants
Northridge, CA 91324

Androgens: Endocrine Physiology and Pharmacology

Stephen J. Winters

INTRODUCTION

Androgens are used in clinical medicine primarily to treat hypogonadal androgen-deficient men. The observation that a lipid extract of the urine of normal adult men decreased urinary nitrogen excretion in orchidectomized dogs (Kochakian 1935) followed within a few years by the isolation of testosterone and the finding that it caused nitrogen retention and muscle growth in hypogonadal men (Kenyon et al. 1938) has led eugonadal men to use various androgens to increase muscle growth and strength. Androgens stimulate many other target tissues in addition to skeletal muscle, however, and, when androgens are administered in pharmacological dosages, undesirable effects may occur in those tissues. Although all androgens function by activating seemingly identical intracellular receptors, differences in absorption and metabolism of androgen preparations may lead to unequal actions on individual target issues. The purpose of this chapter is to compare the physiology of testosterone with the pharmacological information available for the testosterone derivatives currently in clinical use. An understanding of the similarities and differences among these compounds should aid in our approach to androgen use and misuse (Wilson and Griffin 1980).

TESTOSTERONE PHYSIOLOGY

Testosterone is the principal androgen in males. Approximately 95 percent of the testosterone in adult men is produced by the Leydig cells of the testis; the remaining 5 percent is produced directly or indirectly by the adrenal glands. During early fetal development, the placenta produces human chorionic gonadotropin, which enters the fetal circulation and stimulates testosterone secretion. Only late in the first trimester does the pituitary develop. Secretion of the pituitary gonadotropins luteinizing hormone (LH) and follicle-stimulating hormone (FSH) begins in the second trimester. The principal stimulus to the fetal gonadotroph, as in the adult, appears to be gonadotropin releasing hormone (GnRH), which is produced in the anterior

113

hypothalamus. Pituitary gonadotropin secretion declines in late fetal life and decreases further in the neonate such that, by 2 to 4 months of age, little testosterone is produced. The ability of administered GnRH to stimulate LH and FSH release in children suggests that these changes are due to a decline in GnRH secretion, However, GnRH cannot be studied directly in humans, since it is present in undetectable amounts, except in the hypothalamus and in hypothalamic-pituitary portal blood. There is presently no known mechanism to explain the decrease in GnRH secretion during childhood, although studies in nonhuman primates indicate that it also occurs in castrated animals and is therefore independent of testicular factors (Plant 1980).

Figure 1 is a diagram of the interrelationships between the hypothalamus, pituitary, and testes. GnRH secretion occurs primarily from the anterior hypothalamus in the region of the arcuate nucleus where it appears to be coupled to discharges of excitatory neurons. Numerous hormones and neurotransmitters have been found to influence GnRH release under different conditions. GnRH stimulates the synthesis, glycosylation, and release of LH and FSH (Clayton 1987). LH and FSH stimulate Leydig cells and Sertoli cells within seminiferous tubules, respectively. Gonadotropin secretion is also negatively regulated by Leydig cell steroids (Plant 1986) and by inhibin, a glycoprotein produced by Sertoli cells.

GnRH secretion reawakens at the time of puberty. LH and FSH levels increase and testis growth commences. Testosterone levels begin to rise at age 12 and reach adult levels at approximately age 16. Gonadotropin secretion exhibits a striking diurnal rhythm in early puberty with elevated levels of LH and testosterone at night (Boyar et al. 1972). In adult men, it is more difficult to demonstrate a diurnal rhythm for LH, although testosterone levels are highest at about 8 a.m. and are about 35 percent lower in the late afternoon to early evening (Spratt et al. 1988). Direct analysis of GnRH in hypothalamic blood in experimental animals and the tracking of GnRH secretion by measuring moment-to-moment changes in circulating LH concentrations indicate that GnRH secretion is episodic and that LH pulses generally follow GnRH secretory episodes. LH pulses in adult men appear to occur every 60 to 100 minutes. The estimate of frequency depends upon the blood-sampling protocol and the method used to analyze hormone-secretory events. This mode of intermittent secretion is needed for pituitary gonadotrophs to function normally (Belchetz et al. 1978). Unlike the situation in many lower animals, including nonhuman primates, striking fluctuations in testosterone levels are not observed in the peripheral blood in men, although a pulsatile pattern of testosterone release can be identified in spermatic vein blood (Winters and Troen 1986).

Although there is no male climacteric comparable to the dramatic hormonal changes that occur in women, aging is associated with a series of endocrine changes in men. Serum testosterone levels decline and LH and FSH levels

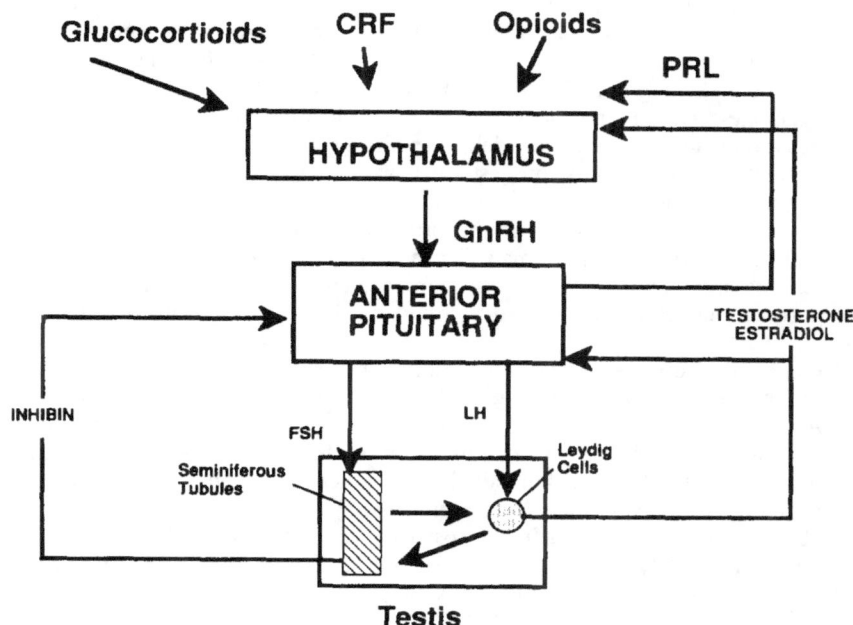

FIGURE 1. *Interrelationships between the hypothalamus, pituitary, and testes*

rise, indicating testicular damage. Responses to GnRH are also altered, revealing an additional abnormality of the hypothalamic-pituitary unit (Winters and Troen 1982). Androgen negative feedback is increased, and there is a blunting of the normal diurnal rhythm in testosterone secretion. Impotence is common in older men, as is a decrease in skeletal and muscle mass. Finally, sperm production declines (Neaves et al. 1984). It is sometimes difficult, however, to separate changes due to aging from changes resulting from illness and medications taken by older adults or from social changes.

TESTOSTERONE BIOSYNTHESIS, TRANSPORT, AND METABOLISM

Testosterone is a steroid hormone with 19 carbons synthesized from cholesterol (Miller 1988) through a pathway summarized in figure 2. The major portion of precursor cholesterol in humans is produced in Leydig cells from acetate and is stored in lipid droplets. There is no evidence for the delivery of circulating cholesterol bound to lipoproteins to the testis via the low-density lipoprotein (LDL) receptor. Cholesterol is converted in mitochondria to pregnenolone, which is in turn transported to the endoplasmic reticulum and its surrounding cytoplasm (microsomes). Pregnenolone is converted to testosterone in three steps: **17α** hydroxylation and C17-20 side-chain cleavage, which are catalyzed by the same enzyme, and reduction of the 17-keto group. Two possible pathways exist for the synthesis of testosterone from pregnenolone; one is through **17α** hydroxypregnenolone to dehydroepiandrosterone (the delta-5 pathway) and the second is through progesterone, **17α** hydroxy progesterone, and androstenedione (the delta-4 pathway). Incubation of human testicular microsomes with radiolabeled pregnenolone and examination of the products formed suggest that the delta-5 pathway predominates in man (Yanaihara and Troen 1972). Most of the testosterone produced is released immediately into the circulation. The normal production rate of testosterone in adult men is about 6 mg per day.

Circulating testosterone is bound tightly by a serum glycoprotein of hepatic origin, sex-hormone-binding globulin (SHBG), and weakly by albumin. Approximately 1 to 2 percent of the circulating testosterone is thought to be unbound. The binding to albumin is of such low affinity, however, that this pool is believed to be functionally equivalent to unbound testosterone. Testosterone is thought to enter target cells by simple diffusion (figure 3). The 50 percent of the circulating testosterone in normal men that is bound tightly to SHBG probably does not enter cells, although some evidence to the contrary has been presented. Changes in the concentrations of SHBG will therefore influence the measured total testosterone level as well as the proportion of the testosterone in serum that can enter target cells.

Figure 4 is a diagram outlining the metabolism of testosterone. Testosterone is metabolized by the liver to the 17 keto-steroids **5α**-androsterone and **5β**-etiocholanolone, which are excreted in urine. The total 17 keto-steroids in the urine of normal adult men is 5 to 25 mg over 24 hours. Testosterone derivatives constitute a small percentage of the total urinary 17 keto-steroids, which also include the metabolites of androstenedione and dehydroepiandrosterone produced by the adrenal cortex. Testosterone is metabolized to a series of 3, 15, and 16 hydroxylated polar compounds, which are excreted in the urine, and is conjugated to sulfuric and glucuronic acids, which are excreted in the urine and bile. A small amount (<250 μg per day) of testosterone is excreted unmetabolized in the urine. Testosterone is bioconverted in certain target tissues to the active compounds **5α**--dihydrotestosterone (DHT) and estradiol, as discussed below.

TESTOSTERONE ACTION ON TARGET CELLS

Testosterone influences the function of its target cells by binding to a high-affinity intracellular receptor protein (figure 3). Complementary DNA sequences to androgen receptors have been recently obtained (Lubahn et al. 1988), facilitating the study of the structure and biological actions of the receptor. The androgen receptor is a protein of approximately

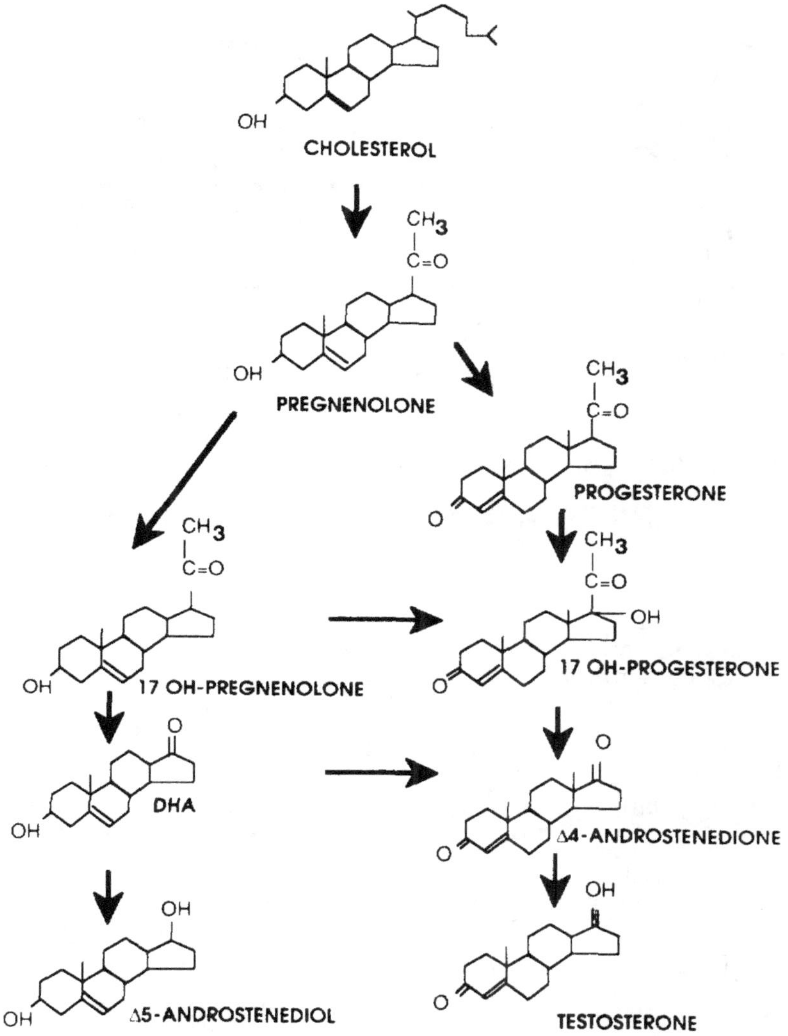

FIGURE 2. *Pathways of testosterone biosynthesis in the human*

120 kilodaltons coded in humans by genes located on the X-chromosome. Based upon physicochemical and kinetic properties, the androgen receptor appears to be identical in all androgen target cells. However, the concentration of receptors in target tissues varies widely. Evidence to date suggests that, by binding to the receptor, testosterone dissociates the active monomer from a larger inactive protein. The receptor is thus activated and capable

SCHEMATIC DIAGRAM OF
ANDROGEN ACTION AT ITS TARGET CELLS

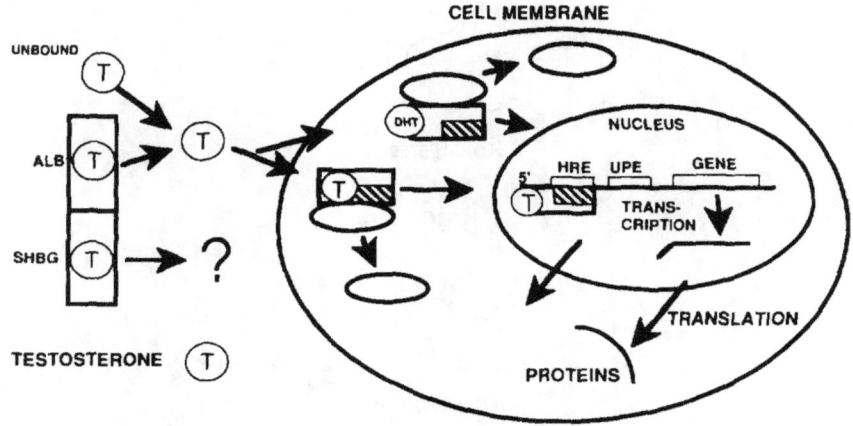

FIGURE 3. *Schematic model of androgen action in target cells*

PATHWAYS FOR THE METABOLISM
OF TESTOSTERONE

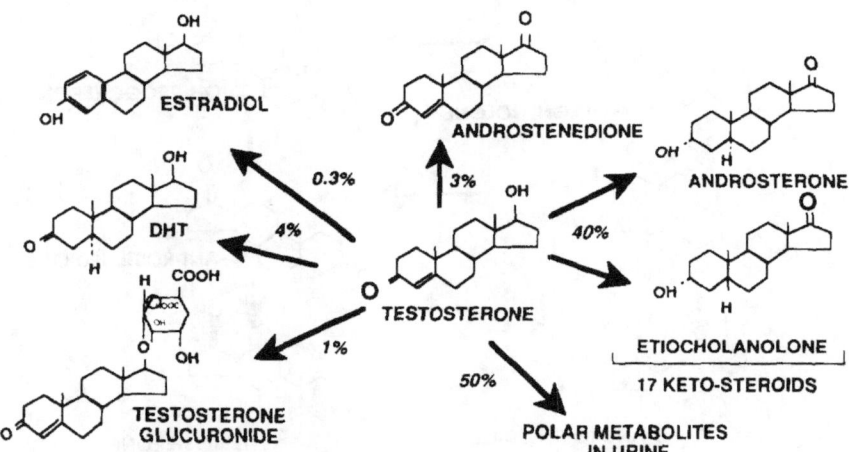

FIGURE 4. *The metabolic pathways for testosterone*

of binding to nucleotide sequences known as the hormone-response element. Nuclear binding increases RNA and protein synthesis and, in some tissues, DNA synthesis. Upstream promoter elements at the 5' flanking region bind intracellular proteins that regulate the rate of transcription. These intracellular events appear to be similar to those for the other steroid hormones

118

including glucocorticoids, mineralocorticoids, estrogens, progestins, thyronines, and vitamin D (Carson-Jurica et al. 1990).

Androgens probably influence the action of most cells (Mooradian et al. 1987). A list of selected androgen target tissues and the biological actions of androgens on these cells is presented in table 1. Classically, the actions of testosterone have been divided into those that are androgenic, i.e., promoting the development and maintenance of male secondary sex characteristics (virilizing), and anabolic, i.e., assimilating nutritive matter into living substances (muscle promoting). However, the limitations of this classification are evident upon inspection of the many actions of testosterone that are neither androgenic nor anabolic.

TABLE 1. *Functions of androgens in various target tissues*

Target Tissue	Function of Androgen
Testes	Spermatogenesis

Sex-Accessory Glands
    prostate, seminal vesicles,
    epididymis, penis
	Growth and secretions

Skin, Hair, Sebaceous Glands	Hair growth, secretions

Muscle
    skeletal
    cardiac
    smooth
	
	Hypertrophy
	Increase contractility

Central Nervous System	Libido
Hypothalamus/Pituitary	GnRH, LH, and FSH secretion
Liver	Enzymes and secreted proteins
Kidney	Enzymes
Larynx	Growth
Hemapoietic Organs	Erythropoiesis
Immune System	Lymphoid involution
Salivary Glands	Pheromones
Breast	Inhibit glandular development
Bone	Promote mineralization

In certain target tissues, such as prostate, seminal vesicles, and pubic skin, testosterone is irreversibly and nearly completely metabolized to DHT, and it is DHT that primarily binds to the androgen receptor. In other target tissues, such as kidney, testis, and skeletal muscle, which contain little

5α-reductase, testosterone interacts with the receptor directly. Although there is no clear explanation for the presence of testosterone 5α-reductase in only certain androgen target tissues, the significance of testosterone 5α-reductase is underscored by the existence of a clinical syndrome of ambiguous external genitalia in patients who lack normal testosterone 5α-reductase activity (Peterson et al. 1977). DHT is 2.5 to 10 times more potent than testosterone in bioassays and binds with two to three times higher affinity (K_D=0.25 to 0.50 nM) to the androgen receptor than does testosterone (K_D=0.4 to 1.0 nM). In this way, 5α reduction appears to locally amplify the actions of testosterone in selected target tissues. Because DHT is present in the circulation of adult men in levels (30 to 80 ng/dl) about one tenth those of testosterone, circulating DHT has little influence on target tissues compared to testosterone.

Not only is little DHT produced by skeletal muscle, but DHT is also further metabolized to the weak androgen 5α-andrcstane-3,17β diol by the cytosolic enzyme 3α-hydroxysteroid oxidoreductase (Warrenski and Almon 1983). This bioconversion limits the action of DHT in skeletal muscle as well as the action of other androgens metabolized by this enzyme. By contrast, the action of 5α-reduced androgens is sustained in prostate, which contains considerable 5α-reductase and little 3α- and 3β-hydroxysteroid oxidoreductase activity. In this way, target tissue metabolism modifies the actions of androgens unequally among target tissues. This concept is schematically represented in figure 5.

Estradiol is a second product of testosterone with biological activity. Approximately one-fourth of the estradiol produced in men is secreted directly by the testes, and the remainder is produced from circulating testosterone in liver and fat cells (MacDonald et al. 1979). The physiological actions of estrogens in men are largely unknown. Estrogens increase the synthesis of several hepatic proteins, including SHBG, thyroid-binding globulin, and lipoproteins; estradiol may be important in mediating some aspects of male sexual behavior (Pardridge et al. 1982). Estrogen administration or increased estrogen secretion by a tumor of the adrenal gland or testis suppresses gonadotropin and testosterone secretion, producing hypogonadism and feminization.

CLINICAL EFFECTS OF ANDROGENS

Male sexual differentiation occurs during the first trimester of fetal life. The urogenital sinus and external genitalia develop identically in both sexes by the eighth week of gestation and have the capacity to differentiate into either male or female structures. Testosterone induces differentiation of the internal (Wolffian) ducts. The urethral folds fuse to form a phallic urethra, the labialscrotal swellings fuse to form a scrotum, and the prostate and bulbourethral glands form as outgrowths of the urogenital sinus. Descent of the testes into the scrotum occurs during the third trimester. There is

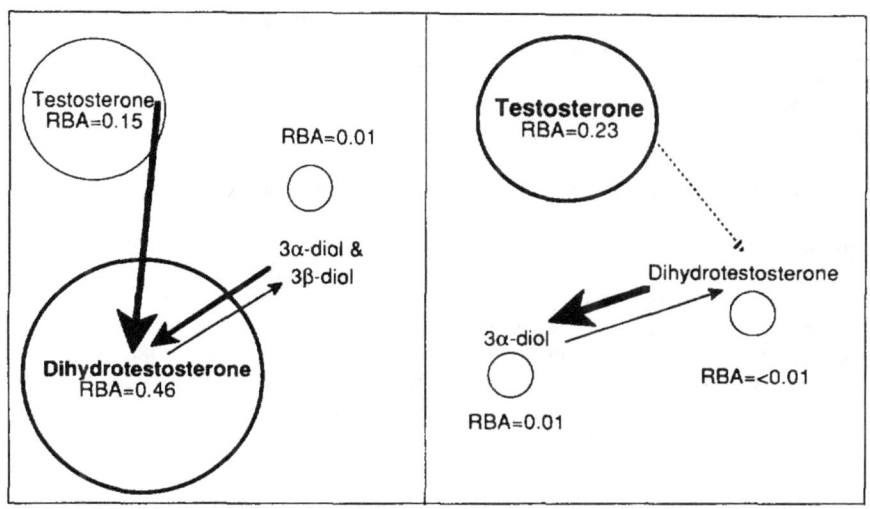

PROSTATE   SKELETAL
                        MUSCLE

FIGURE 5. *A comparison of the relative androgen receptor-binding affini-*
ties and intracellular metabolism of testosterone, DHT, and
5α- androstane-3α,17β diol (3α-diol) in rat prostate and
skeletal muscle

NOTE: Relative binding affinity was studied using (^{3}H)methyltrienolone as the radiolabeled ligand
         and setting the EC_{50} of nonlabeled methyltrienolone equal to 1.0.

SOURCE: Data from Saartok et al. 1984.

accumulating evidence that behavioral masculinization also begins during
fetal life.

Thereafter, the reproductive system is relatively quiescent until puberty, at
which time testosterone secretion increases, and a complex series of physical and behavioral changes produce the adult male phenotype. The testes
grow to adult size between ages 11 and 16, and the production of sperm
commences (Nielsen et al. 1986). The scrotum darkens and becomes rugat-
ed. Beard and body hair growth are stimulated, and sebaceous gland development occurs, increasing the production of sebum producing an adult body
odor and acne. The phallus enlarges. Growth and development of the
prostate and seminal vesicles permit the production of semen. The larynx
enlarges, the vocal cords thicken, and the voice deepens. Adult sexual

behavior begins. There is an increase in the linear growth rate known as the adolescent growth spurt. Accelerated growth is maintained for about 2 years and is accompanied by skeletal maturation. Fusion of epiphyseal growth plates usually occurs by age 17, terminating longitudinal growth. Skeletal muscles grow, and there is an increase in total body water, indicating a relative decline in body fat.

In adult men, testosterone sustains these secondary sex characteristics and increases male sexual behavior. Testosterone stimulates erectile potency, although the details of its interaction with the neural and vascular mechanisms for this effect are uncertain. Testosterone is also an important spermatogenic hormone, which affects both Sertoli and myoid cells within the seminiferous tubule. Androgens influence bone metabolism, since androgen deficiency is associated with osteoporosis (Greenspan et al. 1986). Finally, androgens stimulate erythropoiesis by increasing renal erythropoietin production and by directly affecting bone marrow cells; androgen-deficient men are frequently mildly anemic.

CLINICAL USE OF ANDROGENS

Androgens are used in clinical medicine to treat adult men with androgen deficiency owing to either an abnormality of the testes or of the hypothalamus-pituitary axis (Wilson and Griffin 1980). The goal of therapy is to restore libido and potency and to stimulate the expression of secondary sex characteristics. Because of etythropoietic actions, androgens have been used in patients with the anemia of chronic renal failure (Neff et al. 1981) and in patients with aplastic anemia. Androgens are used to prevent attacks of hereditary angioneurotic edema because androgens stimulate the production of an inhibitor of the activated first component of complement, which is deficient in these individuals (Gelfand et al. 1976). Patients with insufficient protein synthesis and excessive protein breakdown, such as those with malignancies, bums, major trauma, and chronic illnesses such as AIDS, have also been treated with androgens.

In women, androgens have been used in the treatment of osteoporosis, endometriosis, fibrocystic disease of the breast, and breast cancer. In the pediatric population, androgens are used in boys with congenital micropenis. Most boys born with a small phallus will have hypogonadism as adults. A much more common problem in pediatric endocrinology is the young teenager with short stature and delayed puberty. Some of these short children have a disturbance in pituitary hormone secretion or systemic illness, whereas others are normal short children. Androgens are given to these teenagers to stimulate linear growth and to accelerate the clinical features of puberty. The use of androgens in children and women is limited, however, by the undesirable side effects of virilization.

ANDROGEN PREPARATIONS

The structures of androgens currently used in clinical medicine are diagrammed in figure 6. Natural testosterone taken orally or injected intramuscularly is rapidly cleared by the liver and is therefore ineffective clinically. Esterification of testosterone at the 17-hydroxyl position produces compounds with increased lipid solubility. These derivatives, administered by intramuscular injection in oil, represent the most commonly prescribed androgens today. The solubility and rate of absorption of these compounds varies depending upon the fatty acid chain. After they leave the depot, the esters are rapidly metabolized to free steroid, which interacts with target tissues. The testosterone released is also available for bioconversion to DHT and estradiol.

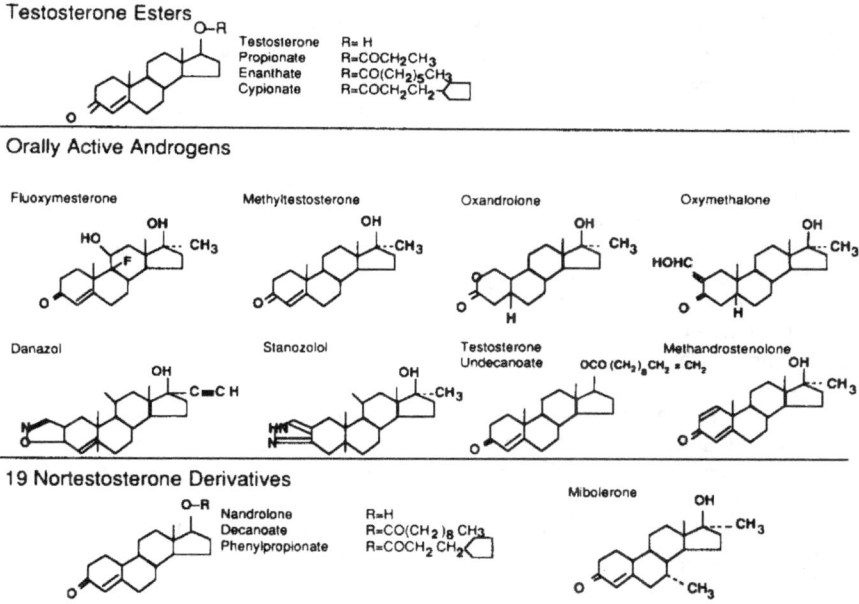

FIGURE 6. *Androgens used orally and parenterally*

Testosterone esters in clinical use in the United States are propionate, cypionate (Depo-testosterone, Virilon IM), and enanthate (Delatestryl, Testaval). Testosterone propionate at a dose of 50 mg sustains physiologic testosterone levels for 36 to 48 hours (Fujioka et al. 1986). Because of its short duration of action, this ester is of limited clinical usefulness. Doses of 200 mg of testosterone enanthate (Snyder and Lawrence 1980) or cypionate (Nankin et al. 1986) maintain normal serum testosterone levels for 10 to 14 days. These doses generally produce supraphysiological levels of both testosterone and estradiol for 1 to 3 days. The increase in estradiol levels may produce gynecomastia in some testosterone-treated men. Both the peak and trough levels are monitored in treated patients because the hormone levels produced and the clinical responses vary among individuals. Long-acting testosterone esters are well tolerated by patients and in replacement dosages are free of side effects. Because the hormone profiles produced do not mimic physiological levels, alternative delivery systems including transdermal, buccal, and longer acting injectable formulations are currently under study.

Several testosterone derivatives are available for oral use. Most are alkylated at the 17α position, as this change produces compounds that are more slowly metabolized by the liver. Oral testosterone derivatives available in the United States include methyltestosterone (Android, Metandren, Oreton methyl, Testred, Virilon), fluoxymesterone (Halotestin), and danazol (Danacrine). Stanozolol (Stromba, Winstral) is not licensed in the United States for clinical use but is used in veterinary medicine. These androgens are not metabolized to testosterone, but rather interact directly with the androgen receptor. These steroids are also neither metabolized to estradiol nor to DHT. Since they tend to bind less tightly to the receptor than does testosterone (Saartok et al. 1984), they tend to be less biologically active. In sufficient dosages, however, they inhibit LH, FSH, and testosterone secretion (Vigersky et al. 1976; Small et al. 1984). The 17α~alkylated androgens elevate serum levels of haptoglobin, orosomucoid, and plasminogen (Barbosa et al. 1971) and reduce the circulating concentrations of SHBG and thereby total testosterone, thyroid-binding globulin and thereby total 1-thyroxine levels, and vitamin-D-binding globulin and 25 hydroxy vitamin D levels. 17-Alpha methylated androgens also reduce HDL cholesterol and increase LDL cholesterol (Haffner et al. 1983).

Manufacturers' recommendations indicate that oral androgens can be given in a single daily dose or three to four times per day. Recommended doses do not generally produce complete androgenization in hypogonadal men, however, perhaps because these compounds bind weakly to androgen receptors and cannot be metabolized to DHT. Further, the absence of convenient assays for these compounds in serum together with the difficulty associated with determining the appropriate end point for assessing bioactivity limits their clinical usefulness. Finally, 17-alkyl androgens are associated with idiosyncratic liver disease. Accordingly, oral androgens are generally reserved for patients who do not tolerate intramuscular injections, such as children and those with bleeding disorders. Testosterone undecanoate (Sustanon), available in Europe, has a long aliphatic side chain resulting in its adsorption into lymphatics bypassing the liver. The ester linkage is broken, and unconjugated testosterone is present in the circulation. This androgen must be given three times daily (Gooren 1986).

Deletion of the 19 methyl group of testosterone produces 19-nortestosterone. This change increases the growth-promoting effect on the levator ani muscle relative to that of seminal vesicles (Hershberger et al. 1953). This has been termed the anabolic-androgenic index. Like DHT, 19-nortestosterone is more planar than testosterone, increasing its receptor-binding affinity. However, it binds with similar affinity to androgen receptors in skeletal muscle and in prostate (Saartok et al. 1984). 19-Nortestosterone is not converted to DHT in tissues containing 5α-reductase but instead is converted to 5α-dihydro-19-nortestosterone, a compound that binds less tightly to androgen receptors than does DHT (Bergink et al. 1985). Together, these factors could explain the diminished effect of 19-nortestosterone relative to testosterone on androgen target tissues containing 5α-reductase (e.g., seminal vesicles) together with a greater effect than testosterone on tissues containing little or none of this enzyme, e.g., levator ani and skeletal muscle (Toth et al. 1982). Further, 19-nortestosterone has limited affinity for serum SHBG. Therefore, a greater fraction of circulating 19-nortestosterone than testosterone would be available to all androgen target tissues according to the free-hormone hypothesis.

Of the 19-nortestosterone derivatives, only nandrolone decanoate (Deca-Durabolin) and nandrolone phenylpropionate are licensed for clinical use in the United States. The dimethyl derivative $7\alpha,17\alpha$ dimethyl nortestosterone (mibolerone) binds more tightly to androgen receptors than does 19-nortestosterone and is used in animals. A radioimmunoassay for nandrolone has been developed (Wijnand et al. 1985). Peak levels of 2.0 to 6.5 ng/ml are produced by 12 hours and decline by 50 percent over 7 days after intramuscular injections of 100 to 200 mg of the decanoate ester. The hexoxyphenylpropionate ester has a longer circulating half-life of 21 days (Belkien et al. 1985). Nandrolone derivatives are frequently used by athletes for their anabolic properties. Other androgen target tissues are also influenced by nandrolone, however, when it is taken in sufficient dosage. Nandrolone hexoxyphenylpropionate was given to normal men at a dose of 100 mg twice weekly for 10 weeks. Testis size declined by 50 percent, and all men became azoospermic. These changes were reversed within 16 to 30 weeks of discontinuing treatment (Schurmeyer et al. 1984). There are a few case reports, however, suggesting that recovery of gonadotropin secretion may be incomplete with prolonged high-dose treatment. Nandrolone may also adversely affect the testis directly, as a profound decrease in serum total and free testosterone levels unassociated with a decline in serum LH concentrations has also been reported (Bijlsme et al. 1982).

Oxandrolone (Anavar) was also developed in an effort to dissociate androgenie from anabolic actions. This compound is 17α methylated, slowing its hepatic metabolism, and is modified in the A ring with the substitution of an oxygen for carbon in position 2. Data in rats indicated that this drug had less than 5 percent of the activity of testosterone propionate to stimulate prostate, seminal vesicle, and levator ani growth when both drugs were administered intramuscularly in oil. However, oxandrolone was only 50 to 70 percent as active as methyltestmterone in stimulating seminal vesicle and prostate growth but 110 percent as active in increasing levator ani weight when each was given orally (Lennon and Saunders 1964). Differences in absorption and distribution kinetics as well as the availability of testosterone but not oxandrolone or methyltestosterone for 5α-ıreduction may have influenced these results. Oral oxandrolone has been used to increase linear growth in short children. Although mean height velocity is often initially accelerated, there is no convincing evidence that ultimate height is increased (Marti-Henneberg and Niirianen 1975). As with other anabolic steroids, the clinical use of this compound has not resulted in selected effects on growth. At a dose of 0.1 mg/kg per day, this drug has antigonadotropic actions in children, as testis growth in treated teenagers was reduced compared to an untreated control group (Marti-Henneberg and Niirianen 1975). At a dose of 5 mg per day, oxandrolone had a greater antigonadotropic effect in adult men than did 10 mg of methyltestosterone, based upon suppression of urinary 17-ketosteroid excretion (Fox et al. 1962).

Oxymetholone has also been used to stimulate linear growth in children with similar results. A recent study has verified that intramuscular testosterone enanthate in low doses will also accelerate short-term growth velocity without compromising final adult height (Richman and Hirsch 1988). Methandrostenolone (Dianabol) is another androgen commonly taken for its anabolic properties. The manufacture of methandrostenolone has recently been discontinued in the United States.

CONCLUSION

Testosterone probably affects most cells in the body. However, it is sexual behavior, phenotypic changes, and bone mineral metabolism that are most evidently adversely influenced by androgen deficiency. Androgen treatment of hypogonadal men can restore these abnormalities to normal and is currently most effectively accomplished with long-acting parenteral esters of testosterone.

The availability of preparations with selective actions of testosterone, such as the stimulation of linear growth in children, the restoration of muscle mass in catabolic patients, or the induction of Cl inhibitor in women with hereditary angioedema, would represent an important pharmacological advance. However, such compounds are not presently available. Although the various androgens in clinical use, including those reported to have enhanced anabolic action compared to testosterone, stimulate identical androgen receptors in all target tissues, differences exist in plasma transport, hepatic clearance, and target-tissue metabolism among these compounds. In particular, tissue distribution of 5α-ıreductase appears to be important in explaining differences in dose-response curves among androgen target tissues. Further studies of intracellular androgen metabolism are needed to better understand the many actions and controversies surrounding the efficacy and safety of androgen treatment for conditions other than androgen deficiency.

REFERENCES

Barbosa, J.; Seal, U.S.; and Doe, R.P. Effects of anabolic steroids on haptoglobin, orosomucoid, plasminogen, fibrinogen, transferrin, ceruloplasmin, a,-antitrypsin, ß-glucuronidase, and total serum proteins. *J Clin Endocrinol Metab* 33:388-398, 1971.

Belchetz, P.E.; Plant, T.M.; Nakai, Y.; Keogh, E.J.; and Knobil E. Hypophysial responses to continuous and intermittent delivery of hypothalamic gonadotropin-releasing hormone. *Science* 202:631-633, 1978.

Belkien, L.; Schurmeyer, T.; Hano, R.; Gunnarsson, P.O.; and Nieschlag, E. Pharmacokinetics of 19-nortestosterone esters in normal men. *J Steroid Biochem* 22:623-629, 1985.

Bergink, E.W.; Geelen, J.A.A.; and Turpijn, E.W. Metabolism and receptor binding of nandrolone and testosterone under in vitro and in vivo conditions. *Acra Endocrinol* 110(Suppl 271):31-37, 1985.

Bijlsma, J.W.J.; Duursma, S.A.; Thijssen, J.H.H.; and Huber, 0. Influence of nandrolone decanoate on the pituitary gonadal axis in males. *Acta Endocrinol* 101:108-112, 1982.

Boyar, R.; Finkelstein, J.W.; Roffwarg, H.; Kapen, S.; Weitzman, E.; and Hellman, L. Synchronization of augmented luteinizing hormone secretion with sleep during puberty. *N Engl J Med* 287:582-586, 1972.

Carson-Jurica, M.A.; Schrader, W.T.; and O'Malley, B.W. Steroid receptor family: Structure and functions. *Endocr Rev* 11:201-220, 1990.

Clayton, R.N. Gonadotropin-releasing hormone: from physiology to pharmacology. *Clin Endocrinol (Oxf)* 26:361-384, 1987.

Fox, M.; Minot, A.S.; and Liddle, G.W. Oxandrolone: A potent anabolic steroid of novel chemical configuration. *J Clin Endocrinol Metab* 22:921-924, 1962.

Fujioka, M.; Shinohara, Y.; Baba, S.; Irie, M.; and Inoue, K. Pharmacokinetic properties of testosterone propionate in normal men. *J Clin Endocrinol Metab* 63:1361-1364, 1986.

Gelfand, J.A.; Sherins, R.J.; Alling, D.W.; and Frank, M.M. Treatment of hereditary angioedema with danazol. *N Engl J Med* 295:1444-1448, 1976.

Gooren, L.J.G. Long-term safety of the oral androgen testosterone undecanoate. *Int J Androl* 9:21-26, 1986.

Greenspan, S.L.; Neer, R.M.; Ridgway, E.C.; and Klibanski, A. Osteoporosis in men with hyperprolactinemic hypogonadism. *Ann Intern Med* 104:777-782, 1986.

Haffner, S.M.; Kushwaha, R.S.; Foster, D.M.; Applebaum-Bowden, D., and Hazzard, W.R. Studies on the metabolic mechanism of reduced high density lipoproteins during anabolic steroid therapy. *Metabolism* 32:413-420, 1983.

Hershberger, L.G.; Shipley, E.G.; and Meyer, R.K. Myotropic activity of 19-nortestosterone and other steroids determined by modified levator ani muscle method. *Proc Soc Exp Biol Med* 83:175-180, 1953.

Kenyon, A.T.; Sandiford, I.; Bryan, A.H.; Knowlton, K., and Koch, F.C. The effect of testosterone propionate on nitrogen, electrolyte, water and energy metabolism in eunuchoidism. *Endocrinology* 23:135-153, 1938.

Kochakian, C.D. Effect of male hormone on protein metabolism of castrate dogs. *Proc Soc Exp Biol Med* 32:1064-1065, 1935.

Lennon, H.D., and Saunders, F.J. Anabolic activity of 2-ox9-17α-methyl-dihydrotestosterone (oxandrolone) in castrated rats. *Steroids* 4:689-697, 1964.

Lubahn, D.B.; Joseph, D.R.; Sullivan, P.M.; Willard, H.F.; French, F.S.; and Wilson, E.W. Cloning of human androgen receptor complementary DNA and localization to the X chromosome. *Science* 240:327-330, 1988.

MacDonald, P.C.; Madden, J.D.; Brenner, P.F.; Wilson, J.D.; and Siiteri, P.K. Origin of estrogen in normal men and in women with testicular feminization. *J Clin Endocrinol Metab* 49:905-916, 1979.

Marti-Henneberg, C., and Niirianen, A.K. Oxandrolone treatment of constitutional short stature in boys during adolescence: Effect on linear growth, hone age, pubic hair, and testicular development. *J Pediatr* 86:783-788, 1975.

Miller, W.L. Molecular biology of steroid hormone synthesis. *Endocr Rev* 9:295-318, 1988.

Mooradian, A.D.; Morley, J.E.; and Korenman, S.G. Biological actions of androgens. *Endocr Rev* 8:1-28, 1987.

Nankin, H.R.; Lin, T.; and Osterman, J. Chronic testosterone cypionate therapy in men with secondary impotence. *Fertil Steril* 46:300-307, 1986.

Neaves, W.B.; Johnson, L.; Porter, J.C.; Parker, C.R., Jr.; and Petty, C.S. Leydig cell numbers, daily sperm production, and serum gonadotropin levels in aging men. *J Clin Endocrinol Metab* 55:756-763, 1984.

Neff, M.S.; Goldberg, J.; Slifkin, R.F.; Eiser, A.R.; Calamia, V.; Kaplan, M.; Baa, A.; Gupta, S.; and Mattoo, N. A comparison of androgens for anemia in patients on hemodialysis. *N Engl J Med* 304:871-875, 1981.

Nielsen, C.T.; Skakkebaek, N.E.; Richardson, D.W.; Darling, J.A.B.; Hunter, Wm.; Jorgensen, M.; Nielsen, A.; Ingerslev, O.; Keiding, N.; and Muller, J. Onset of the release of spermatozoa (spermarche) in boys in relation to age, testicular growth, pubic hair, and height. *J Clin Endocrinol Metab* 62:532-535, 1986.

Pardridge, W.M.; Gorski, R.A.; Lippe, B.M.; and Green, R. Androgens and sexual behavior. *Ann Intern Med* 96:488-501, 1982.

Peterson, R.E.; Imperato-McGinley, J.; Gautier, T.; and Sturla, E. Male pseudohermaphroditism due to steroid 5α-reductase deficiency. *Am J Med* 62:170-191, 1977.

Plant, T.M. The effects of neonatal orchidectomy on the developmental pattern of gonadotropin secretion in the male rhesus monkey (Macaca mulatta). *Endocrinology* 106:1451-1454, 1980.

Plant, T.M. Gonadal regulation of hypothalamic gonadotropin-releasing hormone release in primates. *Endocr Rev* 7:75-88, 1986.

Richman, R.A.; and Kirsch, L.R. Testosterone treatment in adolescent boys with constitutional delay in growth and development. *N Engl J Med* 319:1563-1567, 1988.

Saartok, T.; Dahlberg, E.; and Gustafsson, J.-A. Relative binding affinity of anabolic-androgenic steroids: Comparison of the binding to androgen receptors in skeletal muscle and in prostate, as well as to sex-hormone binding globulin. *Endocrinology* 114:2100-2106, 1984.

Schurmeyer, Th.; Knuth, U.A.; Belkien, L.; and Nieschlag, E. Reversible azoospermia induced by the anabolic steroid 19-nortestosterone. *Lancet* 1:417-420, 1984.

Small, M.; Beastall, G.H.; Semple, C.G.; Cowan, R.A.; and Forbes, C.D. Alteration of hormone levels in normal males given the anabolic steroid stanozolol. *Clin Endocrinol* 21:49-55, 1984.

Snyder, P.J., and Lawrence, D.A. Treatment of male hypogonadism with testosterone enanthate. *J Clin Endocrinol Metab* 51:1335-1339, 1980.

Spratt, D.I.; O'Dea, L.; Schoenfeld, D.; Butler, J.; Rao, P.N.; and Crowley, W.F., Jr. Neuroendocrine-gonadal axis in men: Frequent sampling of LH, FSH, and testosterone. *Am J Physiol* 254:E658-666, 1988.

Toth, M., and Zakar, T. Relative binding affinities of testosterone, 19-nortestosterone and their 5α-ιreduced derivatives to the androgen receptor and to other androgen-binding proteins: A suggested role of 5α-reductive steroid metabolism in the dissociation of "myotropic" and "androgenic" activities of 19-nortestosterone. *J Steroid Biochem* 17:653-660, 1982.

Vigersky, R.A.; Easley, R.B.; and Loriaux, D.L. Effect of fluoxymesterone on the pituitary-gonadal axis: The role of testosterone-estradiol binding globulin. *J Clin Endocrinol Metab* 43:1-9, 1976.

Warrenski, J., and Almon, R.R. Effect of castration on the metabolism of androgens in rat skeletal muscle. *Int J Biochem* 15:1149-1153, 1983.

Wijnand, H.P.; Bosch, A.M.G.; and Donker, C.W. Pharmacokinetic parameters of nandrolone (19-nortestosterone) after intramuscular administration of nandrolone decanoate (Deca-Durabolin) to healthy volunteers. *Acta Endocrinol* 110(Suppl 271):19-30, 1985.

Wilson, J.D. Androgen abuse by athletes. *Endocr Rev* 9:181-199, 1988.

Wilson, J.D., and Griffin, J.E. The use and misuse of androgens. *Metabolism* 29:1278-1295, 1980.

Winters, S.J., and Troen, P. Episodic luteinizing hormone (LH) secretion and the response of LH and follicle-stimulating hormone to LH-releasing hormone in aged men: Evidence for coexistent primary testicular insufficiency and an impairment in gonadotropin secretion. *J Clin Endocrinol Metab* 55:560-565, 1982.

Winters, S.J., and Troen, P. Testosterone and estradiol are co-secreted episodically by the human testis. *J Clin Invest* 78:870-873, 1986.

Yanaihara, T., and Troen, P. Studies of the human testis. I. Biosynthetic pathways for androgen formation in human testicular tissue in vitro. *J Clin Endocrinol Metab* 34:783-792, 1972.

ACKNOWLEDGMENTS

This work supported in part by U.S. Public Health Service grant R01 HD 19546 from the National Institutes of Health. Philip Troen, M.D., provided helpful suggestions in the development of this chapter.

AUTHOR

Stephen J. Winters, M.D.
Associate Professor of Medicine
Division of Endocrinology
University of Pittsburgh School of Medicine
Montefiore Hospital
3459 Fifth Avenue
Pittsburgh, PA 15213

The Androgen-Induced Phenotype

C. Wayne Bardin, James F. Catterall, and Olli A. Jänne

INTRODUCTION

Early studies on the action of testosterone emphasized that this steroid influences almost every organ in the body. Actions on reproductive tracts were called androgenic, while those on other organs were termed anabolic (Mainwaring 1977; Kochakian 1984). These designations were the first attempt to characterize the diverse effects of testosterone and other steroids with similar structures (Bardin and Catterall 1981). Androgen receptors were initially identified in prostate, seminal vesicle, and other reproductive tissues. Subsequent studies showing that antiandrogens could compete with testosterone and its reduced metabolite, 5α-dihydrotestosterone (DHT), for receptor binding sites clearly associated these receptors with the action of androgens (Jänne and Bardin 1984). The ultimate proof, however, that androgen receptors were an essential link between the steroid and the androgen-induced phenotype was the identification of receptor mutants in the rat and the mouse that were insensitive to many of the effects of testosterone and other androgens (Bardin et al. 1973). Studies on these animals, and ultimately in men (Keenan et al. 1974) with similar receptor abnormalities, emphasized that both the androgenic and the anabolic effects of testosterone were mediated by the androgen receptor.

In view of the fact that many of the diverse effects of androgens were mediated via a common receptor protein, it was perplexing that their actions were so diverse and their effectiveness so varied on tissues. Part of the reason why some steroids appear to have more androgenic than anabolic activity relates to their ability to undergo metabolism either to a 5α-reduced product with enhanced biological potency or to an estrogen that may be antiandrogenic (Bardin and Catterall 1981). Thus, in reproductive tissues and skin, testosterone is metabolized by 5α-reductase to DHT, which is five times more potent than testosterone, whereas there is very little 5α-reductase activity in most nonreproductive tissues, and testosterone per se is the active intracellular androgen. In addition, testosterone in some tissues can be aromatized to estrogens, which can, in turn, either oppose the action of androgen or exert anabolic effects via estrogen receptors (Bardin and

131

Catterall 1981). These observations suggest that part of the differential effects of one androgen on multiple tissues or of multiple androgens on the same tissue result from tissue- and steroid-specific differences in androgen metabolism.

Testosterone metabolism cannot, however, explain all of the variable responses to androgens observed in different tissues. The general concept of androgen action holds that interaction of testosterone, DHT, or other anabolic steroids with the androgen receptor changes its conformation and allows it to bind to hormone regulatory elements adjacent to or within androgen-responsive genes (Beato 1987). Such steroid response elements are able to interact with other regulatory elements and tissue-specific factors. Diversity of the receptor-mediated responses will, therefore, be generated by the nature of the steroid bound to the receptor, the structure of regulatory DNA motifs that regulate individual genes, and the tissue-specific factors that are present. All these factors determine whether a gene will be responsive to androgen in a given tissue and, if so, the magnitude of the ensuing response. Finally, it will be the variable tissue-specific responses of multiple genes along with the kinetics of mRNA and protein turnover that will eventually determine the androgen-dependent phenotype of an individual.

In the present chapter, a scheme of androgen action will be reviewed that attempts to illustrate (1) how androgen receptor levels relate to androgen action; (2) how the androgen-induced phenotype is produced; and (3) why differential sensitivity of genes is necessary to explain differences in phenotype. These concepts will be reviewed in line with research from our own and other laboratories. An attempt to refer to all of the relevant articles on this subject must await a more comprehensive treatise.

Most of the experiments reported here have been conducted using mouse kidney, as this androgen-responsive tissue has a number of features that make it particularly amenable to study. These include the facts that testosterone rather than DHT is the active intranuclear androgen; mRNA kinetics are easily studied, as RNA synthesis is not interrupted by successive rounds of DNA replication as it is in prostate, in which androgens are mitogenic; and there are established genetic variants of mice that demonstrate differences in the magnitude of response of individual genes to testosterone and other hormones (Bardin et al. 1973; Catterall et al. 19%). To study the androgen-induced events in mouse kidney, a number of genes were cloned and cDNAs prepared for measurement of mRNA levels. These genes include those coding for kidney androgen-regulated protein (KAP), ornithine decarboxylase (ODC), and ß-glucuronidase (ß-Gluc). Androgens stimulate accumulation of KAP, ODC, ß-Glut mRNAs, and the rates of synthesis of the respective proteins in the epithelial cells of the proximal tubule.

THE RELATION OF ANDROGEN RECEPTOR LEVELS TO ANDROGEN ACTION

The notion that the amount of androgen receptor in a tissue might determine the magnitude of androgenic response probably arose from the observation that some individuals with receptor defects have reduced receptor levels associated with an incompletely androgenized phenotype. Such a conclusion appeared to be supported by observations showing a linear relationship between the dose of testosterone and the amount of occupied nuclear androgen receptor in responsive tissues (Van Doom et al. 1976). These results led to the expectation that there would also be a linear relationship between the number of occupied nuclear androgen receptors and the accumulation of some androgen-induced gene products. Such an expectation appeared to be fulfilled, provided that receptor levels were related to a single androgen-induced product. Once multiple responses were examined in the same cell, then a clear relationship to androgen receptor levels was not obvious (Pajunen et al. 1982). This is illustrated by the results of an experiment shown in figure 1, in which a large single dose of testosterone was administered to mice, and the accumulation of ODC, KAP, and ß-Glut mRNAs was plotted relative to nuclear androgen receptor levels. ODC mRNA levels rose rapidly after hormone administration and plateaued at a high level by 20 hours. KAP mRNA levels also increased rapidly but plateaued at a much lower level. The rise in ß-Glut mRNA was not observed until 24 hours, and the peak response was observed only after a continuous administration of androgen for about 3 weeks (Watson and Catterall 1986). Thus, there was dissociation between the slope of the response and the magnitude of the response (Catterall et al. 1986).

A similar dissociation was also shown in a study that compared serum testosterone levels, nuclear androgen receptors per cell, and ODC activity in intact male mice of eight different genetic backgrounds (Melanitou et al. 1987). Even though serum testosterone concentration varied over a tenfold range, there was no correlation between the steroid levels and the nuclear androgen receptor concentrations across mouse strains. For example, the C57BL/6J mice, which had the lowest serum testosterone levels, had the same nuclear receptor concentrations as RF/J mice, which had the highest circulating testosterone levels. In spite of this, the renal ODC activity in RF/J mice was five times higher than that of C57BL/6J animals. Examination of the other six strains confirmed that there was no correlation between the concentration of nuclear androgen receptors and ODC activity. Another illustration of how nuclear androgen receptors do not strictly relate to the biologic response of a given gene is demonstrated by the fact that agents such as testosterone, medroxyprogesterone acetate, and a nonsteroidal antiandrogen, flutamide, can all occupy similar numbers of androgen receptors but can, respectively, markedly stimulate, modestly stimulate, or inhibit the response of an individual gene (Kontula et al. 1985; Bullock 1983).

133

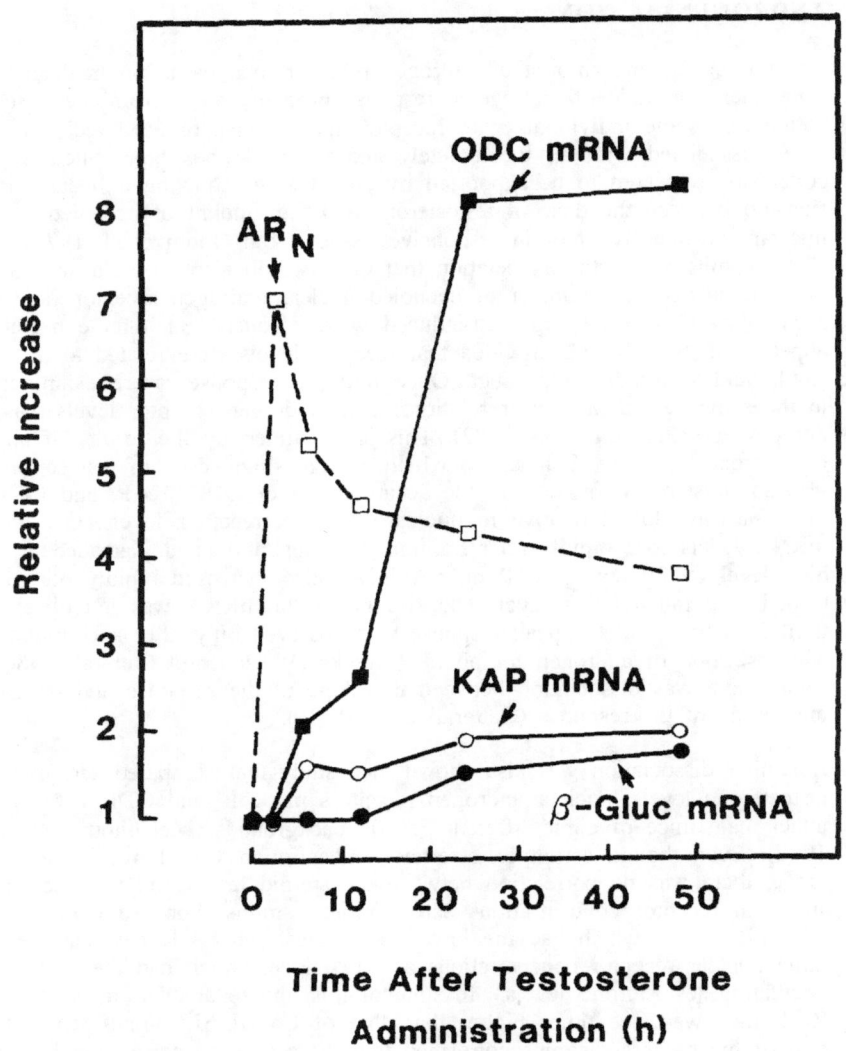

FIGURE 1. *Changes in accumulation of mRNAs coding for ODC, KAP, ß-Gluc, and nuclear androgen receptors (AR,) in mouse kidney after a single dose of testosterone (10 mg)*

NOTE: All values are expressed relative to those of untreated female mice.

We infer from these observations that the concentration of occupied androgen receptors in a cell is correlated, at least in some cases, directly with the response in a single gene product. However, the number of occupied nuclear receptors cannot be correlated with differential responses of two genes within the same cell, of one gene in different cell types, of one gene in the same cell type of animals with different genetic backgrounds, or of two hormones, such as androgen and progestin, that mediate response on the same gene via the same receptor.

THE ANDROGEN-INDUCED PHENOTYPE

The phenotype is defined as the manifest characteristics of a cell, organ, or organism collectively, including all traits that result from heredity and environment. The androgen-induced phenotype would be those characteristics of an organism that are dependent upon testosterone-induced differentiation or growth. In an attempt to explain the difference in the phenotype between individual men, investigators have attempted to relate prostate size, muscle mass, magnitude of aggression, etc., to testosterone levels in blood or tissue. There are, however, marked variations in phenotype among individuals that are exposed to the same testosterone concentrations and environmental factors. Although these differences have been attributed to genetic variation, this postulate has been difficult to confirm in humans. Some verification for such a proposal was derived from responses of various inbred strains of mice to graded doses of androgens. Kidneys of such animals were removed, and mRNA concentrations for KAP, ODC, and ß-Gluc were measured. Concentrations of these three mRNAs are representative of an androgen-dependent phenotype for the epithelial cells of renal proximal tubules. Four androgen phenotypes are illustrated for both A/J and C57BR/cdJ mice in figure 2. The amounts of three different mRNAs are shown by Northern blot analysis for the two strains of mice exposed to four vastly different testosterone levels. These phenotypes are those for animals exposed to doses of testosterone found in normal females (~0.4 µg/day), normal males (4 µg/day), 10 times the normal male secretion rate (40 µg/day), and 50 times the normal male secretion rate (200 µg/day).

The relative amounts of the three mRNAs that comprise the four phenotypes are strikingly different. Simulated dose-response curves of the three mRNAs to various doses of testosterone in A/J and C57BR/cdJ mice are illustrated in figure 3. In this figure, the testosterone production rate is displayed against the percent of the maximal response for the three mRNAs. The testosterone production rate of normal males is taken as 4 µg/day, emphasizing that, in most species, males produce approximately 10 times more testosterone than females. A series of vertical lines defines the phenotypes for a given dose of testosterone as each intersects the three response curves. For example, in A/J mice the phenotype of renal cells stimulated by the physiological level of testosterone is characterized by KAP and ß-Gluc mRNA levels that are 20 percent and 7.5 percent of maximal, and ODC

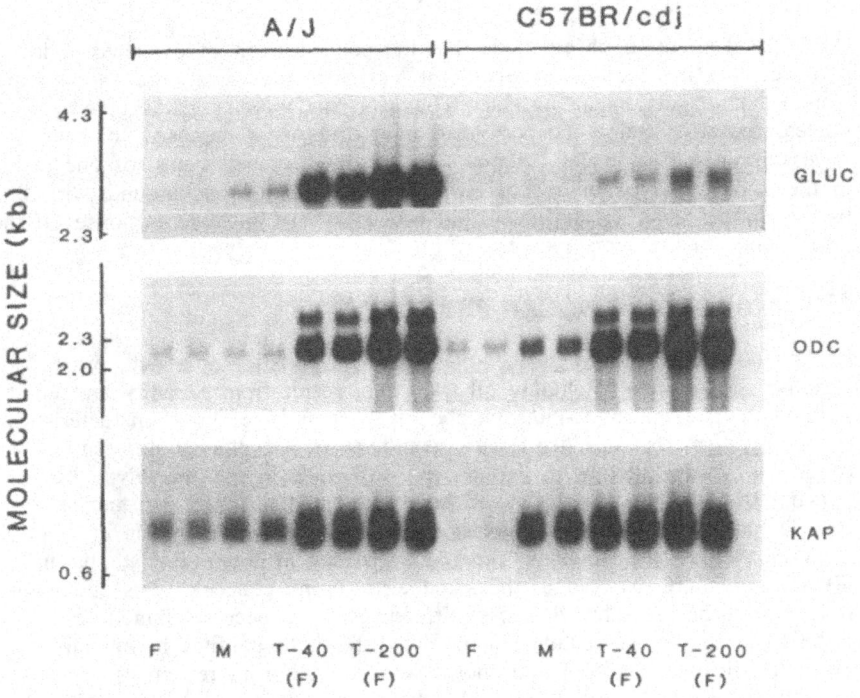

FIGURE 2. *Concentrations of β-Gluc, ODC, and KAP mRNAs in kidneys of two inbred strains of mice exposed to different doses of testosterone*

KEY: F=intact female mice; M=intact male mice; T-40=female mice treated for 5 days with implants releasing 40 µg testosterone per day; T-200=female mice treated for 5 days with implants releasing 200 µg testosterone per day.

NOTE: Each sample was analyzed in duplicate, and the filters hybridized successively with cDNAs specific for each of the three mRNAs.

mRNA levels that are not different from those in the uninduced females. By contrast, in C57BR/cdJ mice, the male phenotype is characterized by stimulation of KAP, ODC, and ß-Gluc mRNA accumulation to levels that are 50 percent, 12 percent, and 5 percent of maximal, respectively. Not only is the magnitude of the response for each gene different between the two strains, but the ordering of the dose-response curves for each of the three genes is dissimilar. Thus, the possible androgen-induced phenotypes for the mouse kidney can be illustrated by an ordered series of curves that describe the responses of all the different mRNAs and proteins that increase in this organ in response to androgens. The fact that each response curve can be genetically regulated offers tremendous opportunity for diversity.

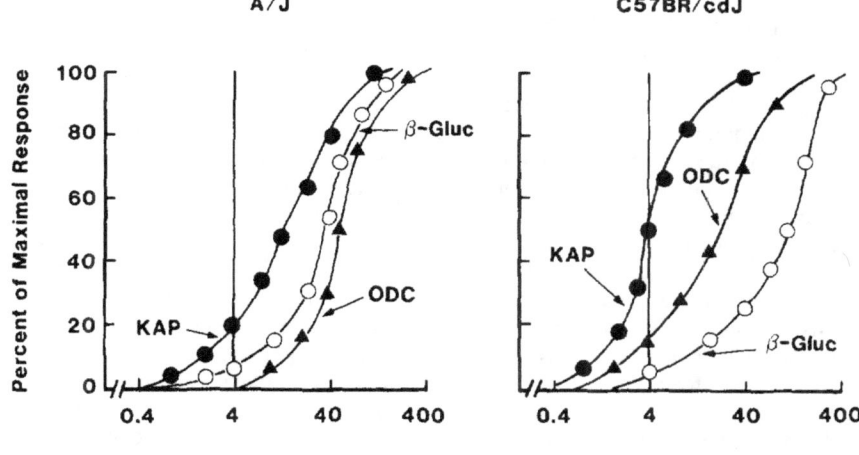

FIGURE 3. *Hypothetical dose-response curves for the expression of ß-Gluc, ODC, and KAP genes in two strains of mice exposed to different doses of testosterone*

NOTE: The vertical line illustrates the situation when testosterone production rate is approximately that of intact male mice.

When these and other observations are applied to the androgen-induced phenotype in humans, the following predictions are warranted: (1) clinical phenotypes are defined by the sum of multiple androgen-induced responses; (2) differences in phenotype between individuals result from how individual dose-response curves are ordered as well as from other environmental factors such as exercise; (3) physiological androgen levels do not maximally express the male phenotype; and (4) the response to androgens in most species is based upon the log of the steroid dose, and, as a consequence, a significant change in the phenotype may require a three- to tenfold increase in the circulating testosterone concentration, depending upon what percent of the maximal response is already archived by physiological hormone levels.

DIFFERENTIAL SENSITIVITY OF ANDROGEN-RESPONSIVE GENES

Studies on the mechanism of androgen action now provide insight into the reasons for the genetic diversity between individuals with different genotypes. Genetic regulation of ß-Gluc, an acid hydrolase present in lysosomes and endoplasmic reticulum of virtually all tissues, serves as a good example to illustrate this point. Genetic studies led to the identification of four genes in the ß-Gluc genetic complex *(Gus)* (Swank et al. 1978). The ß Gluc structural gene, *Gus-s,* has five well-characterized alleles that code for electrophoretic and thermostability variants of the enzyme protein. In addition to *Gus-s,* three regulatory loci have been described. These have all been shown to be linked closely to *Gus-s.* The *Gus-t* locus regulates the temporal development of enzyme activity in various tissues. This locus is unique among the regulators of the *Gus* complex because it appears to encode a *trans*-acting factor. A second regulatory locus of the Gus complex, *Gus-u,* controls the synthesis of ß-Gluc in all tissues at all stages of development. This is a *cis*-acting systemic regulator. Finally, a third regulatory locus, *Gus-r,* acts *cis* to control the response of the structural gene, *Gus-s,* to androgens. There are two alleles of *Gus-r,* and mouse strains are divided into two haptotypes based on their response to androgens. In strains of mice carrying the *Gus-r^b* allele, ß-Gluc activity rises slowly in response to testosterone and reaches a plateau at approximately 3 weeks of treatment. Strains carrying the *Gus-r^a* allele exhibit a more rapid and a much higher maximum response. The responses to androgen administration of the A/J strain with the *Gus-r^a* allele and the C57BL/6J strain with the *Gus-r^b* allele are shown in figure 4.

The nature of the *Gus-r* locus and its location within the DNA either adjacent to or remote from the structural gene for ß-Gluc is currently being intensely investigated by several laboratories. Direct cloning of *Gus-r* will be difficult, since there is no Gus-r-encoded gene product. It is assumed by many that the *Gus-r* locus will be found near the site of initiation of transcription of the Gus-s gene. If this assumption is correct, then characterization of the Gus-s transcription unit and sequences flanking it will provide means to identify Gus-r. However, comparison of sequences encompassing about 2,500 nucleotides of DNA flanking the two alleles has revealed no significant differences (unpublished results). It is also possible that *Gus-r* is located within Gus-s, possibly as part of an intervening sequence. It is interesting that the only major difference between the structures of *Gus-s^a* and *Gus-s^b* is a 206-base pair element in intervening sequence 4 of *Gus-s^a* that is absent in *Gus-s^b* (D'Amore et al. 1988). The relationship, if any, between this element and Gus-r function is not known. Alternatively, *Gus-r* may represent a tissue- and gene-specific enhancer, possibly acting at a distance from *Gus-s.* In the latter two cases, characterization of *Gus-r* is also approachable by cloning and sequencing of Gus-s and its flanking DNA from mouse strains carrying the *Gus-r^a* and *Gus-r^b* alleles. Ultimately, however, a correlation must be made between structural variation and allelic *Gus-r* regulatory function.

On the basis of observations on other hormone-responsive genes, it is assumed, but not proven, that *Gus-r* is a hormone-response element interacting with the androgen receptor, similar to those that have been identified as DNA-binding sites for glucocorticoid, progesterone, and estrogen receptors, which are other members of the receptor gene superfamily. The fact that

138

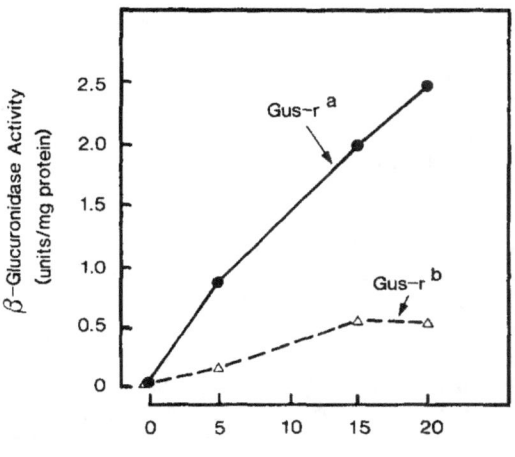

FIGURE 4. *Androgen-related increase in renal β-Gluc activity in mice carrying* Gus-r[a] *and* Gus-r[b] *regulatory alleles of the β-Gluc gene*

there can be multiple hormone regulatory elements for a single steroid receptor associated with a given gene, that these DNA motifs can regulate either negatively or positively, and that they can interact with a variety of tissue-specific transcription factors offers the possibility for variable sensitivity between different hormone-responsive genes in the same individual. Regulatory elements may also show genetic diversity, as is the case with the *Gus-r* locus, which provides one possible explanation for dissimilar responses to androgens of the same gene in two individuals. This, in turn, will explain the enormous diversity in phenotype that is observed among men.

REFERENCES

Bardin, C.W.; Bullock, L.P.; Sherins, R.J.; Mowszowicz, I.; and Blackbum, W.R. Androgen metabolism and mechanism of action in male pseudohermaphroditism: A study of testicular feminization. *Recent Prog Horm Res* 29:65-109, 1973.

Bardin, C.W., and Catterall, J.F. Testosterone, a major determinant of extragenital sexual dimorphism. *Science* 211:1285-1294, 1981.

Beato, M. Induction of transcription by steroid hormones. *Biochim Biophys AcTa* 910:95-102, 1987.

Bullock, L.P. Androgen and progestin stimulation of omithine decarboxylase activity in the mouse kidney. *Endocrinology* 112:1903-1909, 1983.

Catterall, J.F.; Kontula, K.K.; Watson, C.S.; Seppanen, P.J.; Funkenstein, B.; Melanitou, E.; Hickok, N.J.; Bardin, C.W.; and Janne, O.A. Regulation of gene expression by androgens in murine kidney. *Recent Prog Horm Res* 42:71-109, 1986.

D'Amore, M.A.; Gallagher, P.M.; Korfhagen, T.R.; and Ganschow, R.E. Complete sequence and organization of the murine ß-glucuronidase gene. *Biochemistry* 27:7131-7140, 1988.

Jänne, O.A., and Bardin, C.W. Androgen and antiandrogen receptor binding. *Annu Rev Physiol* 46:107-118, 1984.

Keenan, B.S.; Mayer, W.J., III; Hadjian, A.J.; Jones, H.W.; and Migeon, C.J. Syndrome of androgen insensitivity in man: Absence of 5α-dihydrotestosterone binding protein in skin fibroblasts. *J Clin Endocrinol Metab* 38:1143-1146, 1974.

Kochakian, C.D. *How It Was. Anabolic Action of Steroids and Remembrances.* Birmingham: University of Alabama School of Medicine, 1984.

Kontula, K.K.; Seppanen, P.J.; Van Duyne, P.; Bardin, C.W.; and Jänne, O.A. Effect of a nonsteroidal antiandrogen, flutamide, on androgen receptor dynamics and ornithine decarboxylase gene expression in mouse kidney. *Endocrinology* 116:226-233, 1985.

Mainwaring, W.I.P. *The Mechanism of Action of Androgens.* New York: Springer-Verlag, 1977.

Melanitou, E.; Cohn, D.A.; Bardin, C.W.; and Jänne, O.A. Genetic variation in androgen regulation of omithine decarboxylase gene expression in inbred strains of mice. *Mol Endocrinol* 1:266-273, 1987.

Pajunen, A.E.I.; Isomaa, V.V.; Jänne, O.A.; and Bardin, C.W. Androgenic regulation of omithine decarboxylase activity in mouse kidney and its relationship to changes in cytosol and nuclear androgen receptor concentrations. *J Biol Chem* 257:8190-8198, 1982.

Swank, R.T.; Paigen, K.; Davey, R.; Chapman, V.; Labarca, C.; Watson, G.; Ganshow, R.; Brandt, E.J.; and Novak, E. Genetic regulation of mammalian glucuronidase. *Recent Prog Horm Res* 34:401-436, 1978.

Van Doom, E.; Craven, S.; and Bruchovsky, N. The relationship between androgen receptors and the hormonally controlled responses of rat ventral prostate. *Biochem J* 160:11-21, 1976.

Watson, C.S., and Catterall, J.F, Genetic regulation of androgen-induced accumulation of mouse renal ß-glucuronidase mRNA. Endocrinology 118:1081-1086, 1986.

ACKNOWLEDGMENT

This work was supported in part by U.S. Public Health Service grant HD 13541 from the National Institutes of Health.

AUTHORS

C. Wayne Bardin, M.D.
Vice President and Director

James F. Catterall, Ph.D.
Scientist

Olli A. Jänne, M.D., Ph.D.
Senior Scientist and Associate Division Director

Center for Biomedical Research
The Population Council
1230 York Avenue
New York, NY 10021

Reappraisal of the Health Risks Associated With the Use of High Doses of Oral and Injectable Androgenic Steroids

Karl E. Friedl

INTRODUCTION

> A price is paid for a beard and the presence of functional
> testes. Inheritance, ageing, and other factors determine what
> the cost will be to the individual. (Hamilton 1948, p. 315)

Many athletes, especially bodybuilders, powerlifters, and football players, are reported to use androgenic steroids for physical and psychological advantage. The specific benefits and the ethics of such benefits have been heatedly debated. Meanwhile, due to the absence of substantive scientific data on the health risks, proponents of androgen use by athletes claim an advantageous "benefit-to-risk ratio" (Hatfield 1984). Their opponents make equally unfounded claims (Miller 1987) with gross exaggerations such as "six athletes died as a consequence of their steroid use in 1984 alone" *(USA Today* 1987, p. 6C). Such overwrought lay reviews predominate by default because scientists and physicians have had little interest in the medical problems of athletes who choose to medicate themselves in drug regimens that defy any scientific rationale. The scare tactics of negative reviews are unlikely to be effective in discouraging the abuse of androgens by athletes (Wade 1972), but they do undermine legitimate applications of androgens and contribute to the paranoia that impedes reliable investigation of androgen abuse.

This chapter reviews the health risks associated with the use of synthetic androgens by adult men on the basis of primary-source reports of studies and cases published in the medical literature. Extrapolation of this information to the health risks that may be faced by self-medicating athletes using very high ("mega") doses is still tenuous; very high dose androgen may

142

produce effects through other, nonandrogenic, actions, as discussed by Jänne (this volume).

SUSPECTED RISKS AND THE UNKNOWN DENOMINATORS

Much of the attention lavished by the public press on adverse effects of androgens is based on case reports generated when significant morbidity or mortality is involved. The published cases are summarized in table 1.

TABLE 1. *Summary of case reports of significant morbidity or mortality in athletes with associated androgen use*

Age	Disease	Outcome	Description of Use	Reference
38 BB	Wilm's tumor	Death from cancer with metastases	Possibly high-dose methandrostenolone	Prat et al. 1977
26 BB	Hepatocellular carcinoma	Death from cancer with metastases	Many androgens for 4 years	Overly et al. 1984
37 BE	Hepatocellular adenoma	Surgical resection and recovery	Oxymetholone 100 mg/d for 5 years	Goldman 1985
40 BB	Adenocarcinoma of prostate	Death from cancer with metastases	15 cycles of many androgens in 20 years	Roberts and Essenhigh 1986
27 BB	Hepatocellular adenoma	Death from hemorrhage	Anabolic steroids for at least 3 years	Creagh et al. 1988
34 BB	Cerebrovascular thrombosis	Partial recovery	Cycles of anabolic steroids for 4 years	Frankle et al. 1988
32 BB	Cerebrovascular thrombosis (?) and cardio-myopathy	Partial recovery	Many androgens since age 16; stopped 4 months before second cardiovascular accident	Mochizuki and Richter
22 PL	Myocardial infarction	Recovery	IM and oral androgens for 6 weeks	McNutt et al. 1988

KEY: BB=bodybuilder; PL=powerlifter.

Even the rare conditions, such as hepatic adenoma (Pelletier et al. 1984) and Wilm's tumor (Scully et al. 1981) have also been observed in adult men not known to be using any androgens. In some cases, other likely causes of the disease are present, For example, a 22-year-old elite power-lifter with myocardial infarction weighed 330 pounds and had a serum cholesterol of 596 mg/dl (McNutt et al. 1988). Inexplicably, these cases nearly all involve bodybuilders.

A common aspect of these athlete case reports is the inadequate description of their drug use. More to the point, in each of the four cases resulting in death, the use of androgens appeared to be a chance discovery that gave the case report current relevance. Other athletes with significant morbidity may conceal their drug use when complications arise. No systematic study of the medical risks of androgen use by any athletes has ever been conducted, and even the population of adult athletes at risk remains undefined.

The doses used by athletes range from levels that may make them hypogonadal to the more frequently documented doses that far exceed any experienced in clinical medicine. For example, replacement doses of testosterone enanthate for a hypogonadal man average 75 to 100 mg per week; doses of 200 to 250 mg per week have been used in male contraceptive trials and in the treatment of oligospermia with suppression-rebound therapy; and doses reportedly used by athletes for a cycle of use lasting 6 weeks or more have exceeded 1 g per week (Yesalis et al. 1988). Oxymetholone, an orally active 17-alkylated androgen, is used at high doses of 150 mg per day in the treatment of life-threatening anemias, and this dose is comparable to that used by some athletes, with other androgens used in addition (Friedl and Yesalis 1989). Methandrostenolone, which is estimated to give full replacement in hypogonadal men at 15 mg a day (Liddle and Burke 1960), has been administered in doses of 100 mg a day to athletes (Hervey et al. 1975), with doses up to 300 mg a day reportedly used by some athletes for several years (Freed et al. 1975). Although generally used for short durations of several weeks at a time by bodybuilders (Friedl and Yesalis 1989), powerlifters have been reported to use high doses of androgens continuously for up to 7 years (Cohen et al. 1988). A summary of the most frequently used drugs based on survey reports is presented in table 2.

The wide variety of doses and drug combinations employed by athletes makes it difficult to pinpoint the agent responsible for an adverse effect. More reliable information on androgen effects is available from male contraceptive trials that use greater than replacement doses of androgens and from therapeutic treatment of specific disease such as aplastic anemias with high-dose androgen treatment and male hypogonadism with replacement-dose treatment. Even replacement-dose treatments yield adverse effects because of nonandrogenic properties of the synthetic steroids, such as 17-alkylated testosterone, and some of these effects will be common to the androgen-abusing athletes.

Two main categories of androgens are considered here: orally active androgens alkylated at the 17-carbon position, which are therefore afforded some protection against first-pass hepatic clearance, e.g. oxandrolone, oxymetholone, methandrostenolone, and stanozolol, and parenterally administered nonmethylated androgens with a 17b-ester, e.g., testosterone enanthate and nandrolone decanoate. A few exceptions to these two principal categories, such as mesterolone, testosterone undecanoate, and methenolone, so far appear to be compounds of lesser significance in the epidemiology of androgen abuse by athletes.

144

TABLE 2. *Summary of androgens and associated drugs used by athletes, or&red by ranked frequency of use within surveys*

Androgen	Number of Reported Users								
	A	B	C	D	E	F	G	H	I
Total Users	32	50	24	8	7	17	22	15	?
Oral Use									
Methandrostenolone	26	7	x	16	6		16	14	
Oxandrolone	19	5	x	19				12	
Stanozolol	(5)	3	(x)	17		5	5	8	
Oxymetholone	5	2	x	3		2		6	
Ethylestrenol	5			3					
Methyltestosterone	1			1		4		1	
Methenolone Acetate		1		1				3	(2)
Fluoxymesterone				2				1	
Other								3	1
Parenteral Use									
Testosterone Esters	14-22	9	x	20	7	1	16	12	5
Nandrolone Esters	24-30	5	x	8	7	6-8	5	8	
Methenolone Esters	7			1				4	(2)
Stanozolol	(5)		(x)		4			6	
Testosterone (Aqueous)		1						5	
Boldenone Undecylenate			x					4	
Methandriol Dipropionate	1			6					
Other	3							1	
Other (Nonsteroidal)									
Chorionic Gonadotropin	x	x	x			x			
Growth Hormone			x			x		x	
Diuretics	x					x		x	
Thyroid Hormones	x					x			
Testolactone/Tamoxifen				x					
Others			x					x	x

KEY: A=several U.S. gyms; Strauss et al. 1983.
  B=St. Louis—8 powerlifters and 4 bodybuilders; Hurley et al. 1984.
  C=Chicago—22 competitive bodybuilders, powerlifters; Frankle et al. 1984.
  D=Phoenix—19 bodybuilders, 2 powerlifters, 3 other; Burkett & Falduto 1984.
  E=Finland-nationally ranked athletes; Alen & Rahkila 1984.
  F=Glasgow, Scotland—bodybuilders; McKillop 1987.
  G=Cape Town, South Africa—powerlifters; Cohen et al. 1988.
  H=1987 US. Powerlifting Federation Championship; Yesalis et al. 1988.
  1=1984 Olympics-positive drug screens; Catlin et al. 1987.
  ( )=oral or injected use not specified for stanozolol or methenolone, each of which have been administered by either route by athletes.
  x=use indicated but unquantified.

145

17-ALKYLATED ANDROGEN SUPPRESSION OF HDL-CHOLESTEROL (HDLC)

The single significant adverse effect that has been clearly established for androgen self-administration by athletes is the alteration in serum lipids, most dramatically a reduction in serum HDLC. This begins within a few days after the start of use and generally recovers within approximately a month after cessation. Figure 1 illustrates this change in a 23-year-old university student who injected testosterone cypionate and ingested stanozolol in one cycle (left shaded area), quit steroids for several months, and then began a cycle of oral methandrostenolone and injected nandrolone decanoate (right shaded area). Sex-hormone-binding globulin (SHBG) changes parallel

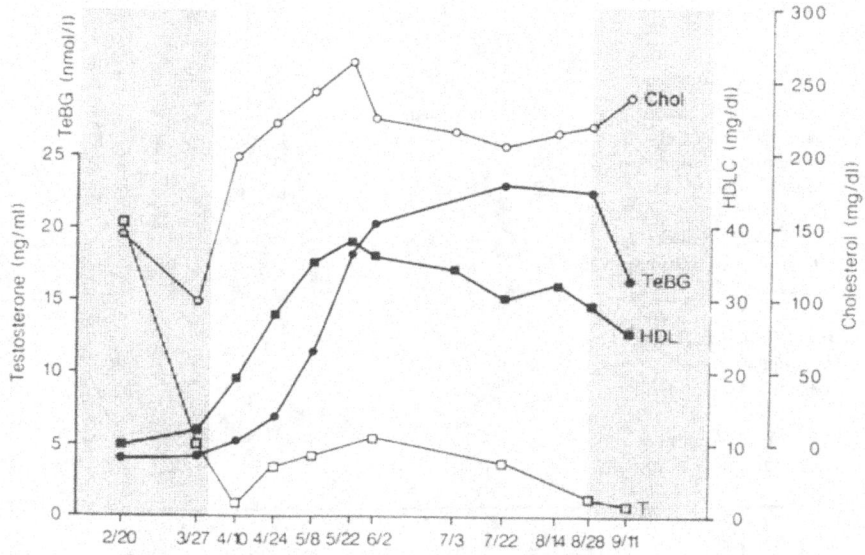

FIGURE 1. *Serum cholesterol, HDLC, SHBG, and testosterone concentrations during and between two cycles of androgen self-administration in a 23-year-old university student, an amateur bodybuilder*

the changes in HDLC. The consistency of this decrease in HDLC is evident from a summary of nine different lipid surveys in table 3. Profound reductions into the single-digit mg/dl concentrations were observed in individuals in several of the studies (Hurley et al. 1984; Costill et al. 1984). This reduction in HDLC is largely due to a reduction of the HDLC-2 subfraction and the accompanying apolipoprotein AI, as an apparent

TABLE 3. *Serum lipid measurements with and without androgen self-administration in athletes (mg/dl±SE)*

Athletes (n); Androgens Used	Chol Off	Chol On	Trig Off	Trig On	HDLC Off	HDLC On	LDLC Off	LDLC On	Chol/HDLC Off	Chol/HDLC On	Reference
PL (vs C) (9) oxy, meth, T?	(204) ±8	218 ±16			(45) ±1	17* ±2			(4.6) ±0.4	16.4* ±3.8	Costill et al. 1984
PL, BB (12) many	185 ±8	232* ±23	80 ±9	90 ±9	51 ±4	23* ±2	117 ±9	188* ±22	3.6	10.1	Hurley et al. 1984
Elite PL (5) oxan+meth+ND, TE	200 ±11	223 ±26			52 ±10	16* ±3			3.8	13.9	Peterson and Fahey 1984
BB (11), PL (3) meth+TE, ND	210 ±13	209 ±15	120 ±14	153 ±28	61 ±4	29* ±2	125 ±10	150* ±12	3.4	7.2	Webb et al. 1984
BB, PL, W (5) meth, st-V, NP, T?	205 ±29	201 ±31	101 ±12	113 ±27	47 ±4	21* ±4			4.2 ±0.9	9.1* ±5.0	Alen et al. 1985
PL (vs C) (5) meth+TC	(176) ±14	183 ±12	(93) ±18	93 ±12	(50) ±6	26* ±4	(108) ±14	138 ±11	(3.7) ±0.4	8.2* ±2.0	Kantor et al. 1985
BB (5), W (1) many	184 ±13	158 ±16	69 ±16	72 ±10	43 ±5	15* ±7	127 ±14	129 ±14	3.1 ±0.5	12.4* ±4.9	Friedl and Plymate, unpublished manuscript, 1986**
PL (vs C) (9) meth, m, TC, ND	(183) ±9	291* ±29			(52) ±4	24* ±3			3.5	12.1	Cohen et al. 1986
BB (16) many	216 ±60	260 +108	123 ±71	129 ±81	46 ±2	23* ±3	154 ±15	222* ±27	4.7	11.3	Lenders et al. 1988

*p<.05.
**All used meth or oxan+oxy or flu+TC or st-V; all used tamoxifen.

KEY: BB=bodybuilder; PL=powerlifter; W=wrestler; C=control; flu=fluoxymesterone; m=methenolone; meth=methandrostenolone; oxan=oxandrolone; oxy=oxymetholone; ND=nandrolone decanoate; st-V=stanozolol; T?=testosterone ester; TC=testosterone cypionate. Values in parentheses are from a reference control group.

NOTE: The decline in HDLC with androgen administration is consistent across studies; all used 17-alkylated androgens with or without injectable androgens. Oral androgens were generally used alone or in conjunction with injected androgens; duration of use ranged from 4 to 26 weeks.

consequence. of the induction of hepatic triglyceride lipase activity (HTGLA) (Kantor et al. 1985; Lenders et al. 1988; Applebaum et al. 1987). The substantial reduction in HDLC is generally offset by an increase in low-density lipoprotein cholesterol (LDLC), with no net alteration in total cholesterol, although in two reports total cholesterol also increased (Hurley et al. 1984; Cohen et al. 1986). In each of these nine studies, 17-alkylated androgens were used by the athletes, with or without the addition of parenteral androgens.

The altered balance of cholesterol fractions in self-medicating athletes suggests that these individuals are at substantially increased risk for coronary heart disease. Coronary artery disease tripled in middle-aged men in the

Framingham Heart Study with antecedent HDLC measurements of less than 25 mg/dl, compared to the incidence in men starting with a mean level of 50 mg/dl (Gordon et al. 1977). Other studies have suggested that the level of apolipoprotein AI, which decreases markedly in the self-medicating athletes, is an even better discriminator of coronary artery disease (Maciejko et al. 1983), while serum LDLC and the associated apolipoprotein B appear to be more important determinants of the production and reversal of vascular lesions (Nessim et al. 1983). In one study, reduced HDLC was the single factor identified (with normal gonadal steroid levels) that distinguished men at low risk for heart disease who still develop heart disease (Heller et al. 1983). Whether or not an androgen-induced change in this risk factor in this group produces a detectable increase in heart disease in athletes remains to be established. At least while they are still engaged in athletics, these men tend to be nonsmokers, exercise intensively, and maintain relatively low body fat, thereby minimizing other risk factors for heart disease; most of these men also maintain normal total cholesterol levels. Androgen-induced alteration may actually reduce other risk factors. For example, the substantial niacinlike reduction in serum lipoprotein a (Lp(a)), demonstrated with stanozolol administration (Albers et al. 1984), may signify a reduction in risk of ischemic heart disease (Schriewer et al. 1984) and cerebrovascular disease (Jurgens and Koltringer 1987). The case-reported increase in left ventricular mass among strength athletes using androgens (McKillop et al. 1986) plays an unknown role in heart disease.

To date there is only one published case of heart disease in a young androgen-using athlete (McNutt et al. 1988). As previously described, other predisposing factors were clearly present. Another case that was reportedly investigated demonstrated a familial risk: a 27-year-old steroid user who died of heart disease had a father who had died at age 32 of heart disease (Cowart 1987). The role of other drug use in such cases also needs to be carefully considered; the bodybuilder depicted in figure 1 eventually admitted to a history of intravenous drug use (unspecified) under questioning by a physician in connection with a diagnosis of hepatitis. Thus, if an increased incidence of heart disease in androgen-using athletes emerges, it is likely to be detected only in a properly designed epidemiological study with careful control of the potential confounders.

The HDLC depression observed so consistently in self-medicating athletes is not an obligatory consequence of androgen use. It is also not readily apparent that studies with synthetic androgens explain the sex differences in serum lipids and heart disease (Godsland et al. 1987; Nordoy et al. 1979). Early studies demonstrating opposing effects of estrogens and androgens on the HDLC/LDLC ratio were all based on methyltestosterone administration (Russ et al. 1955; Furman et al. 1958; Oliver and Boyd 1956). Once this effect of methyltestosterone was ascribed to an androgenic effect, the premise was reversed, with the suggestion that HDLC depression could serve as an index of androgenicity (Furman et al. 1957). Thus, it was concluded that 17-alkylated androgens such as methyltestosterone and methylnortestosterone were highly potent androgens, while up to 100 mg per day sublingual testosterone had little androgenic potency because of nonsignificant decrements in HDLC (Furman et al. 1957). A similar absence of effect on HDLC was discovered for testosterone propionate (Oliver and Boyd 1956), and parenteral administration of androsterone was found to reduce only the LDLC fraction (Cohen et al. 1971).

Subsequent studies in normolipid subjects have failed to demonstrate a clinically significant reduction in HDLC with androgen ester administration in doses that are markedly androgenic (table 4). Thus, while 17-alkylated androgens such as stanozolol, oxandrolone (Hazzard et al. 1984), and methyltestosterone reduce HDLC by approximately half, the administration of nandrolone and testosterone esters has little or no effect.

TABLE 4. *Serum lipid concentrations before and during androgen administration in normolipidemic volunteers (mg/dl±SE)*

Androgen/Dose Exposure (n)	Chol Bef	Chol Dur	Trig Bef	Trig Dur	HDLC Bef	HDLC Dur	LDLC Bef	LDLC Dur	Reference
MeT (varied) (10)	199 ±9	197 ±11			46 ±4	28* ±2	149 ±8	166 ±3	Russ et al. 1955
Stan 6 mg/day 4 weeks (2M, 4F)	237 ±25	232 ±46	126 ±51	120 ±36	59 ±18	29* ±7	160 ±36	181* ±42	Haffner et al. 1983
TC 400 mg/week 3 weeks (6)	202 ±10	175* ±10	109 ±17	89* ±17	49 ±4	42* ±4			Crist et al. 1985
TC 100 mg/week 3 weeks (8M, 1F)	174 ±7	180 ±7			49 ±1	43* ±1			Crist et al. 1986
ND 100 mg/week 3 weeks (xover)	174 ±7	192 ±8			49 ±1	41* ±2			Crist et al. 1986
MeT 40 mg/day 12 weeks (6)	182 ±13	208 ±24	107 ±17	145 ±48	46 ±5	30* ±5	115 ±8	150 ±18	Friedl et al. 1990
TE 280 mg/week 12 weeks (6)	170 ±13	189 ±10	89 ±11	87 ±10	45 ±4	42 ±3	108 ±12	120 ±13	Friedl et al. 1990
Stan 6 mg/day 6 weeks (11)	182 ±16	192 ±22	133 ±21	111* ±21	45 ±3	30* ±2	111 ±14	143* ±12	Thompson et al. 1989
TE 200 mg/week 6 weeks (xover)	191 ±15	171* ±14	131 ±15	148 ±24	43 ±2	39* ±2	121 ±14	102* ±11	Thompson et al. 1989

*p<.05.

KEY: MeT=methyltestosterone; stan=stanozolol; TC=testosterone cypionate; TE=testosterone enanthate.

NOTE: 17-Alkylated androgen-treated groups show the greatest decreases in HDLC. Mixed sex subjects are indicated with counts of each; Crist et al. (1986) was a crossover design that included placebo; Thompson et al. (1989) was a crossover design.

This difference is explained by the induction of HTGLA demonstrated for methyltestosterone or stanozolol, with no effect on this enzyme by testosterone enanthate in the same studies (Friedl, submitted for publication; Thompson et al. 1989). Induction of HTGLA may be specific to the 17-alkyl-substituted androgens and may not be due to an androgenic effect at all, but a simpler explanation is that it reflects an alteration in the androgen—estrogen balance in the presence of an androgen that is not readily aromatized to estrogen, since estrogen has an opposite effect, suppressing HTGLA (Applebaum et al. 1977; Tikkanen et al. 1982). Testosterone enanthate administration results in a large increase in estrogen, while a lesser proportion of methyltestosterone is aromatized, and only to 17a-methylestradiol, which appears to be a weak estrogen (Ryan 1963; Dimick et al. 1961; Feenstra et al. 1983). Further evidence for this role of estrogen comes from a study with coadministration of the aromatase inhibitor, testolactone, with testosterone enanthate. This suppresses the normally observed increase in estradiol following administration of the enanthate and produces a modest but significant reduction in HDLC that does not occur with testosterone enanthate alone (Fried et al. 1990, Friedl et al. 1988).

Paradoxically, the reduction in serum lipids by androgens suggested possibilities for clinical use in the treatment of hypertriglyceridemia (Stone 1963; Sachs and Wolfman 1968; Howard and Furman 1962); this was suggested by observations that triglycerides tend to be elevated by estrogens and could be reduced by androgens (Howard and Furman 1962; Kim and Kalkhoff 1975), but the benefit of a reduction in serum triglycerides that occurs in some patients is offset by the atherogenic shift in HDLC/LDLC produced at the same time (Hazzard et al. 1984).

Androgens have long been suspected of a role in heart disease because of gender differences in the disease incidence, but estrogens may be involved. Serum estrogens are higher and testosterone is reduced in men with coronary artery disease (Chute et al. 1987; Hamalainen 1985) although such alterations may be secondary to illness and stress (Plymate et al. 1987; Friedl et al. 1988). Estrogens increase apolipoprotein AI secretion; but at a substantially higher dose, estrogens also increase apolipoproteins B and E (Tam et al. 1986). Although male patients treated with estrogens in the Coronary Drug Project did not show a change in the rate of myocardial infarction, the risk of venous thromboembolism approximately doubled (Coronary Drug Project Research Group 1973). The case reports of stroke in two athletes (Frankle et al. 1988; Mochizuki and Richter 1988) and one additional case of a young hypogonadal man self-administering very high doses of testosterone (Nagelberg et al. 1986) are consistent with a role of estrogen in thrombotic stroke (Collaborative Group for the Study of Stroke in Young Women 1975). Increased estrogenicity is supported by the occurrence of gynecomastia in some androgen-using athletes, including one of the athletes with stroke (Frankle et al. 1988); presumably, this is a result of aromatization of high doses of androgen, but it may also result from an altered hepatic clearance of steroid (Friedl and Yesalis 1989).

Hyperinsulinemia and impaired glucose tolerance has been reported with methandrostenolone (Woodard et al. 1981; Landon et al. 1962), oxymetholone (Landon et al. 1962) and for athletes self-administering several androgens (Cohen and Hickman 1987). Such an effect may adversely affect serum HDLC (Stalder et al. 1981), and it has been suggested from epidemiological observations that testosterone increases risk of heart disease through an effect on insulin (Lichtenstein et al. 1987). Alternatively, it may count as an additional independent risk factor, additive to the HDLC reduction. This effect has not been duplicated with androgen esters (Friedl et al. 1989; Swerdloff et al. 1978; Landon et al. 1963), including injected methenolone acetate, a 1-methylated androgen (Landon et al. 1963). In one recent report, a Klinefelter's patient whom the authors claimed was receiving parenteral methyltestosterone (250 mg every 3 weeks), developed glucose intolerance and acanthosis nigricans (Shuttleworth et al. 1987), again supporting the contention that the effect on glucose tolerance is specific to 17-alkylation and is not simply a consequence of the route of androgen administration.

OTHER SERUM PROTEIN ALTERATIONS RELATED TO 17-ALKYLATION

17-alkylated androgen-induced changes like those observed with HTGLA have also been obtained for other functionally diverse proteins produced by the liver (Barbosa et al. 1971a; Barbosa et al. 1971b). Some of these changes are what make the 17-alkylated androgens clinically useful, such as the stimulation of complement Cl inhibitor activity and complement C4 in the treatment of angioedema. On the other hand, hemostatic alterations, coupled with an increased hematocrit in some athletes (Alen 1985), could conceivably lead to thromboembolytic disorders including stroke and myocardial infarction, or increased fibrinolytic activity (Feamley and Chakrabarti 1964; Feamley and Chakrabarti 1962) may account for an apparent tendency for androgen-associated hepatic tumors to rupture. Some of these hemostatic changes may be more structure-related than simply 17-alkyl substitution; seven different 17-alkylated androgens produced increases in plasminogen (while no esters did), but only oxymetholone, oxandrolone, and norethandrolone also produced decreases in fibrinogen (Barbosa et al. 1971a). On the other hand, Kruskemper reported increases in clotting factors with any methylated androgens, but this did not occur with testosterone propionate (Kuskemper 1968) while a net increase in fibrinolytic activity is reported in some patients with either oral androgen administration (Feamley and Chakrabarti 1964) or parenteral testosterone propionate (Feamley and Chakrabarti 1962). Small but statistically significant increases in systolic blood pressure have been reported with androgen use in athletes (Freed et al. 1975; Lenders et al. 1988) and these may also represent alterations in hepatic proteins similar to that observed in some susceptible women with oral contraceptive use (Vessey et al. 1976).

SHBG is reduced by both 17-alkylated androgens and the esters, but the 17-alkylated androgens are more potent in this effect (Stone 1963), perhaps reflecting the difference in androgen-estrogen balance produced with these two classes of androgens (Ruokonen et al. 1985; Belgorosky and Rivorola 1985; Chetkowski et al. 1986). The physiological significance of a reduction in SHBG and the consequent increase in free and albumin-bound testosterone is uncertain, as many of the synthetic androgens have a reduced binding affinity (Saartok et al. 1984) and would be little affected; alternatively, the SHBG-bound steroid may be important for some actions (Reese et al. 1988).

The mechanism of this regulation is more complex than simply a change in the rate of protein secretion by hepatocytes, because, *in vitro,* androgens and estrogens both stimulate SHBG (Lee et al. 1987). As suggested by studies of thyroxine-binding globulin (Ain and Refetoff 1988), an increase in the androgen-estrogen ratio may result in secretion of a less glycosylated form of the binding protein, with a reduced circulation half-time. In this way, thryoxine-binding globulin levels are reduced by oral or sublingual methyltestosterone, while sublingual testosterone propionate and injected nandrolone phenylpropionate have no effect (Barbosa et al. 1971b), again suggesting a structural specificity, in this case perhaps related to the ability to aromatize to potent estrogen.

The moderate increases in serum aspartate aminotransferase (AST, SGOT) and alanine aminotransferase (ALT, SGPT) activities noted in androgen-using athletes (Alen 1985) may reflect hepatocellular necrosis or, less likely, cholestasis, but the elevation has been reported to be a transient phenomenon even with continued use (Wynn et al. 1961; Petera et al. 1962). For example, Petera et al. (1962) found that methyltestosterone (30 mg per day) produced a peak rise in both SGOT and SGPT levels after approximately 10 to 12 days administration to 40 patients, and, with continued therapy, the levels declined again. No such enzyme rise occurred if patients were treated with testosterone propionate (25 mg per day) either by oral or parenteral routes of administration. Kruskemper (1968) also found increased serum transaminase levels only with 17-alkylated androgens and no increase with testosterone propionate or even with an orally administered 1-methylated androgen. The pathological significance of this transient increase is unknown.

CHOLESTATIC JAUNDICE: DISRUPTION OF MICROFILAMENTS?

In 1952, Lloyd-Thomas and Sherlock used methyltestosterone to treat pruritis associated with obstructive jaundice and found that the jaundice

152

deepened in five of their seven cases (Lloyd-Thomas and Sherlock 1952). This, and several cases of jaundice in hypogonadal men replaced with methyltestostetone (Werner 1947; Werner et al. 1950), led to the association of cholestatic jaundice with 17-alkylated androgen administration; subsequent cases were reported primarily for patients treated with methyltestosterone (Brick and Kyle 1952; Bonner and Homburger 1952; Wood 1952; Almaden and Ross 1954; Kaplan 1956; Koszalka 1957) and norethandrolone (Dunning 1958; Schaffner et al. 1959; Shaw and Gold 1960; Gordon et al. 1960; Gilbert et al. 1963) but also with stanozolol (Evely et al. 1987), methyl-not-testosterone (Peters et al. 1958), and methandrostenolone (Wynn et al. 1961). Foss and Simpson (1959) summarized 42 case reports in 1959, and cases reiterating this association continue to appear in the literature 30 years later (Lucey and Moseley 1987).

One case of jaundice with testosterone enanthate administration occurred during pregnancy (Gill et al. 1986), making this connection with androgen esters uncertain, since the same form of cholestatic jaundice is an established consequence of pregnancy for some women (Svanborg and Ohlsson 1959). However, recurrent jaundice of pregnancy has been attributed to an abnormal response to high circulating levels of estrogen in subjects with a familial history (Reyes et al. 1981), and this effect is conceivably enhanced by the addition of a readily aromatizable androgen.

Androgen-related cholestasis ranges in frequency from very few patients with even histological evidence of disease (Cicardi et al. 1983; Westaby et al. 1977; Kory et al. 1959) to 17.3 percent of patients evolving an overt jaundice (Pecking et al. 1980). This form of cholestatic drug reaction generally lacks histological features of inflammation and necrosis and is characterized by a bland accumulation of bile in cells and canaliculi (Foss and Simpson 1959). Recovery typically occurs within several weeks after drug cessation, and jaundice does not necessarily recur in these patients with reinstitution of treatment (Werner et al. 1950; Pecking et al. 1980).

Death is a highly unlikely consequence: the reports of death with cholestatic jaundice that have been attributed to 17-alkylated androgen administration (summarized in table 5) have all occurred in elderly or very ill patients, including two patients with metastatic carcinomas and at least one suspected of suffering from severe viral hepatitis; in four of these cases, the medication was continued until the death of the patient because it was not recognized as a potential agent of the cholestasis.

Intrahepatic cholestasis can be produced with norethandrolone infusion in rats, and the primary defect appears to be a disruption of microfilaments similar to the action produced with cytochalasin B (Phillips et al. 1978). This suggests that reduced bile transport and hepatocyte structural changes that lead to cholestasis are mediated through this single mechanism. Reduced transport may be an early marker of hepatic dysfunction, since it

TABLE 5. *Summary of case reports of deaths attributed to androgen-induced cholestatic jaundice by the authors or later reviewers*

Age/Sex	Disorder Treated	Androgen Used/ Dose/Exposure	Cause of Death	Reference
60 M	"to improve healing and protein anabolism" (metastatic disease)	methyl-testosterooe(sl) 30 mg/d, 10 weeks	'obstructive jaundice"	Koszalka 1957
62 M	"therapeutic trial" (metastatic disease and angina, treated with I-131-induced myxedema)	methyl-nortestosterone 6 to 25 mg/d, for 18 weeks	? ? (histology: "resolving jaundice")	Peters et al. 1958
43 M	corticosteroid-induced osteoporosis	norethandrolone 30 mg/d, 23 weeks	cholestasis and peliosis	Gordon et al. 1960
57 F	anorexia (result of 'pancreatic insufficiency")	norethandrolone 20 mg/d, 42 weeks	*severe viral hepatitis" with cholestasis and peliosis	Gordon et al. 1960
74 M	osteoporosis and hemiplegia	norethandrolone 30 mg/d, 30 weeks	sepsis and intrahepatic cholestasis	Gilbert et al. 1963

appears to precede cholestasis and jaundice. Thus, in one anemia study, 254 patients were randomized to one of four oral androgens (norethandrolone, methandrostenolone, oxymetholone, and the 6-methylated methenolone); 35 percent of patients had signs of abnormal liver function, including reduced bromosulfophthalein (BSP) uptake, but only 17.3 percent had overt jaundice (Pecking et al. 1980). Similarly, Kory et al. (1959) noted abnormal BSP retention in 74 percent of 47 patients treated with norethandrolone (25 or 50 mg a day), but liver biopsies from seven of the patients with poor BSP retention times yielded normal tissue, with only one demonstrating a minimal bile stasis and focal necrosis.

Hypercholesterolemia is also a marker of cholestasis, and there may be a relation to hypercholesteremia, which has been reported for some androgen-using athletes (Cohen et al. 1988).

PELIOSIS HEPATIS: AN UNKNOWN ETIOLOGY

Peliosis hepatis is a potentially life-threatening hepatic lesion characterized by a spectrum of microscopic to grossly visible blood-filled cysts in the liver, with or without endothelial lining (Kalra et al. 1976). Originally recognized as a very rare disease associated with fatal pulmonary tuberculosis (Zak 1950), Burger and Marcuse (1952) proposed a relationship between peliosis hepatis and androgen treatment in 1952 with a case report. Since then, more than 70 cases have been reported in association with androgen administration (Gordon et al. 1960; Kintzen and Silny 1960; Bernstein et al. 1971; Port et al. 1971; Bagheri and Boyer 1974; Ogg and Cattell 197.5; Kew et al. 1976; Paradinas et al. 1977; Nadell and Kosek 1977; Groos et al. 1974; Taxy 1978; Wakabayashi et al. 1984; Nuzzo et al. 1985; Karasawa et al. 1979; Bird et al. 1979), and this has included cases of splenic peliosis (Taxy 1978; Slater et al. 1981; Fouquette and Lefebvre 1976). Wakabayashi et al. (1984) performed autopsies on 47 patients with aplastic anemia and found peliosis in 7 of 19 patients who had been treated with oxymetholone or methenolone and in only 1 of 28 patients not treated with androgens. In an American series of patients with wasting disorders, Karasawa et al. (1979) found that of nine postmortem peliosis cases, five of the patients had received androgens. In the Westaby series (Westaby et al. 1977) of 60 transsexual women and impotent men treated with MeT (150 mg per day) for up to 5 years, 9 patients had sinusoidal dilatation and 3 patients had cyst formation, suggestive of potential prepeliotic lesions. Although the patients in this series were free of symptoms, a later case report described peliosis hepatis and liver tumor rupture requiring emergency surgery in one of the transsexuals following 7 years of continuous androgen treatment. In a 3-to-5-year followup of many of the patients from this series and others on various androgens, Lowdell and Murray-Lyon (1985) found hepatic abnormalities (based on liver scans and colloid uptake) only in the patients still using methyltestosterone, with resolution of abnormalities in those who had stopped using methyltestosterone, and essentially normal livers in those using sublingual or parenteral steroids.

Most reported cases of androgen-associated peliosis involve patients treated with 17-alkylated androgens including fluoxymesterone (Kintzen and Silny 1960; Nuzzo et al. 1985), norethandrolone (Gordon et al. 1960; Ogg and Cattell 1975) oxymetholone (Nadell and Kosek 1977; Groos et al. 1974), methenolone (Wakabayashi 1974), and methyltestosterone (Bird et al. 1979). Peliosis is not clearly associated with androgen esters; however, Turani et al. (1983) reported peliotic lesions in postmortem study of a series of six chronic renal failure patients who received only androgen esters for an average of more than 3 years. Saheb (1980) found no peliosis in postmortem examinations of 52 dialysis patients, but these patients had a much shorter exposure to testosterone enanthate (up to 250 mg a week for 5 months).

Peliosis may not be readily diagnosed by standard laboratory studies and is usually discovered either as occult disease in postmortem examination or, rarely, as a result of symptomatic hemorrhage. At least five patients died from internal hemorrhage resulting from their peliosis (Bagheri and Boyer 1974; Nadell and Kosek 1977; Taxy 1978), but internal hemorrhage is also a frequent cause of death in severe anemias. In nine other cases, death from hepatic failure was attributed to the existing peliosis (Gordon et al. 1960; Bernstein et al. 1971; Bagheri and Boyer 1974; Nadell and Kosek 1977); in several of these cases, metastatic disease and severe cholestasis may have been more directly responsible for patient death. One case of histologically diagnosed peliosis hepatis was followed after androgen withdrawal, and complete recovery was observed (Nadell and Kosek 1977).

Peliosis has also been observed in a woman treated with tamoxifen (Loomus et al. 1983), a drug that is also used by some androgen-abusing athletes in an attempt to prevent the side effect of gynecomastia (Friedl and Yesalis 1989). Although this represents only a single case, it is unusual, since this is such a rare disorder, and it may indicate a role of an androgenic-estrogenic component in this disorder.

Paradinas et al. (1977) have proposed a mechanism that may explain occurrence of cholestasis and peliosis hepatis through a single pathogenic mechanism. Based on microscopic evaluation of biopsy material from the Westaby series of patients treated with methyltestosterone, they propose that 17-alkylated androgens specifically produce hepatocyte hyperplasia; the enlarged hepatocytes then encroach on the hepatic venous system, occluding vessels and perhaps also blocking bile canaliculi to produce cholestasis or peliotic sinusoids.

ANDROGEN-ASSOCIATED TUMORS: A PECULIAR FORM OF HEPATOCELLULAR CARCINOMA

Just as with heart disease, a male predominance of hepatocellular carcinoma has led to a suspected involvement of androgen, and this has been supported by animal studies with castration and androgen replacement (Vesselinovitch and Mihailovich 1967). Since the first suggestion of a relation between androgen treatment and hepatic tumors (Bernstein et al. 1971), at least 91 cases of androgen-associated tumors have been reported in the medical literature. Most of these cases were identified by collecting all reports indexed in five DIALOG data bases: Biosis (for 1969), Cancerlit (for 1963), Embase (for 1974), Medline (for 1966), and Scisearch (for 1974); additional cases were gleaned from bibliographies of identified reports.

Of the 91 cases, 48 were discarded because they were not histologically demonstrated or because they were demonstrated to be patients with Fanconi's anemia. Hereditary anemias such as Fanconi's syndrome carry an increased incidence of malignant neoplasia (Schaison et al. 1983), and there may be a predisposition to the development of hepatic tumors in this group (Cattan et al. 1974a; Cattan et al. 1974b), with such tumors emerging more frequently when lives are extended by androgen therapy.

For the 43 remaining cases, the diagnoses were reportedly established through microscopic evaluation of tumor material obtained through biopsy, surgical resection, or at postmortem examination. This included 28 cases recognized antemortem (or through death as a direct consequence of the disease) (table 6). Another eight cases represented occult disease, detected

156

TABLE 6. *Summary of case reports of histologically diagnosed hepatic tumors associated with androgen administration*

Year Diag-nosed	Age al Diag-nosis	Diag-nosis	FP	Androgens Used Dose	Duration	Reason Used	Means of Discovery	Treatment of Tumor	Survival	References/Case
Death Due to Hepatic Failure or Tumor Rupture										
(76)	17M	HCA	-	oxy 50	68 m	apl anemia	hemoperitoneum		*0	Lesna et al. 1976
76	50M	CLC	-	oxy 100-300	24 m	anemia	pain	M	*4wk	Stromeyer et al. 1979
79	71M	HCC	-	oxy 50;ND 100	36 m	nephrectomy	pain		*1m	Zevin et al. 1981
83	26M	HCC	+	(several)	48 m	athlete	malaise/anorexia	M	*3 m	Overly et al. 1984
88	27M	HCA	-	unspecified	36 m	athlete	hemoperitoneum		*0 m	Creagh et al. 1988
Successful Treatment and/or Regression of Hepatic Tumor										
61	44M	HCC	-	MeT 50	11 yr	cryptorchid	pain	1b,2,4 R	22 yr	Drew 1984
67	33M	HCC	-	MeT 50+TP 12	8 yr	cryptorchid	pain/anorexia	1b M? R	66 m	Farrell et al. 1975/3
70	40M	HCC	-	MeT 50	72 m	hypopituitar	pain/fever	1b,2 R	14 yr	Farrell et al. 1975; McCaughan et al. 1985/2
71	18F	HCC	-	oxy 150-250	28 m	apl anemia	laporotomy	1	*8 m	Johnson et al. 1972/2
71	6F	HCC	-	oxy 30-100	41 m	apl anemia	pain	1 R	*8 m	Johnson et al. 1972/1
72	25M	HCC	-	MeT 50	60 m	hypogonadism	pain/fever	4 R	48 m	Goodman and Laden 1977
73	68M	HCC	-	MeT ?	30 yr	impotence	pain	?,2,4		Ziegenfuss and Carabasi 1973
74	33M	HCC		oxy 150	64 m	par noct hem	pain	1 R	10 yr	Farrell et al. 1975; McCaughan et al. 1985/1
75	19M	HCA	-	oxy ?	36 m	par noct hem	hemoperitoneum	?,2	-	Bruguera 1975
75	30F	HCA	+	MeT 150	37 m	transsexual	pain/anorexia	1,2	-	Westaby et al. 1977; Coombes et al. 1977
75	19M	HCA		meth 65	36 m	par noct hem	hemoperitoneum	?,2		Hernandez-Nieto et al. 1977
(75)	29M	HCC	-	MeT 25-60	11 yr	craniopharyng	hemoperitoneum	1,2	18 m	Boyd and Mark 1977

TABLE 6. (continued)

Year Diagnosed	Age at Diagnosis	Diagnosis	FP	Androgens Used Dose	Duration	Reason Used	Means of Discovery	Treatment of Tumor	Survival	References/Case
(77)	7M	HCC	-	oxy ?	60 m	sider anemia	?	?,2		Ishak 1979/2
78	51M	HCC	-	MeT 150	20 yr	hypogonadism	hemoperitoneum	1,2,3 R	24 m	Cocks 1981; Westaby et al. 1983
78	28M	HCA	-	MeT 40	10 yr	hypogonadism	hemoperitoneum	1 R	48 m	Westaby et al. 1983/1
78	58M	HCA	-	MeT 50	10 yr	hypogonadism	pain	1	124 m	Westaby et al. 1983/2
(78)	39F	HCA	-	MeT 150	84 m	transsexual	hemoperitoneum	?,2	-	Bird et al. 1979
79	16M	HCC	-	oxy 75	72 m	apl anemia	pain/fever	1,2 R	6 m	Treuner et al. 1980
(82)	49M	HCA	-	MeT 50	25 yr	hypopituitar	hemoperitoneum	1,3	42 m	Lewis et al. 1986
82	29M	HCA	-	oxy 150-300	44 m	apl anemia	pain/fever	1b,2 R	3 m	Lyon et al. 1984
(83)	68M	CLC	-	ND 100	24 m	gen weakness	hemoperitoneum	?,2	-	Turani et al. 1983/11
83	32M	HCA	-	TE 250/2wk	11 yr	Alports synd	liv funct tests	1	6 m	Carrasco et al. 1985
85	37M	HCA		oxy 100	60 m	athlete	pain/vomiting	?,2	-	Goldman 1985

*Death reported.

KEY: HCA=hepatocellular adenoma; HCC=hepatocellular carcinoma; CLC=cholangiocarcioma (or mixed with HCC); FP=alpha fetoprotein within normal limits (-) or above normal limits (+). Androgens orally administered in mg/day: MeT=methyl testosterone, oxy=oxymetholone, meth=methandrostenolone; androgens injected in mg/week: ND=nandrolone decanoate, TE=testosterone enanthate. Apl=aplastic, sider=siderde+stic, par noct hem=paroxysmal nocturnal hematuria. Pain usually described as right upper quadrant or epigastric; hemoperitoneum in all cases, severe abdominal pain. 1=withdrawn from androgen 1b=with- drawn >1 year after diagnosis or androgen reinstated, 2=partial or complete tumor excision, 3=tumor dearterialization 4=chemotherapy (usually 5-FU). R=apparent regression of tumor. M=metastatic; survival=known survival after diagnosis.

NOTE: Not listed in table are four cases of hepatic angiosarcoma, three cases of focal nodular hyperplasia, and eight cases of occult disease discovered in postmortem examination.

only in postmortem examinations and unrelated to the cause of death (Turani et al. 1983; Ishak 1979; Sale and Lerner 1977; Chandra et al. 1984; Bakker et al. 1976; Sugiyama et al. 1982; Meadows et al. 1974). The remaining cases were minority diagnoses of nonepithelial tumors: four hepatic angiosarcomas (Falk et al. 1979) and three focal nodular hyperplasias (Kessler et al. 1976; Sweeney and Evans 1976; Alberti-Flor et al. 1984).

The earliest known case with an androgen association (Drew 1984) typifies the liver tumors that have been described. In 1961, hepatocellular carcinoma (HCC) was diagnosed in a 44-year-old man presenting with a right upper quadrant abdominal mass. The multinodular tumor was partially resected, and he was given treatments of 5-fluorouracil. This patient was alive 22 years later with no complaints of liver dysfunction.

The androgen-associated tumors do not behave as cancers, although they may present with cytological characteristics of HCC (Sweeney and Evans 1975; Anthony 1975; Johnson 1975); in some cases, this has led authors to construct incongruous diagnoses such as "benign" HCC or "malignant" adenoma (Goldman 1985). In another case, the authors concluded that they had nodules with both HCC and hepatocellular adenoma (HCA), which suggested the possibility that HCA can transform into HCC (Boyd and Mark 1977). That these are benign tumors is indicated by the long survival following diagnosis, the absence of metastases, and the absence of elevated alpha fetoprotein (FP) production. Nearly all of the reported cases are also negative for serum hepatitis surface antigen and lack evidence of an associated cirrhosis, which is found with many of the more typical HCC cases, in the absence of known exogenous androgen exposure (Peters 1976). That they are androgen related is supported by the finding that tumor regression occurred in more than half of the cases with followup observation following androgen withdrawal, with no other treatment (or only partial tumor excision). Although regarded as a subgroup of HCC, cholangiocarcinoma, by itself or in association with HCC, was associated with a much poorer prognosis compared to the other androgen-related tumors; two of these three tumors demonstrated malignant behavior.

The associated drug was largely determined by the condition being treated. The median time of androgen exposure before diagnosis was 5 years, with a range of latency between 2 and 30 years. All patients with severe anemias had exposure to oxymetholone, usually at a dose of at least 100 mg a day, and all androgen-deficient patients received methyltestosterone, usually at a dose of 50 mg per day. Only two cases were associated with exclusive use of androgen esters, and Carrasco et al. (1984) were unable to demonstrate the androgen dependence in their patient (Carrasco et al. 1985). Whether or not methyltestosterone and oxymetholone are the still preferred drugs is uncertain, as drug production figures are not readily forthcoming from the producers; however, the superiority of parenteral androgens in the treatment of anemia has been promoted (Neff et al. 1981), and the use of methyltestosterone for replacement therapy has fallen into disfavor (Nieschlag 1982). On the other hand, methyltestosterone is manufactured by 14 of the 28 legitimate U.S. androgen manufacturers, and, for 12 of these companies, this is the only androgen produced (Food and Drug Administration, personal communication). Anemia patients, of which androgen-deficient patients may be a part, may be more predisposed to tumor formation, and they are already at greater risk through transfusional hemosiderosis (Steinherz et al. 1976); however, these are also the two main groups of patients who would receive the majority of legitimate androgen treatments and are probably not overrepresented.

The three most recent case reports comprise all the reports of liver tumors in androgen-using athletes. These include one who died from a metastatic carcinoma (Overly et al. 1984), one who died from internal hemorrhage following the rupture of an adenoma (Creagh et al. 1988) and another who apparently survived following surgical resection of an adenoma (Goldman 1985). In the case reported by Overly et al. (1984), the features are typical of the better known malignant HCC, including high serum levels of FP synthesized by the carcinoma, and the aggressive biological behavior of the tumor with metastasis and short time to death. The median survival time for this disease may be as short as 1 month, with very few patients expected to live beyond 1 year (Lai et al. 1979); in contrast, most patients with androgen-associated tumors survive following successful treatment or with only withdrawal of androgen treatment. The Overly case (Overly et al. 1984) also included cholangiole involvement, seen in only two other patients in these cases (one of which also metastasized). Thus, this cancer case does not bear the characteristics that are typical of the androgen-associated tumors.

These reports are selective for the more extreme and symptomatic cases and for current issues, e.g., steroid-using athletes. This may explain why 10 of these cases were diagnosed after internal hemorrhage brought the case to medical attention (24 of 28 presented with acute abdominal pain). The majority of tumors may remain undetected because they do not rupture and the patients remain unsymptomatic. Cases of such occult disease have been described from careful postmortem examinations of androgen-treated patients (Turani et al. 1983; Ishak 1979; Sale and Lerner 1977; Chandra et al. 1984; Bakker et al. 1976; Sugiyama et al. 1982; Meadows et al. 1974). On the other hand, in 31 cases of HCA in males collected from the literature by Pelletier et al. (1984), all three associated with androgen use ruptured. It could be suggested that 17-alkylation does not produce more tumors than the androgen esters but simply increases the likelihood of discovery through rupture. Turani et al. (1983) have described tumors and peliosis associated with nonalkylated androgens in a mostly postmortem series; however, this still remains an isolated finding. The high rate of adenoma rupture and hemorrhage in women using oral contraception, compared to women with HCA not using oral contraceptives, is particularly associated with the use of

160

17-alkyl-substituted progestagens with some androgenic activity (Klatskin 1977). This data suggests a structural specificity; although this too could reflect selective reporting.

In our series, peliosis was not consistently present with the tumors (it was described in half of the cases), and it has been suggested that necrotic lesions described as peliosis may be more representative of the vascular ectasia frequently seen with tumors (Peters 1976). As an example, in the case of the athlete who died following tumor rupture (Creagh et al. 1988) the liver surrounding the adenomas was described as hyperplastic with ectatic sinusoids but was apparently devoid of peliotic cysts.

The occurrence of androgen-related tumors appears to be considerably higher than the rate of hepatic tumors associated with female oral contraceptive steroids; within 5 years of the first case report associating oral contraceptives with liver tumors, at least 117 cases had been documented in the literature, with perhaps 100 more claimed; 92 percent of these were benign tumors, for which fewer than 400 cases had been reported in women since 1937 (Klatskin 1977). Oral-contraceptive-related tumors are rare relative to the size of the population at risk; at least 30 million women are estimated to be currently using contraceptive steroids in the United States alone. The prevalence of androgen use, even with inclusion of androgen abusers, is not reasonably expected to come close to this, nor is exposure during the past 30 years likely to rival oral contraceptive exposures. In patients with severe anemia surviving 2 years with androgen treatment, the incidence was 2 benign tumors in 137 patients (Pecking et al. 1980; Joint Group for the Study of Aplastic and Refractory Anemias 1981); previously, Hemandez-Nieto et al. (1977) reported tumor rupture in a patient from the larger sample of 429 patients originally enrolled in this same series (3 patients out of 429), although many of these patients have had a shorter exposure to androgens. In the Westaby study of 60 female-to-male transsexuals and impotent men treated with high-dose methyltestosterone (Westaby et al. 1977; Coombes et al. 1977). only one HCA was detected, although Bird et al. (1979) later reported a case with tumor rupture in another transsexual from the same series (2 patients out of 60). Thus, the incidence of hepatic tumors may be estimated to be 1 to 3 percent within 2 to 8 years of exposure of greater-than-replacement doses of 17-alkylated androgen; occult disease undoubtedly drives this incidence higher.

Hepatic angiosarcoma has also been associated with androgen use in one retrospective epidemiological study. In a review of 168 cases of histologically confirmed cases of hepatic angiosarcoma, 4 cases with some previous androgen exposure (3.1 percent) were identified from a review of medical records (Falk et al. 1979). The connection with androgen exposure remains unconfirmed, with no new androgen-associated cases reported since the latest of the four case deaths in 1974, and at least one of those four patients was exposed to isoniazid, another proposed agent of hepatic angiosarcoma (Daneshmend and Bradfield 1979). Three cases of focal nodular hyperplasia (Kessler et al. 1976; Sweeney and Evans 1987; Alberti-Flor 1974) have also been reported in patients with androgen exposure, in two cases with only 3 and 6 months of androgen exposure, thus leaving the role of androgen open to question.

Androgens do not appear to be in themselves mutagenic but may enhance effects of carcinogens and promote tumor formation (Lesna and Taylor 1986; Anderson and Rossof 1979). In animal studies, doses of androgenic steroids (AS) 400 to 600 times the equivalent human dose are given over most of the life span of the animal. These steroids cause liver growth (hyperplasia and hypertrophy) without tumors and are not mutagenic in the Ames test (lngerowski et al. 1981). In mice, nandrolone decanoate (600 mg/kg a week for 6 weeks) did not produce liver tumors, but if it followed exposure to dimethylnitrosamine, which is known to produce liver cancer in rodents, the expected tumor formation was markedly enhanced (Lesna and Taylor 1986).

ANDROGENS AS POTENTIAL CONTRACEPTIVES: REVERSIBLE INFERTILITY

Androgen treatment in normal men will produce oligo- or azoospermia through suppression of gonadotropins, and most, if not all, will be rendered infertile after weeks or months of continuous high-dose exposure (Swerdloff et al. 1978; Mauss et al. 1975; Matsumoto 1988). Since the major portion of the testis is composed of seminiferous tubules and developing germ cells, this reduction in the population of developing germ cells decreases testicular size by a measurable 15 to 35 percent (Lichtenstein et al. 1987; Palacios et al. 1981). Since the normal cycle of sperm development from spermatogonia to mature spermatid in the testis takes 64 days, it is not surprising that the recovery with cessation of steroid may take 6 months or more for some men; some androgens with long half-times will have an even more extended effect. There are no documented cases of irreversible sterility occurring in healthy men with initially normal sperm count as a result of As use.

High-dose AS use has been used in the opposite sense as well, in an attempt to restore fertility in men with low sperm count through a well recognized but poorly understood rebound that occurs following several months of high-dose AS sperm suppression (Rowley and Heller 1972; Chamy and Gordon 1978). Up to 60 percent of patients with below normal spermatogenic activity but otherwise normal seminiferous epithelia show at least a temporary improvement in their sperm counts, and, in some patients, this is a permanent improvement. Norethandrolone, testosterone esters, and mesterolone have all been used in rebound therapy and appear to improve pregnancy success rates. Nevertheless, there has been no study of the

162

reproductive axis in men who previously used high doses of androgens for several years.

CONCLUSION

From the evidence of studies of androgen administration, it is not readily apparent that significant adverse health effects can be attributed to androgens as a general class; however, the 17-alkyl-substituted androgens have certain established consequences, all involving the liver. The 17-alkylated androgens produce a consistent and substantial reduction in HDLC/LDLC fractions, possibly increasing the risk of heart disease, although this outcome remains to be demonstrated in androgen users. Cholestatic jaundice has been observed in frequencies ranging from none to 17 percent in various categories of 17-alkylated-androgen-treated patients, but is readily reversed when androgen treatment is stopped. Peliosis hepatis clearly occurs in association with 17-alkylated androgen use, but with unknown frequency. Hepatic tumors are rare in men but occur with a frequency as high as 1 to 3 percent with 17-alkylated-androgen treatment with a latency of 2 to 30 years, Nearly half of these discovered tumors rupture, although a yet larger proportion of benign disease may remain undetected. In two cases, including one of a self-medicating bodybuilder, rupture proved fatal. In the absence of effects reported in association with 17-alkylated androgens, there would be few reports of androgen adverse effects, even though the clinical use of injected androgen esters appears to be widespread.

Several case reports involving death or significant illness in athletes who were thought to be self-administering androgens suggest the possibility of other adverse effects that have not been commonly associated with androgen doses in the clinical range. Foremost among these reports are several cases of stroke reported in two bodybuilders and a third in a hypogonadal man with unsupervised high-dose androgen self-administration. Previously unobserved adverse consequences may emerge from extraordinarily high-dose androgen actions through effects related to crossover interactions with non-androgenic receptors and to the unusually high serum levels of some metabolites, including estrogens. These effects may become apparent only with prospective study of androgen abusers.

What these findings mean to current efforts to reduce the abuse of androgens by athletes is that *some* aspects of a standard smoking-cessation type educational approach may not be useful, since there are few direct health consequences, other than cosmetic effects such as acne (Strauss and Pochi 1963; Kiraly et al. 1988) and gynecomastia (Friedl and Yesalis 1989), that can be used to dissuade these athletes from androgen use. There are also certain problems with athletes discovering that the injectable esters may carry less health risk than the orally active 17-alkylated androgens if this causes more athletes to shift to the abuse of injectable androgens. This introduces all the risks associated with self-injection by nonmedically trained individuals using materials that are largely procured through unreliable black market sources, ranging from localized sepsis (Rastad et al. 1985) to hepatitis and AIDS (Sklarek et al. 1984). This may also lead to much higher dose administration of these more potent and longer lasting compounds, and such use may introduce a new set of adverse actions not previously encountered.

Thus, the question remains open: Hamilton (1948) suggested that there was a price to pay for virilization, and studies of androgen administration in men are not yet adequate to determine if additional androgen exacts a higher price in health consequences. Clearly, 17-alkyl substitution in an androgen introduces properties producing health risks that should not be ascribed to androgenic actions. It may be speculated that more serious side effects such as stroke may occur at very high doses, even with androgen esters, through estrogenic metabolites or by actions of nonphysiological receptor binding.

REFERENCES

Ain, K.B., and Refetoff, S. Relationship of oligosaccharide modification to the cause of serum thyroxine-binding globulin excess. *J Clin Endocrinol Metab* 66:1037-1043, 1988.

Albers, J.J.; Taggart, H.McA.; Applebaum-Bowden, D.; Haffner, S.; Chesnut, C.H., III; and Hazzard, W.R. Reduction of lecithin-cholesterol acyltransferase, apolipoprotein D and the Lp(a) lipoprotein with the anabolic steroid stanozolol. *Biochim Biophys Acta* 795:293-296, 1984.

Alberti-Flor, C.C.; Iskandarani, M.; Jeffers, L.; Zappa, R.; and Schiff, E.R. Focal nodular hyperplasia associated with the use of a synthetic anabolic androgen. *Am J Gastroenterol* 79:150-151, 1984.

Alen, M. Androgenic steroid effects on liver and red cells. *Brit J Sports Med* 19:15-20, 1985.

Alen, M., and Rahkila, P. Reduced high-density lipoprotein-cholesterol in power athletes: Use of male sex hormone derivates, an atherogenic factor. *Int J Sports Med* 5:341-342, 1984.

Alen, M.; Rahkila, P.; and Marniemi, J. Serum lipids in power athletes self-administering testosterone and anabolic steroids. *Int J Sports Med* 6:139-144, 1985.

Almaden, P.J., and Ross, S.W. Jaundice due to methyl testosterone therapy: *Case report. Ann Intern Med* 40:146-152, 1954.

Anderson, K.M., and Rossof, A.H. The influence of androgens on tumor development. In: Kellen, J.A., and Hilf, R., eds. influences of *Hormones in Tumor Development.* Vol II. Boca Raton, FL: CRC Press, Inc., 1979. 214 pp.

Anthony, P.P. Hepatoma associated with androgenic steroids. *Lancet* 1685-686, 1975.

Applebaum, D.M.; Goldberg, A.P.; Pykalisto, O.J.; Brunzell, J.D.; and Hazzard, W.R. Effect of estrogens on postheparin plasma lipolytic activity: Selective decline in hepatic triglyceride lipase. *J Clin Invest* 59:601-608, 1977.

Applebaum, D.M.; Haffner, S.; and Hazzard, W.R. The dyslipoproteinemia of anabolic steroid therapy: Increase in hepatic triglyceride lipase precedes the decrease in high density lipoprotein-2 cholesterol. *Metabolism* 36:949-952, 1987.

Bagheri, S.A., and Bayer, J.L. Peliosis hepatis associated with androgenic-anabolic steroid therapy-a severe form of hepatic injury. *Ann Intern Med* 81:610-618, 1974.

Bakker, K.; Brouwers, T.M.; Houthoff, H.J.; and Postma, A. Liver lesions resulting from the protracted use of anabolic steroids and oral contraceptives [Dutch]. *Ned Tijdschr Geneesk* 120:2214-2220, 1976. Dialog file 159, item CARC/77003800.

Barbosa, J.; Seal, U.S.; and Doe, R.P. Effects of anabolic steroids on haptoglobin, orosomucoid, plasminogen, fibrinogen, transferrin, ceruloplasmin, a1-antitrypsin, b-glucuronidase and total serum proteins. *J Clin Endocrinol* 33:388-398, 1971a.

Barbosa, J.; Seal, U.S.; and Doe, R.P. Effects of anabolic steroids on hormone-binding proteins, serum cortisol and serum nonprotein-bound cortisol. *J Clin Endocrinol* 32:232-240, 1971b.

Belgorosky, A., and Rivorola, M.A. Sex hormone binding globulin response to testosterone: An androgen sensitive test. *Acta Endocrinol* 109:130-138, 1985.

Bernstein, M.S.; Hunter, R.L.; and Yachnin, S. Hepatoma and peliosis hepatis developing in a patient with Fanconi's anemia. *N Engl J Med* 284:1135-1136, 1971.

Bird, D.; Vowles, K.; and Anthony, P.P. Spontaneous rupture of a liver cell adenoma after long term methyltestosterone: Report of a case successfully treated by emergency right hepatic lobectomy. *Br J Surg* 66:212-213, 1979.

Bonner, C.D., and Hornburger, F. Jaundice of the hepatocellular type during methyl testosterone therapy: Report of two cases. *Bull N Engl Med Center* 14:87-89, 1952.

Boyd, P.R., and Mark, G.J. Multiple hepatic adenomas and a hepatocellular carcinoma in a man on oral methyltestosterone for eleven years. *Cancer* 40:1765-1770, 1977.

Brick, I.B., and Kyle, L.H. Jaundice of hepatic origin during the course of methyl testosterone therapy. *N Engl J Med* 246:176-179, 1952.

Bruguera, M. Hepatoma associated with androgenic steroids. *Lancet* 1:1295, 1975.

Burger, R.A., and Marcuse, P.M. Peliosis hepatis: Report of a case. *Am J Clin Pathol* 22:569-573, 1952.

Burkett, L.N., and Falduto, M.T. Steroid use by athletes in a metropolitan area. *Phys Sportmed* 12:69-74, 1984.

Carrasco, D.; Pallardo, L.; Prieto, M.; Moll, J.L.; Cruz, J.M.; and Berenguer, J. Hepatic adenomata and androgen treatment. *Ann Intern Med* 100:316, 1984.

Carrasco, D.; Prieto, M.; Pallardo, L.; Moll, J.L.; Cruz, J.M.; Munoz, C.; and Berenguer, J. Multiple hepatic adenomas after long-term therapy with testosterone enanthate: Review of the literature. *J Hepatol* 1:573-578, 1985.

Catlin, D.H.; Kammerer, R.C.; Hatton, C.K.; Sekera, M.H.; and Merdink, J.L. Analytical chemistry at the games of the XXIIIrd Olympiad in Los Angeles, 1984. *Clin Chem* 33:319-327, 1987.

Cattan, D.; Kalifat, R.; Wautier, J.L.; Meignan, S.; Vesin, P.; and Piet, R. Fanconi's anemia and primary carcinoma of the liver [French]. *Arch Fr Mal App Dis* 63:141-48, 1974a.

Cattan, D.; Vesin, P.; Wautier, J.; Kalifat, P.; and Meighan, S. Liver tumors and steroid hormones. *Lancet* 1:878, 1974b.

Chandra, R.S.; Kapur, S.P.; Kelleher, J., Jr.; Luban, N.; and Patterson, K. Benign hepatocellular tumors in the young. A clinicopathologic spectrum. *Arch Pathol Lab Med* 108:168-171, 1984.

Chamy, C.W., and Gordon, J.A. Testosterone rebound therapy: A neglected modality. *Fertil Steril* 29:64-68, 1978.

Chetkowski, R.J.; Meldrum, D.R.; Steingold, K.A.; et al. Biologic effects of transdermal estradiol. *N Engl J Med* 314:1615-1620, 1986.

Chute, C.G.; Baron, J.A.; Plymate, S.R.; Kiel, D.P.; Pavia, A.T.; Lozner, E.C.; O'Keefe, T.; and MacDonald, G.J. Sex hormones and coronary artery disease. *Am J Med* 83:853-859, 1987.

Cicardi, M.; Bergamaschini, L.; Tucci, A.; Agostoni, A.; Tomaghi, G.; Coggi, G.; Colombi, R.; and Viale, G. Morphologic evaluation of the liver in hereditary angioedema patients on long-term treatment with androgen derivatives. *J Allergy Clin Immunol* 72:294-298, *1983.*

Cocks, J.R. Methyltestosterone-induced liver-cell tumours. *Med J Aust* 2:617-619, 1981.

Cohen, J.C.; Faber, W.M.; Benade, A.J.S.; and Noakes, T.D. Altered serum lipoprotein profiles in male and female power lifters ingesting anabolic steroids. *Phys S'rtsmed* 14:131-136, 1986.

Cohen, J.C., and Hickman, R. Insulin resistance and diminished glucose tolerance in powerlifters ingesting anabolic steroids. *J Clin Endocrinol Metab* 64:960-963, 1987.

Cohen, J.C.; Noakes, T.D.; and Benade, A.J.S. Hypercholesteremia in male power lifters using anabolic-androgenic steroids. *Phys Sportsmed* 16:49-56, 1988.

Cohen, W.D.; Higano, N.; Robinson, R.W.; and le Beau, R. Changes in serum lipids and urinary ketostetoids during oral and intramuscular administration of androsterone. *J Clin Endocrinol* 21:1208-1217, 1971.

Collaborative Group for the Study of Stroke in Young Women. Oral contraceptives and stroke in young women. *JAMA* 231:718, 1975.

Coombes, G.B.; Reiser, J.; Paradinas, F.J.; and Bum, I. An androgenic-associated hepatic adenoma in a transsexual. *Br J Surg* 65:869-870, 1977.

Coronary Drug Project Research Group. The coronary drug project: Findings leading to discontinuation of the 2.5-mg/day estrogen group. *JAMA* 226:652-657, 1973.

Costill, D.L.; Pearson, D.R.; and Fink, W.J. Anabolic steroid use among athletes: Changes in HDL-C levels. *Phys Sportsmed* 12:113-117, 1984.

Cowart, V. Steroids in sports: After four decades, time to return these genies to bottle? *JAMA* 257:421-427, 1987.

Creagh, T.M.; Rubin, A.; and Evans, D.J. Hepatic turnouts induced by anabolic steroids in an athlete. *J Clin Pathol* 41:441-443, 1988.

Crist, D.M.; Peake, G.T.; and Stackpole, P.J. Alphalipoproteinemic effects of androgenic-anabolic steroids in athletes. *Ann Sport Med* 2:125-128, 1985.

Crist, D.M.; Peake, G.T.; and Stackpole, P.J. Lipemic and lipoproteinemic effects of natural and synthetic androgens in humans. *Clin Exper Pharmacol Physiol* 13:513-518, 1986.

Daneshmend, T.K., and Bradfield, J.W.B. Hepatic angiosarcoma associated with androgenic-anabolic steroids. *Lancet* 2:1249, 1979.

Dimick, D.F.; Heron, M.; Baulieu, E.E.; and Jayle, M.F. A comparative study of the metabolic fate of testosterone, 17a-methyltestosterone, 19-nortestosterone, 17a-methyl-19-nor-testosterone and 17a-methyl-estr-5(10)-ene-17b-ol-3-one in normal males. *Clin Chim Acta* 6:63-71, 1961.

Drew, E.J. Androgen related primary hepatic carcinoma in a patient on long term methyltestosterone therapy. *J Abdom Surg* 26:103-106, 1984.

Dunning, M.F. Jaundice associated with norethandrolone (Nilevar) administration. *JAMA* 167:1242-1243, 1958.

Evely, R.S.; Triger, D.R.; Milnes, J.P.; Low-Beer, T.S.; and Williams, R. Severe cholestasis associated with stanozolol. *Br Med J* 294:612-513, 1987.

Falk, H.; Thomas, L.B.; Popper, H.; and Ishak, K.G. Hepatic angiosarcoma associated with androgenic-anabolic steroids. *Lancet* 2:1120-1123, 1979.

Farrell, G.C.; Joshua, D.E.; Uren, R.F.; Baird, P.J.; Perkins, K.W.; and Kronenberg, H. Androgen-induced hepatoma. *Lancet* 1:430-432, 1975.

Fearnley, G.R., and Chakrabarti, R. Increase of blood fibrinolytic activity by testosterone. *Lancet* 2:128-132, 1962.

Fearnley, G.R., and Chakrabarti, R. The pharmacological enhancement of blood fibrinolytic activity with special reference to phenformin. *Acta Cardiol* 19:1-13, 1964.

Feenstra, A.; Vaalburg, W.; Nolten, G.M.J.; Reiffers, S.; Talma, A.G.; Wiegman, T.; van der Molen, H.D.; and Woldring, M.G. Estrogen receptor binding radiopharmaceuticals: II. Tissue distribution of 17a-methyl-estradiol in normal and tumor bearing rats. *J Nucl Med* 24:522-528, 1983.

Foss, G.L., and Simpson, S.L. Oral methyltestosterone and jaundice. *Br Med J* 1:259-263, 1959.

Fouquette, B., and Lefebvre, R. Hepatic and splenic peliosis [French]. *Rev Franc Gastroenterol* 117:15-18 1976.

Frankle, M.A.; Cicero, G.J.; and Payne, J. Use of androgenic anabolic steroids by athletes. *JAMA* 252:482, 1984.

Frankle, M.A.; Eichberg, R.; and Zachariah, S.B. Anabolic androgenic steroids and a stroke in an athlete: *Case* report. *Arch Phys Med Rehabil* 69:532-633, 1988.

Freed, D.L.J.; Banks, A.J.; Longson, D.; and Burley, D.M. Anabolic steroids in athletics: Crossover double-blind trial on weightlifters. *Br Med J* 2:471-473, 1975.

Friedl K.E.; Hannan, C.J., Jr.; Jones, R.E.; Kettler, T.M.; and Plymate, S.R. Serum lipid and sex hormone binding globulin changes in men after administration of 17a-methyltestosterone, testosterone enanthate, and testosterone enanthate with testolactone. *Clin Res* 36:122A, 1988.

Friedl K.E.; Hannan, C.J., Jr.; Jones, R.E.; and Plymate, S.R. High-density lipoprotein cholesterol is not decreased if aromatized androgen is administered. *Metabolism* 39:69-74, 1990.

Friedl K.E.; Jones, R.E.; Hannan, C.J., Jr.; and Plymate, S.R. The administration of pharmacological doses of testosterone or 19-nortestosterone to normal men is not associated with increased insulin secretion or impaired glucose tolerance. *J Clin Endocrinol Metab* 68:971-975, 1989.

Friedl K.E., and Plymate, S.R. Parallel changes of HDL-cholesterol and testosterone-binding globulin in bodybuilders with self-administration of anabolic steroids. Unpublished manuscript, 1986.

Friedl, K.E.; Plymate, S.R.; Bernhard, W.N.; and Mohr, L.C. Elevation of plasma estradiol in healthy men during a mountaineering expedition. *Horm Metab Res* 20:239-242, 1988.

Friedl, K.E., and Yesalis, C.E. Self-treatment of gynecomastia in bodybuilders who use anabolic steroids. *Phys Sportsmed* 17:67-79, 1989.

Furman, R.H.; Howard, R.P.; Norcia, L.N.; and Keaty, E.C. The influence of androgens, estrogens and related steroids on serum lipids and lipoproteins: Observations in hypogonadal and normal human subjects. *Am J Med* 24:180-97, 1958.

Furman, R.H.; Howard, R.P.; Smith, C.W.; and Norcia, L.N. Comparative androgenicity of oral androgens, determined by steroid-induced decrements in high density (alpha) lipoproteins: Studies utilizing testosterone, methyltestosterone, 19-nortestosterone, 17-methyl nortestosterone and 17-ethyl nortestosterone. *Am J Med* 22:966, 1957.

Gil, V.G.; Lapuerta, J.B.; Garcia, J.P.; and Martin, M.R. A non-C17-alkylated steroid and long-term cholestasis. *Ann Intern Med* 104:135-136, 1986.

Gilbert, E.F.; DaSilva, A.Q.; and Queen, D.M. Intrahepatic cholestasis with fatal termination following norethandrolone therapy. *JAMA* 185:538-539, 1963.

Godsland, I.F.; Wynn, V.; Crook, D.; and Miller, N.E. Sex, plasma lipoproteins, and atherosclerosis: Prevailing assumptions and outstanding questions. *Am Heart J* 114:1467-1503, 1987.

Goldman, B. Liver carcinoma in an athlete taking anabolic steroids. *J Am Osteopath Assoc* 85:56, 1985.

Goodman, M.A., and Laden, A.M.J. Hepatocellular carcinoma in association with androgen therapy. *Med J Aust* 1:220-221, 1977.

Gordon, B.S.; Wolf, J.; Krause, T.; and Shai, F. Peliosis hepatis and cholestasis following administration of norethandrolone. *Am J Clin Pathol* 33:156-165, 1960.

Gordon, T.; Castelli, W.P.; Hjortland, M.C.; Kannel, W.B.; and Dawber, T.R. High density lipoproteins as a protective factor against coronary heart disease: The Framingham Study. *Am J Med* 62:707-714, 1977.

Groos, G.; Arnold, O.H.; and Brittinger, G. Peliosis hepatis after long-term administration of oxymethalone. *Lancet* 1:874, 1974.

Haffner, S.M.; Kushwaha, R.S.; Foster, D.M.; Applebaum-Bowden, D.; and Hazzard, W.R. Studies on the metabolic mechanism of reduced high density lipoproteins during anabolic steroid therapy. *Metabolism* 32:413-420, 1983.

Hamalainen, E. Hyperestrogenemia and increased risk of coronary heart disease in men-an unproved association? *Farmos Diagnostica Newsletters* 6:31-37, 1985.

Hamilton, J.B. The role of testicular secretions as indicated by the effects of castration in man and by studies of pathological conditions and the short lifespan associated with maleness. *Recent Prog Horm Res 3:257-322, 1948.*

Hatfield, F.C. *Bodybuilding: A Scientific Approach.* Chicago, IL: Contemporary Books, Inc., 1984. p. 212.

Hazzard, W.R.; Wahl, P.W.; Gagne, C.; Applebaum-Bowden, D,; Warnick, G.R.; and Albers, J.J. Plasma and lipoprotein lipid responses to four hypolipid drugs, *Lipids* 19:73-79, 1984.

Heller, R.F.; Miller, N.E.; Wheeler, M.J.; and Kind, P.R. Coronary heart disease in "low risk" men. *Atherosclerosis* 49:187-193, 1983.

Hemandez-Nieto, L.; Bruguera, M.; Bombi, J.A.; Camacho, L.; and Rozman, C. Benign liver-cell adenoma associated with long-term administration of an androgenic-anabolic steroid (methandienone). *Cancer* 40:1761-1764, 1977.

Hervey, G.R.; Hutchinson, I.; Knibbs, A.V.; Burkinshaw, L.; Jones, P.R.M.; Nolan, N.G.; and Levell, M.J. "Anabolic" effects of methandienone in men undergoing athletic training. *Lancet* 2:699-702, 1975.

Howard, R.P., and Furman, R.H. Estrogens, androgens, and serum lipids: The enigmatic triad of atherogenesis. *Ann Intern Med* 56:668, 1962.

Hurley, B.F.; Seals, D.R.; Hagberg, J.M.; Goldberg, A.C.; Ostrove, S.M.; Holloszy, J.O.; Wiest, W.G.; and Goldberg, A.P. High-density-lipoprotein cholesterol in bodybuilders v powerlifters: Negative effects of androgen use. *JAMA* 252:507-513, 1984.

Ingerowski, G.H.; Scheutwinkel-Reich, M.; and Stan, H.J. Mutagenicity studies on veterinary anabolic drugs with the salmonella/microsome test. *Mutat Res* 91:93-98, 1981.

Ishak, K.G. Hepatic neoplasms associated with contraceptive and anabolic steroids. *Recent Results Cancer Res* 66:73-128, 1979.

Johnson, F.L. Hepatoma associated with androgenic steroids. *Lancet* 1:1294-1295, 1975.

Johnson, F.L.; Lemer, K.G.; Siegel, M.; Faegler, J.R.; Majerus, P.W.; Hartmann, J.R.; and Thomas, E.D. Association of androgenic-anabolic steroid therapy with development of hepatocellular carcinoma. *Lancet* 2:1273-1276, 1972.

Joint Group for the Study of Aplastic and Refractory Anemias. Long-term follow-up of patients with medullary aplasia [French]. *Ann Med Interne* 132:530-534, 1981.

Jurgens, G., and Koltringer, P. Lipoprotein(a) in ischemic cerebrovascular disease: A new approach to the assessment of risk for stroke. *Neurology* 37:513-515, 1987.

Kalra, T.M.S.; Mangla, J.C.; and DePapp, E.W. Benign hepatic tumors and oral contraceptive pills. *Am J Med* 61:871-877, 1976.

Kantor, M.A.; Bianchini, A.; Bemier, D.; Sady, S.P.; and Thompson, P.D. Androgens reduce HDL2-cholesterol and increase hepatic triglyceride lipase activity. *Med Sci Sports Exerc* 17:462-465, 1985.

Kaplan, A.A. Jaundice due to methyltestosterone therapy. *Gastroenterol* 31:384-390, 1956.

Karasawa, T.; Shikata, T.; and Smith, R.D. Peliosis hepatis: Report of nine *cases. Acta Pathol Jpn* 29:457-469, 1979.

Kessler, E.; Bar-Meir, S.; and Pinkhas, J. Focal nodular hyperplasia and spontaneous hepatic rupture in aplastic anemia treated with oxymetholone [Hebrew]. *Hurefuah* 90:521-524, 1976. Dialog file 173, item 77141380.

Kew, M.C.; van Caller, B.; Prowse, C.M.; Skikne, B.; Wolfsdorf, J.I.; Isdale, J.; Krawitz, S.; Altman, H.; Levin, S.E.; and Bothwell, T.H. Occurrence of primary hepatocellular cancer and peliosis hepatis after treatment with androgenic steroids. *S Afr Med J* 50:1233-1237, 1976.

Kim, H.J., and Kalkhoff, R.K. Sex steroid influence on triglyceride metabolism. *J Clin Invest* 56:888-896, 1975.

Kintzen, W., and Silny, J. Peliosis hepatis after administration of fluoxymesterone. *Can Med Assoc J* 83:860-862, 1960.

Kiraly, C.L.; Alen, M.; Korvola, J.; and Horsmanheimo, M. The effect of testosterone and anabolic steroids on the skin surface lipids and the population of Propionibacteria acnes in young postpubertal men. *Acta Derm Venereol* 68:21-26, 1988.

Klatskin, G. Hepatic tumors: Possible relationship to use of oral contraceptives. *Gastroenterology* 73:386-394, 1977.

Kory, R.C.; Bradley, M.H.; Watson, R.N.; Callahan, R.; and Peters, B.J. A six-month evaluation of an anabolic drug, norethandrolone, in underweight persons: II. Brosulphalein (BSP) retention and liver function. *Am J Med* 26:243-248, 1959.

Koszalka, M.F. Medical obstructive jaundice: Report of death due to methyltestosterone. *Lancet* 77:51-54, 1957.

Kruskemper, H.L. *Anabolic Steroids. New York:* Academic Press, 1968. p. 176.

Lai, C.L.; Wu, PC.; Lam, K.C.; and Todd, D. Histologic prognostic indicators in hepatocellular carcinoma. *Cancer* 44:1677-1683, 1979.

Landon, J.; Wynn, V.; Cooke, J.N.C.; and Kennedy, A. Effects of anabolic steroid, methandienone, on carbohydrate metabolism in man. *Metabolism* 11:501-512, 1962.

Landon, J.; Wynn, V.; Houghton, B.J.; and Cooke, J.N.C. Effects of anabolic steroid, methandienone, on carbohydrate metabolism in man: II. Effect of methandienone on response to glucagon, adrenalin, and insulin in the fasted subject. *Metabolism* 11:513-523, 1962.

Landon, J.; Wynn, V.; and Samols, E. The effect of anabolic steroids on blood sugar and plasma insulin levels in man. *Metabolism* 12:924-935, 1963.

Lee, I.R.; Dawson, S.A.; Wetherall, J.D.; and Hahnel, R. Sex hormone-binding globulin secretion by human hepatocarcinoma cells is increased by both estrogens and androgens. *J Clin Endocrinol Metab* 64:825-831, 1987.

Lenders, J.W.M.; Demacker, P.N.M.; Vos, J.A.; Jansen, P.L.M.; Hoitsma, A.J.; van't Laar, A.; and Thien, T. Deleterious effects of anabolic steroids on serum lipoproteins, blood pressure, and liver function in amateur body builders. *Int J Sports Med* 9:19-23, 1988.

Lesna, M.; Spencer, I.; and Walker, W. Liver nodules and androgens. *Lancet* 1:1124, 1976.

Lesna, M., and Taylor, W. Liver lesions in BALB/C mice induced by an anabolic androgen (Decadurabolin), with and without pretreatment with diethylnitrosamine. *J Steroid Biochem* 24:449-453, 1986.

Lewis, J.L.; Irving, J.D.; Beswick, D.; and Mason, R.C. Successful management of an androgen-induced hepatic adenoma by embolisation of the hepatic artery. *J R Coll Surg Edinburgh* 31:315-316, 1986.

Lichtenstein, M.J.; Yarnell, J.W.G.; Elwood, P.C.; Beswick, A.D.; Sweetnam, P.M.; Marks, V.; Teale, D.; and Riad-Fahmy, D. Sex hormones, insulin, lipids, and prevalent ischemic heart disease. *Am J Epidemiol* 126:647-657, 1987.

Liddle, G.W., and Burke, H.A. Anabolic steroids in clinical medicine. *Helv Med Acta* 27:504-513, 1960.

Lloyd-Thomas, H.G.L., and Sherlock, S. Testosterone therapy for the pruritis of obstructive jaundice. *Br Med J* 2:1289, 1952.

Loomus, G.N.; Aneja, P.; and Bota, R.A. A case of peliosis hepatis in association with tamoxifen therapy. *Am J Clin Pathol* 80:881-883, 1983.

Lowdell, C.P., and Murray-Lyon, I.M. Reversal of liver damage due to long term methyltestosterone and safety of non-17a-alkylated androgens. *Br Med J* 291:637, 1985.

Lucey, M.R., and Moseley, R.H. Severe cholestasis associated with methyltestosterone: A case report. *Am J Gastroenterol* 82:461-462, 1987.

Lyon, J.; Bookstein, J.J.; Cartwright, C.A.; Romano, A.; and Heeney, D.J. Peliosis hepatis: Diagnosis by magnification wedged hepatic venography. *Radiology* 150:647-649, 1984.

Maciejko, J.J.; Holmes, D.R.; Kottke, B.A.; Zinsmeister, A.R.; Dinh, D.M.; and Mao, S.J.T. Apolipoprotein A-I as a marker of angiographically assessed coronary-artery disease. *N Engl J Med* 309:385-389, 1983.

Matsumoto, A.M. Is high dosage testosterone an effective male contraceptive agent? *Fertil Steril* 50:324-328, 1988.

Mauss, J.; Borsch, G.; Bormacher, K.; Richter, E.; Leyendecker, G.; and Nocke, W. Effect of long-term testosterone enanthate administration on male reproductive function: Clinical evaluation, serum FSH, LH, testosterone, and seminal fluid analyses in normal men. *Acta Endocrinol* 78:373-384, 1975.

McCaughan, G.W.; Bilous, M.J.; and Gallagher, N.D. Long-term survival with tumor regression in androgen-induced liver tumors. Cancer 56:2622-2626, 1985.

McKillop, G. Drug abuse in body builders in the West of Scotland. *Scott Med J* 32:39-41, 1987.

McKillop, G.; Todd, I.C.; and Ballantyne, D. Increased left ventricular mass in a bodybuilder using anabolic steroids. *Brit J Sports Med* 20:151-152, 1986.

McNutt, R.A.; Ferenchick, G.S.; Kirlin, P.C.; and Hamlin, N.J. Acute myocardial infarction in a 22-year-old world class weight lifter using anabolic steroids. *Am J Cardiol* 62:164, 1988.

Meadows, A.T.; Naiman, J.L.; and Valdes-Dapena, M. Hepatoma associated with androgen therapy for aplastic anemia. *J Pediatr* 84:109-110, 1974.

Miller, R.W. Athletes and steroids: Playing a deadly game. *FDA Cosum* 21:16-21, 1987.

Mochizuki, R.M., and Richter, K.J. Cardiomyopathy and cerebrovascular accident associated with anabolic-androgenic steroid use. *Phys Sportsmed* 16:109-114, 1988.

Nadell, J., and Kosek, J. Peliosis hepatis. Twelve cases associated with oral androgen therapy. *Arch Parhol Lab Med* 101:405-410, 1977.

Nagelberg, S.B.; Laue, L.; Loriaux, D.L.; Liu, L.; and Sherins, R.J. Cerebrovascular accident associated with testosterone therapy in a 21-year-old hypogonadal man. *N Engl J Med* 314:649-650, 1986.

Neff, M.S.; Goldberg, J.; Slifkin, R.F.; Eiser, A.R.; Calamia, V.; Kaplan, M.; Baez, A.; Gupta, S.; and Mattoo, N. A comparison of androgens for anemia in patients on hemodialysis. *N Engl J Med* 304:871-875, 1981.

Nessim, S.A.; Chin, H.P.; Alaupovic, P.; and Blankenhom, D.N. Combined therapy of niacin, colestipol, and fat-controlled diet in men with coronary bypass: Effect on blood lipids and apolipoproteins. *Arteriosclerosis* 3:568-573, 1983.

Nieschlag, E. Current status of testosterone substitution therapy. *Int J Andrology* 5:225-228, 1982.

Nordoy, A.; Aakvaag, A.; and Thelle, D. Sex hormones and high density lipoproteins in healthy males. *Atherosclerosis* 34:431-436, 1979.

Nuzzo, J.L.J.; Manz, H.J.; and Maxted, W.C. Peliosis hepatis after long-term androgen therapy. *Urology* 25:518-519, 1985.

Ogg, C.S., and Cattell, W. Clinicopathological conference: A patient's life. *Br Med J* 3:209-213, 1975.

Oliver, M.F., and Boyd, G.S. The influence of the sex hormones on the circulating lipids and lipoproteins in coronary sclerosis. *Circulation* 13:82-91, 1956.

Overly, W.L.; Dankoff, J.A.; Wang, B.K.; and Singh, U.D. Androgens and hepatocellular carcinoma in an athlete. *Ann Intern Med* 100:158-159, 1984.

Palacios, A.; McClure, R.D.; Campfield, A.; and Swerdloff, R.S. Effect of testosterone enanthate on testis size. *J Urol* 126:46-48, 1981.

Paradinas, F.J.; Bull, T.B.; Westaby, D.; and Murray-Lyon, I.M. Hyperplasia and prolapse of hepatocytes into hepatic veins during longterm methyltestosterone therapy: Possible relationships of these changes to the development of peliosis hepatis and liver tumors. *Histopathology* 1:225-226, 1977.

Pecking, A.; Lejolly, J.M.; and Najean, Y. Hepatic toxicity of androgen therapy in aplastic anemia. *Nouv Rev Fr Hematol* 22:257-265, 1980.

Pelletier, G.; Frija, J.; Szekely, A.M.; and Clauvel, J.P. Adenoma of the liver in man [French]. *Gastroenterol Clin Biol* 8:269-272, 1984.

Petera, V.; Bobek, K.; and Lahn, V. Serum transaminase (GOT,GPT) and lactic dehydrogenase activity during treatment with methyl testosterone. *Clin Chim Acta* 7:604-606, 1962.

Peters, J.H.; Randall, A.H.; Mendeloff, J.; Peace, R.; Coberly, J.C.; and Hurley, M.B. Jaundice during administration of methylestrenolone. *J Clin Endocrinol Metab* 18:114-115. 1958.

Peters, R.L. Pathology of hepatocellular carcinoma. In: Okuda, K., and Peters, R.L., eds. *Hepatocellular Carcinoma*. New York: John Wiley & Sons, 1976. pp. 107-168.

Peterson, G.E., and Fahey, T.D. HDL-C in five elite athletes using anabolic-androgenic steroids. *Phys Sportsmed* 12:120-130, 1984.

Phillips, M.J.; Oda, M.; and Funatsu, K. Evidence for microfilament involvement in norethandrolone-induced intrahepatic cholestasis. *Am J Pathol* 93:729-744, 1978.

Plymate, S.R.; Vaughan, G.M.; Mason, A.D.; and Pruitt, B.A. Central hypogonadism in burned men. *Horm Res* 27:152-158, 1987.

Port, R.B.; Petasnick, J.P.; and Ranniger, K. Angiogtaphic demonstration of hepatoma in association with Fanconi's anemia. *Am J Roentgenol Radium Ther Nucl Med* 113:82-83, 1971.

Prat, J.; Gray, G.F.; Stolley, P.D.; and Coleman, J.W. Wilms tumor in an adult associated with androgen abuse. *JAMA* 237:2322-2323, 1977.

Rastad, J.; Joborn, H.; Ljunghall, S.; and Akerstrom, G. Gluteal infection in weight lifters after injection of anabolic steroids [Swedish]. *Lakartidningen* 82:3407, 1985. Dialog file 155, item 8639139.

Reese, C.C.; Warshaw, M.L.; Murai, J.T.; and Siiteri, P.K. Alternative models for estrogen and androgen regulation of human breast cancer cell (T47D) growth. *Ann NY Acad Sci* 538:112-121, 1988.

Reyes, H.; Ribalta, J.; Gonzales, C.; Segovia, N.; and Oberhauser, E. Sulfobromophthalein clearance tests before and after ethinyl estradiol administration in women and men with a familial history of intrahepatic cholestasis of pregnancy. *Gastroenterology* 81:226-231, 1981.

Roberts, J.T., and Essenhigh, D.M. Adenocarcinoma of prostate in 40-year-old body-builder. *Lancet* 2:742, 1986.

Rowley, M.J., and Heller, C.G. The testosterone rebound phenomenon in the treatment of male infertility. *Fertil Steril* 23:498-504, 1972.

Ruokonen, A.; Alen, M.; Bolton, N.; and Vihko, R. Response of serum testosterone and its precursor steroids, SHBG and CBG to anabolic steroid and testosterone self-administration in man. *J Steroid Biochem* 23:33-38, 1985.

Russ, E.M.; Eder, H.A.; and Barr, D.P. Influence of gonadal hormones on protein-lipid relationship in human plasma. *Am J Med* 194-24, 1955.

Ryan, K.J. Biogenesis of estrogens. In: Sissakian, N.M., *ed. Proceedings of the 5th International Congress of Biochemistry (Moscow, 1961).* Vol. 7. New York: Pergamon Press, 1963. pp. 381-394.

Saartok, T.; Dahlberg, E.; and Gustafsson, J.A. Relative binding affinity of anabolic-androgenic steroids: Comparison of the binding to the androgen receptors in skeletal muscle and in prostate, as well as to sex hormone-binding globulin. *Endocrinol* 114:2100-2106, 1984.

Sachs, B.A., and Wolfman, L. Effect of oxandrolone *on* plasma lipids and lipoproteins of patients with disorders of lipid metabolism. *Metabolism* 17:400-410, 1968:

Saheb, F. Absence of peliosis hepatis in patients receiving testosterone enanthate. *Hepato-Gastroenterol* 27:432-434, 1980.

Sale, G.E., and Lerner, K.G. Multiple tumors after androgen therapy. *Arch Pathol Lab Med* 101:600-603, 1977.

Schaffner, F.; Popper, H.; and Chesrow, E. Cholestasis produced by the administration of norethandrolone. *Am J Med* 26:249-254, 1959.

Schaison, G.; Leverger, G.; and Yildez, C. Fanconi's anemia: Frequency of leukemic transformation [French]. *Presse Med* 12:1269-1274, 1983.

Schriewer, H.; Assmann, G.; Sandkamp, M.; and Schulte, H. The relationship of lipoprotein(a) (Lp(a)) to risk factors of coronary heart disease: Initial results of the prospective epidemiological study on company employees in Westfalia. *J Clin Chem Clin Biochem* 22:591-596, 1984.

Scully, R.E.; Mark, E.J.; and McNeely, B.U. Weekly clinicopathological exercises: Case 32-1981. *N Engl J Med* 305:331-336, 1981.

Shaw, R.K., and Gold, G.L. Jaundice associated with norethandrolone (Nilevar) therapy. *Ann Intern Med* 52:428-434, 1960.

Shuttleworth, D.; Weavind, G.P.; and Graham-Brown, R.A. Acanthosis nigricans and diabetes mellitus in a patient with Klinefelter's syndrome: A reaction to methyltestosterone. *Clin Exp Dermatol* 12:288-290, 1987.

Sklarek, H.M.; Mantovani, R.P.; Erens, E.; Heisler, D.; Niederman, M.S.; and Fein, A.M. AIDS in a bodybuilder using anabolic steroids. *N Engl J Med* 311:1701, 1984.

Slater D.; Parsons, A.; Platts, M.; and Fox, M. Peliosis in renal failure treated with androgens. *N Engl J Med* 305:345, 1981.

Stalder, M.; Pometta, D.; and Suenram, A. Relationship between plasma insulin levels and high density lipoprotein cholesterol levels in healthy men. *Diabetologia* 21:544-548, 1981.

Steinhetz, P.G.; Canale, V.C.; and Miller, D.R. Hepatocellular carcinoma, transfusion-induced hemochromatosis and congenital hypoplastic anemia (Blackfan-Diamond Syndrome). *Am J Med* 60:1032-1035, 1976.

Stone, M.C. Idiopathic hyperglyceridemia treated with methyl testosterone and methandienone. *Lancet* 1:477-478, 1963.

Strauss, J.S., and Pochi, P.E. III. Hormones and cellular metabolism: The human sebaceous gland: Its regulation by steroidal hormones and its use as an end organ for assaying androgenicity in vivo. *Recent Prog Horm Res* 19:385-444, 1963.

Strauss, R.H.; Wright, J.E.; Finerman, G.A.M.; and Catlin, D.H. Side effects of anabolic steroids in weight-trained men. *Phys Sportsmed* 11:87-%, 1983.

Stromeyer, F.W.; Smith, D.H.; and Ishak, K.G. Anabolic steroid therapy and intrahepatic cholangiocarcinoma. *Cancer* 43:440-443, 1979.

Sugiyama, T.; Akahonai, Y.; Arashi, M.; Hirane, T.; Yachi, A.; Satoh, M.; and Ogawa, K. An autopsy case of hepatocellular adenoma and peliosis hepatis considered to be induced by anabolic steroid therapy for aplastic anemia [Japanese]. *Acta Heparol Jpn* 23:927-933, 1982.

Svanborg, A., and Ohlsson, S. Recurrent jaundice of pregnancy: A clinical study of twenty-two cases. *Am J Med* 27:40-49, 1959.

Sweeney, E.C., and Evans, D.J. Liver lesions and androgenic steroid therapy. *Lancet* 2:1042, 1975.

Sweeney, E.C., and Evans, D.J. Hepatic lesions in patients treated with synthetic anabolic steriods. *J Clin Pathol* 29:626-623, 1976.

Swerdloff, R.S.; Palacios, A.; McClure, R.D.; Campfield, L.A.; and Brosman, S.A. Male contraception: Clinical assessment of chronic administration of testosterone enanthate. *Int J Androl* (suppl) 2:731-47, 1978.

Tam, S.P.; Archer, T.K.; and Deeley, R.G. Biphasic effects of estrogen on apolipoprotein synthesis in human hepatoma cells: Mechanism of antagonism by testosterone. *Proc Natl Acad Sci USA* 83:3111-3115, 1986.

Taxy, J.B. Peliosis: A morphologic curiosity becomes an iatrogenic problem. *Hum Pathol* 9:331-340, 1978.

Thompson, P.D.; Culinane, E.M.; Sady, S.P.; Chenevert, C.; Saritelli, A.L.; Sady, M.A.; and Herbert, P.N. Contrasting effects of testosterone and stanozolol on serum lipoprotein levels. *JAMA* 261:1165-1168, 1989.

Tikkanen, M.J.; Nikkila, E.A.; Kussi, T.; and Sipinen, S. High density lipoprotein-2 and hepatic lipase: Reciprocal changes produced by estrogen and norgestrel. *J Clin Endocrinol Metab* 54:1113-1117, 1982.

Treuner, J.; Niethammer, D.; Flach, A.; Fischbach, H.; and Schenck, W. Hepatocellular carcinoma after oxymetholone treatment [German]. *Med Welt* 31:952-955, 1980.

Turani, H.; Levi, J.; Zevin, D.; and Kessler, E. Hepatic lesions in patients on anabolic androgenic therapy. *Isr J Med Sci* 19:332-337, 1983.

USA Today. Special report: Getting strong, getting hurt: The steroids controversy. January 23, 1987. p. 6C.

Vesselinovitch, S.D., and Mihailovich, N. The effect of gonadectomy on the development of hepatomas induced by urethane. *Cancer Res* 27:1788-1791, 1967.

Vessey, M.; Doll, R.; Peto, R.; Johnson, B.; and Wiggins, P. A long-term follow-up study of women using different methods of contraception-an interim report. *J Biosoc Sci* 8:373-427, 1976.

Wade, N. Anabolic steroids: Doctors denounce them, but athletes aren't listening. *Science* 176:1399-1403, 1972.

Wakabayashi, T.; Onda, H.; Tada, T.; Iijima, M.; and Itoh, Y. High incidence of peliosis hepatis in autopsy cases of aplastic anemia with special reference to anabolic steroid therapy. *Acta Pathol Jpn* 34:1079-1086, 1984.

Webb, O.L.; Laskarzewski, P.M.; and Glueck, C.J. Severe depression of high-density lipoprotein cholesterol levels in weight lifters and body builders by self-administered exogenous testosterone and anabolic-androgenic steroids. *Metabolism* 33:971-975, 1984.

Werner, S.C. Clinical syndromes associated with gonadal failure in men. *Am J Med* 3:52-66, 1947.

Werner, S.C.; Hanger, F.M.; and Kritzler, R. Jaundice during methyl testosterone therapy. *Am J Med* 8:325-331, 1950.

Westaby, D.; Ogle, S.J.; Paradinas, F.J.; Randell, J.B.; and Murray-Lyon, I.M. Liver damage from long-term methyltestosterone. *Lancet* 1(8032):261-263, 1977.

Westaby, D.; Portmann, B.; and Williams, R. Androgen related primary hepatic tumors in non-Fanconi patients. *Cancer* 51:1947-1952, 1983.

Wood, J.C. Jaundice due to methyltestosterone therapy. *JAMA* 150:1484-1486, 1952.

Woodard, T.L.; Burghen, G.A.; Kitabchi, A.E.; and Wihmas, J.A. Glucose intolerance and insulin resistance in aplastic anemia treated with oxymetholone. *J Clin Endocrinol Metab* 53:905-908, 1981.

Wynn, V.; Landon, J.; and Kawerau, E. Studies on hepatic function during methandienone therapy. *Lancet* 169-75, 1961.

Yesalis, C.E.; Herrick, R.T.; Buckley, W.E.; Friedl, K.E.; Brannon, D.; and Wright, J.E. Self-reported use of anabolic-androgenic steroids by elite power lifters. *Phys Sportsmed* 16:91-100, 1988.

Zak, F. Peliosis hepatis. *Am J Pathol* 26:1-15, 1950.

Zevin, D.; Turani, H.; Cohen, A.; and Levi, J. Androgen-associated hepatoma in a hemodialysis patient. *Nephron* 29:274-276, 1981.

Ziegenfuss, J., and Carabasi, R. Androgens and hepatocellular carcinoma. *Lancer* 1:262, 1973.

AUTHOR

Karl E. Friedl, Ph.D.
Captain, Medical Service Corps
Exercise Physiology Division
U.S. Army Research Institute of Environmental Medicine
Natick, MA 01760-5007

Androgen Interaction Through Multiple Steroid Receptors

Olli A. Jänne

INTRODUCTION

Under normal physiological conditions, different classes of steroid hormones initiate distinct actions via binding to their cognate receptor proteins. The specificity of the ensuing biological response relies on several characteristics inherent to the steroid-receptor interaction. First, the steroid-binding specificity of all steroid receptors is relatively strict in that these proteins associate with their cognate physiological steroids with affinities that are usually at least one order of magnitude higher than those for other classes of steroids (Ojasoo and Raynaud 1978). Second, the binding affinity of a given receptor is commensurate with the concentration of its physiological ligand such that the circulating steroid levels are generally close to those required for the half-maximal saturation of the receptor's binding site (Jänne et al. 1978b). Third, steroid metabolism that occurs under physiological conditions does not generate metabolites that are biologically more potent than the parent compound, in cases other than the conversion of testosterone to 5α-dihydrotestcsterone. Finally, the concentration of a receptor within a given target cell is in line with its hormonal responsiveness; the formation of biologically active receptor-steroid complexes is dictated by the law of mass action, a low receptor content permits formation of functionally insufficient amounts of receptor-steroid complexes under physiological ligand concentrations (Jänne and Bardin 1984).

Two main reasons account for deviations from this strict specificity in steroid action: first, a change from a physiological to a pharmacological ligand concentration and, second, modulation of the structure of the steroid in question. In the case of male sex steroids, both natural and synthetic androgens can potentially interact with several separate receptor systems, including those for androgens, estrogens, progestins, and glucocorticoids. In most instances, the interaction of androgens with receptors other than the androgen receptor leads to the expression of the biological action characteristic of the receptor rather than of the androgen; however, this interaction

178

sometimes results in the inhibition of the receptor's function (Samuels and Tomkins 1970). To illustrate some of these observations, results on the interaction of androgens with the uterine progesterone receptors are first reviewed in this chapter.

BINDING OF ANDROGENS TO THE PROGESTERONE RECEPTOR

Table 1 summarizes the relative binding affinities of physiological and synthetic androgens to human and rabbit progestin receptors (Jänne et al. 1978a). All androgens tested, including testosterone and 5α-dihydrotestosterone, competed with progesterone for binding to its receptor. In general, 19-nortestosterone derivatives appear to bind to the progestin receptor better than derivatives of testosterone do (table 1). Two of the androgens, 17α-ethyl-19-nortestosterone and 7α, 17α-dimethyl-19-nortestosterone (figure 1), bound to the progestin receptor with affinities similar to or higher than that of the cognate ligand progesterone. Many of the compounds listed in table 1 have been shown in different bioassays to be more potent androgens than testosterone or 5α-dihydrotestosterone; in addition, several of them (figure 1) are commonly abused by athletes (Wilson 1988). These and other studies (Kontula et al. 1975; Ojasoo and Raynaud 1978) have indicated that most of the structural modifications in the androgens that render them biologically more active (addition of double bonds or hydrophobic substituents, removal of the 19-methyl group) are very similar to the modifications of the progestational molecules required for their improved receptor-binding affinity and biological potency.

TABLE 1. *Relative binding activity of physiological and synthetic androgens to the cytosolic progesterone receptors from human and rabbit uteri*

| Steroid | Relative Binding Affinity* | |
	Human Receptor	Rabbit Receptor
Progesterone	100.0	100.0
Testosterone	1.6	1.6
5α-Dihydrotestosterone	3.3	3.3
19-Nortestosterone	8.9	11.8
6α-Methyl-19-nortestosterone	15.5	19.6
17α-Methyltestosterone	4.6	3.4
17α-Ethyl-19-nortestosterone	130.0	70.1
$7\beta,17\alpha$-Dimethyltestosterone	8.6	6.4
$7\alpha,17\alpha$-Dimethyl-19-nortestosterone	148.0	176.0

*The relative binding affinity was determined according to Kontula et al. (1975).

SOURCE Based on data in Jänne et al. 1978a.

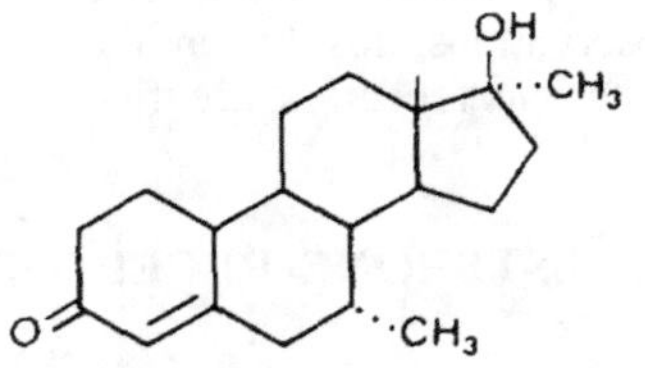

$7\alpha,17\alpha$-Dimethyl-19-nortestosterone (mibolerone)

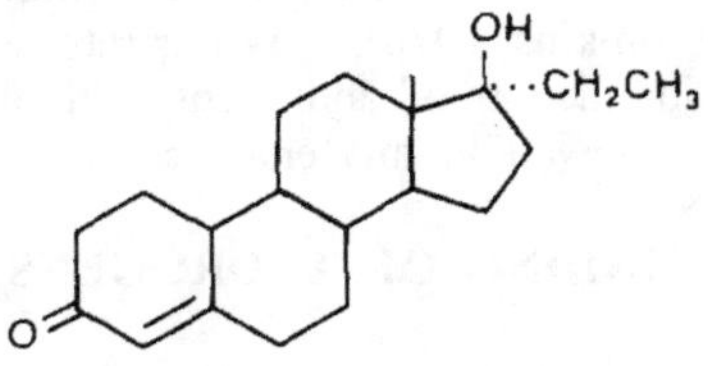

17α-Ethyl-19-nortestosterone (norethandrolone)

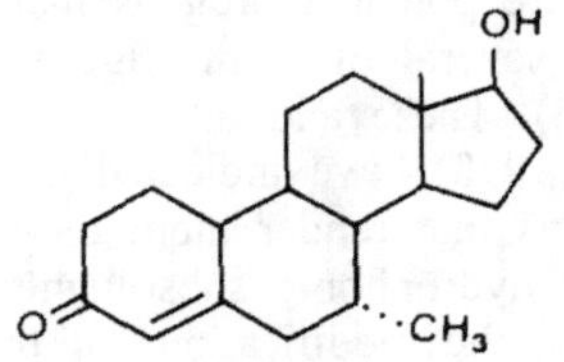

7α-Methyl-19-nortestosterone

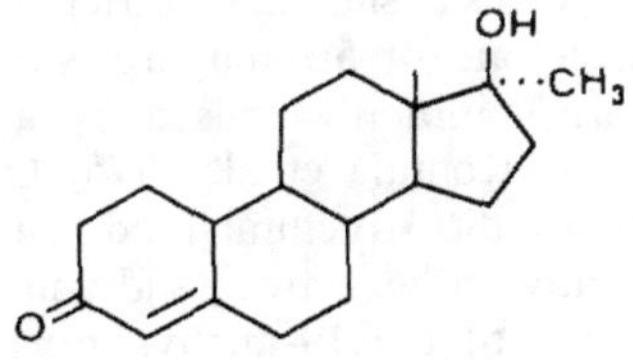

17α-Methyl-19-nortestosterone

FIGURE 1. *Structures of some synthetic androgens known to elicit biological responses via multiple steroid receptors*

PROGESTATIONAL ACTIVITY OF ANDROGENS

To determine whether the binding of androgens to cytosolic progestin receptor had biological consequences, the ability of these proteins to induce uteroglobin, a progesterone-regulated protein in rabbit uterus, was studied (Jänne et al. 1983; Kopu 1981). As illustrated in figure 2, all the androgens induce uteroglobin secretion *in vivo* when administered to rabbits, and the extent of this induction is in good agreement with their ability to interact *in vitro* with the rabbit and human progesterone receptors (table 1). It is of particular note that even the two physiological androgens, testosterone and 5α-dihydrotestosterone, elicit a significant increase in uteroglobin secretion (Jänne et al. 1978a). This response is 1 percent to 3 percent of that brought about by progesterone, when the response is calculated on the molar basis of the steroid administered and, therefore, commensurate with the binding affinity of these androgens to the uterine progestin receptor. Additional studies showed that testosterone and progesterone had similar

180

slopes in their dose-response curves (Jänne et al. 1978a), suggesting that their actions are mediated by a common mechanism.

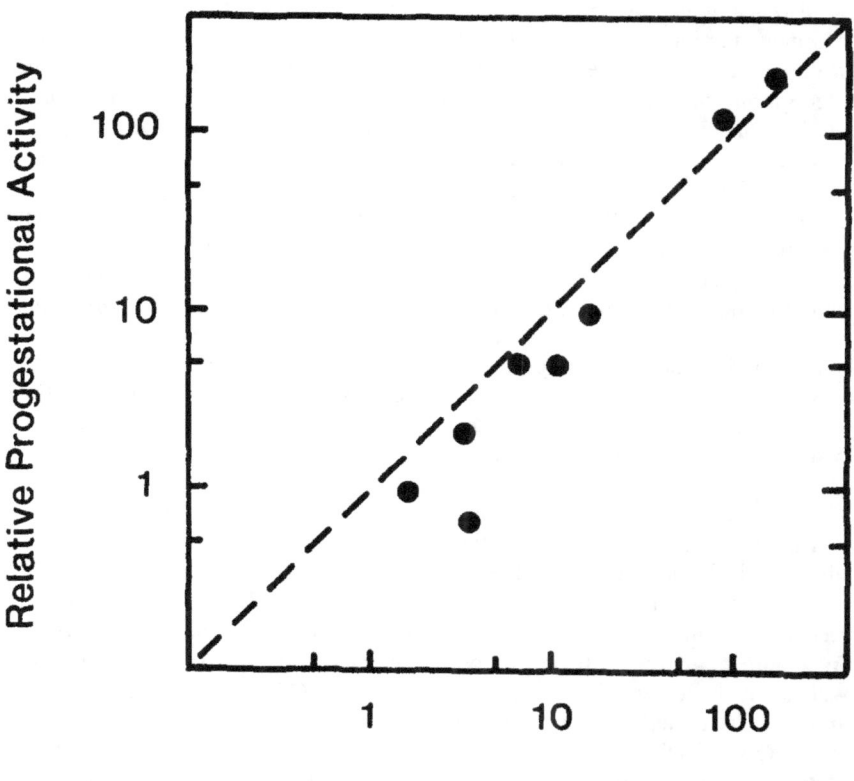

FIGURE 2. *Comparison of the relative progestin receptor-binding activity in vitro to the progestational activity (induction of uteroglobin secretion) in vivo of various androgens*

NOTE: The values are expressed relative to progesterone, which was set at 100 in each case. The dashed line shows the situation when x=y.

SOURCE: Adapted from Jänne et al. 1978a.

Although the above data strongly suggested that uterine androgen and estrogen receptors were not involved in the androgenic regulation of uteroglobin gene expression, additional studies were carried out to substantiate this postulate. In particular, it was important to rule out the participation of the estrogen receptor, since physiological androgens at pharmacological doses are known to interact with this receptor protein (Zava and McGuire 1978; McGuire 1978; Rochefort and Garcia 1979), and since uteroglobin secretion is also stimulated by estradiol to some extent (Jänne et al. 1983). Concomitant administration of antiandrogens such as flutamide or RU 23908 with natural and synthetic androgens was unable to inhibit androgen-induced uteroglobin secretion or accumulation of progesterone receptors in rabbit uterine nuclei (Jänne et al. 1978a; Jänne et al. 1983; Kopu 1981). These data make it very unlikely that androgen receptors are involved, as these nonsteroidal antiandrogens specifically prevent androgen-receptor-mediated events (Liao et al. 1974; Raynaud et al. 1979; Kontula et al. 1985). Simultaneous administration of 5α-dihydrotestosterone and estradiol to rabbits resulted in an estrogen dose-dependent inhibition of uteroglobin secretion and accumulation of uteroglobin mRNA in uterine cells (Kopu 1981; Jänne et al. 1983). This effect was very similar to that observed during a combined administration of progesterone with estradiol (Hemminki et al. 1980) and strongly suggests that androgens and progesterone mediate their actions via the same effector molecule, the progesterone receptor, the function of which is prevented by high doses of estradiol.

The results from these studies illustrate that androgens can modulate endometrial functions through interacting with the uterine progesterone receptor. Physiological androgens are able to do so only when administered at pharmacological doses, as the affinity of these steroids for the progestin receptor is almost two orders of magnitude lower than that of progesterone. By contrast, many synthetic androgens interact with the progestin receptor with a much higher affinity, and some of them (17α-ethyl-l9-nortestosterone and $7\alpha,17\alpha$-dimethyl-19-nortestosterone) can be biologically as potent as progesterone itself. It is of particular note that the rabbit and human progesterone receptors have almost identical steroid-binding specificities (Smith et al. 1974; Kontula et al. 1975; Jänne et al. 1978b); consequently, physiological and synthetic androgens are expected to interfere with the human progesterone-receptor-mediated functions in a manner similar to rabbit uteroglobin gene expression. This interaction does not have to be limited to the uterine tissue, but androgens are expected to interfere with human hypothalamic and pituitary progestin receptors and thus influence gonadotropin release. In this context, it is worth noting that progesterone receptors in different experimental animals have dissimilar ligand-binding specificities (Jänne et al. 1978b), and, therefore, some synthetic androgens may not be able to interact with progestin receptors in all species. This appears to be particularly true for steroids carrying substituents in the D-ring.

INTERACTION OF ANDROGENS WITH ESTROGEN AND GLUCOCORTICOID RECEPTORS

Pharmacological doses of androgens have been shown to elicit hypertrophy with morphological changes similar to those brought about by estrogens in immature rat uterus (Lerner et al. 1966). These experiments utilized aromatizable androgens; therefore, the possibility that the estrogenlike effects of androgens were due to conversion of androgens to estrogens could not be ruled out. The fact that large pharmacological doses of androgens are required for the uterotrophic response to occur suggests that this effect is not mediated by the androgen receptor. By using pharmacological doses of a nonaromatizable androgen, 5α-dihydrotestosterone, Rochefort and Garcia (1979) showed that stimulation of estrogen-specific responses, such as increased protein synthesis and stimulation of the estrogen-induced protein, occurred in immature rat uteri. These responses correlated well with the amount of estrogen receptor translocated to uterine nuclei following 5α-dihydrotestosterone administration. Another estrogen-regulated event, the synthesis of progestrone receptor, has also been shown to be stimulated by pharmacological concentrations of 5α-dihydrotestosterone in cultured human breast cancer cells (Zava and McGuire 1978). Since the above effects are specifically inhibited by concomitant administration of antiestrogens, it is very likely that they result from the interaction of androgens with the estrogen receptor. However, it is not known whether it is 5α-dihydrotestosterone or its reduced metabolites (androstanediols) that bind to the estrogen receptor, since the reduced metabolites have been shown to have higher binding affinity for the estrogen receptor than the parent compound (Poortman et al. 1977).

The estrogenic activity of synthetic androgens appears to be similar to that of the natural androgens (Ojasoo and Raynaud 1978) in that estrogenic effects may be observed only after administration of large doses of these steroids. In view of the above results, it is evident that administration of androgens (natural and synthetic) at very high doses can lead to estrogenic responses in estrogen target tissues. However, aromatization of testosterone derivatives to estrogens and the resulting increase in the circulating estradiol concentrations may be by far more important for the development of feminizing side effects observed during androgen abuse (Wilson 1988).

Physiological and synthetic androgens interact with the glucocorticoid receptor with affinities far below those of natural or synthetic glucocorticoids (Samuels and Tomkins 1970; Rousseau and Schmit 1977; Ojasoo and Raynaud 1978). At pharmacological steroid concentrations, this interaction has significant biological consequences in that potent androgens such as testosterone and 17α-methyltestosterone are antiglucocorticoids (Samuels and Tomkins 1970). In accordance with studies performed using cultured cells, Mayer and Rosen (1975) found that pharmacological doses of androgens act *in vivo* in rat muscle cells to block the catabolic effects of glucocorticoids.

183

Although the detailed mechanisms for this antiglucocorticoid action of androgens are not fully understood, recent studies have indicated that 17α-methyltestosterone competes with glucocorticoids for binding to the 10S cytosolic receptor but does not promote dissociation of the oligomer, and thus inhibits agonist-mediated nuclear actions of the glucocorticoid receptor protein (Raaka et al. 1989).

CONCLUSION

A large body of evidence indicates that all of the potent naturally occurring steroids of each class have relatively short half-lives in blood, have diminished biological activity after 'oral administration, and are inactivated in the enterohepatic circulation. To produce steroids that are orally active and that could be infrequently administered has required modifications of naturally occurring steroid structures. While these alterations have retained the desired biological activity, they have also enhanced the ability of synthetic steroids to interact with multiple receptors and thus exert more than one biological activity, especially when the synthetic steroids are taken at high doses. These phenomena are particularly well illustrated by the spectrum of biological actions exhibited by synthetic androgens. The examples presented in this chapter, androgen action via multiple receptors, describe the phenomenon of hormone action via the "wrong" receptor. It should be reiterated, however, that these effects are observed only with large doses of hormone and occur only very seldom, when the amount of androgen administered is just sufficient to stimulate the male reproductive tract. As a consequence, administration of naturally occurring or synthetic androgens at doses 10 to 100 times higher than those used in treatment of hypogonadal patients, as is the case in self-administration of androgens by athletes (Wilson 1988), will certainly produce biological effects that are not observed at physiological dose levels.

REFERENCES

Hemminki, S.M.; Kopu, H.T.; Torkkeli, T.K.; and Jänne, O.A. Further studies on the role of estradiol in the induction of progesterone-regulated uteroglobin synthesis in the rabbit uterus. *Mol Cell Endocrinol* 17:71-80, 1980.

Jänne, O.A., and Bardin, C.W. Androgen and antiandrogen receptor binding. *Annu Rev Physiol* 46:107-118, 1984.

Jänne, O.; Hemminik, S.; Isomaa, V.; Kokko, E.; Torkkeli, H.; Torkkeli, T.; and Vierikko, P. Progestational activity of natural and synthetic androgens. *Int J Androl* (Suppl) 2:162-174, 1978a.

Jänne, O.; Kontula, K.; Vihko, R.; Feil, P.D.; and Bardin, C.W. Progesterone receptors and regulation of progestin action in mammalian tissues. *Med Biol* 56:225-248. 1978b.

Kontula, K.; Jänne, O.; Vihko, R.; de Jager, E.; de Visser, J.; and Zeelen, F. Progesterone-binding proteins: In vitro binding and biological activity of different steroidal ligands. *Acta Endrocrinol* 78:574-592, 1975.

Kontula, K.K.; Seppänen, P.J.; Van Duyne, P.; Bardin, C.W.; and Jänne, O.A. Effect of a nonsteroidal antiandrogen, flutamide, on androgen receptor dynamics and omithine decarboxylase gene expression in mouse kidney. *Endocrinology* 116:226-233, 1985.

Kopu, H. 5α-Dihydrotestosterone-induced uteroglobin synthesis in rabbit uterus is not inhibited by antiandrogen administration but is prevented by estradiol. *Biochim Biophys Acta* 654:293-296, 1981.

Lemer, L.J.; Hilf, R.; Turkeimer, A.R.; Michel, I.; and Engel, S.L. Effects of hormone antagonists on morphological and biochemical changes induced by hormonal steroids in the immature rat uterus. *Endocrinology* 78:111-124, 1966.

Liao, S.; Howell, D.K.; and Chang, T.M. Action of a non-steroidal anti-androgen, flutamide, on the receptor binding and nuclear retention of 5α-dihydrotestosterone in rat ventral prostate. *Endocrinology* 94:532-540, 1974.

Mayer, M., and Rosen, F. Interaction of anabolic steroids with gluco-corticoid receptor sites in rat muscle cytosol. *Am J Physiol* 229:1381-1386, 1975.

Ojasoo, T., and Raynaud, J.-P. Unique steroid congeners for receptor studies. *Cancer Res* 38:4186-4198, 1978.

Poortman, J.; Vroegindewey-Jie, D.; Thijssen, J.H.H.; and Schwarz, F. Relative binding affinity of androstane and C-19-norandrostane steroids for the estradiol-receptor in human myometrial and mammary cancer tissue. *Mol Cell Endocrinol* 8:27-34, 1977.

Raaka, B.M.; Finnerty, M.; and Samuels H.H. The glucocorticoid antagon-ist 17α-methyltestosterone binds to the 10S glucocorticoid receptor and blocks agonist-mediated dissociation of the 10S oligomer to the 4S deoxy-ribonucleic acid-binding subunit. *Mol Endocrinol* 3:332-341, 1989.

Raynaud, J.-P.; Bonne, C.; Bouton, M.-M.; Lagace, L.; and Labrie, F. Action of a non-steroidal antiandrogen, RU 23908, in peripheral and central tissues. *J Steroid Biochem* 11:93-99, 1979.

Rochefort, H., and *Garcia,* M. Effect of androgens mediated by the oestro-gen receptor in uterus. In: Klopper, A.; Lerner, L.; van der Molen, H.J.; and Sciarra, F., eds. *Research on Steroids,* Vol. VIII. New York: Academic Press, 1979. pp. 323-325.

Rousseau, G.G., and Schmit, J.-P. Structure activity relationships for gluco-corticoids. I: Determination of receptor binding and biological activity. *J Steroid Biochem* 8:911-919, 1977.

Samuels, H.H., and Tomkins, G.M. Relation of steroid structure to enzyme induction in hepatoma tissue culture cells. *J Mol Biol* 52:57-74, 1970.

Smith, H.E.; Smith, R.G.; Toft, D.O.; Neergaard, J.R.; Burrows, E.P.; and O'Malley, B.W. Binding of steroids to progesterone receptor proteins in chick oviduct and human uterus. *J Biol Chem* 249:5924-5932, 1974.

Wilson, J.D. Androgen abuse by athletes. *Endocr Rev* 9:181-199, 1988.

Zava, D.T., and McGuire, W.L. Androgen action through estrogen receptor in a human breast cancer cell line. *Endocrinology* 103:624-631, 1978.

ACKNOWLEDGMENT

This work was supported in part by U.S. Public Health Service grants HD 13541 and DK 37692 from the National Institutes of Health.

AUTHOR

Olli A. Jänne, M.D., Ph.D.
Senior Scientist and Associate Division Director
Center for Biomedical Research
The Population Council
1230 York Avenue
New York, NY 10021

Anabolic-Androgenic Steroids Profoundly Affect Growth at Puberty in Boys

Alan D. Rogol, Paul M. Martha, Jr., and Robert M. Blizzard

INTRODUCTION

Growth at puberty in man (Tanner and Davies 1985) and some animals (Eden 1979) is clearly sexually dimorphic. It has long been surmised that these alterations in linear growth are subserved by augmented gonadal steroid hormone secretion. More recent data (Parker et al. 1984, Link et al. 1986; Mauras et al. 1987; Stanhope et al. 1988) point toward the necessity of increased circulating concentrations of insulinlike growth factor I (IGF-I) (also called somatomedin C); which themselves depend upon augmented growth hormone (GH) secretion. It is the purpose of this chapter to review the evidence for IGF-I and GH secretion during puberty in children whether this process occurs spontaneously or is induced by exogenous gonadal steroid hormone therapy. Although many investigators have contributed to this field, we shall choose most of the specific examples from our own work.

IGF-I

IGF-I levels increase as pubertal development advances in boys and girls (Luna et al. 1982; Rosenfield and Furlanetto 1985). Parker and coworkers (1984) administered testosterone propionate (25 mg intramuscularly (IM) daily for 7 days) to six prepubertal GH-deficient boys. None had increased circulating levels of IGF-I (baseline 0.2 U/ml; after testosterone 0.25 U/ml), although administration of testosterone enanthate markedly increased IGF-I levels in GH-sufficient boys (baseline 0.6 U/ml; after testosterone 1.9 U/ml). GH treatment (0.05 U/kg per day) or the combination of GH and testosterone increased circulating IGF-I levels to 0.84 and 0.87 U/ml, respectively. These data show that testosterone elevates IGF-I concentrations in prepubertal boys who can secrete GH but not in those deemed GH deficient by

classical growth and pharmacological testing criteria. This effect of androgen is considered due to the stimulation of pituitary GH secretion (see
below). Thus, at puberty, physiological concentrations of testosterone may
be responsible for the pubertal IGF-I increase in adolescent boys; however,
since IGF-I levels decline after maximal growth velocity, factors other than
androgenic-anabolic steroid hormones must also play a role.

GROWTH HORMONE

To further define the role of anabolic-androgenic steroid hormones in mediating the rise in IGF-I levels at puberty, we investigated 15 prepubertal
boys, ages 10 to 16.4 years, who had been referred to the Pediatric Endocrinology Clinic at the University of Virginia Health Sciences Center for
evaluation of short stature or delayed sexual development (Link et al. 1986).
Each subject's genital development was stage I (prepubertal) or II (very
early pubertal) based on the method of Tanner (Marshall and Tanner 1970).
GH concentrations were determined every 20 minutes for 24 hours both
before and after treatment with anabolic-androgenic steroids. Following the
baseline study, 10 boys received oxandrolone (Anavar^{tm}), 0.1 mg/kg per day
for 2 months, and 5 boys received testosterone propionate (7.5 mg IM daily
for 7 days) followed by testosterone enanthate (100 mg IM monthly for 3
months). The second GH secretion test occurred within 3 to 5 days after
the third testosterone enanthate injection. The boys receiving oxandrolone
were restudied after a similar therapeutic interval, slightly more than 60
days following the first test.

Although all boys had an increase in their growth rates during treatment,
those receiving testosterone grew twice as fast as the boys in the oxandrolone-treated group (1.2±0.2 cm per month vs. 0.6±0.07 cm per month).
Mean increments above the basal growth rate (approximately 0.4 cm per
month) were 0.84±0.13 cm per month and 0.22±0.12 cm per month,
p=0.002. Mean IGF-I levels before and during therapy are shown in
table 1.

TABLE 1. *IGF-I concentrations before and during treatment*

	IGF-I (U/ml)	
	Pre-R$_x$	2 months on R$_x$
Oxandrolone treatment	0.70±0.2	0.84±0.45
Testosterone treatment	0.82±0.46	2.3±0.4

NOTE: Measurements reflect the mean ± standard deviation.

There was no significant change in the mean IGF-I concentration in the oxandrolone-treated group (mean change, 0.14±0.4 U/ml; p=.31). However, there was a marked increase of 1.52±0.6 U/ml in the mean IGF-I concentration of the testosterone-treated group (p=.007). To determine if the increase in IGF-I concentration in the testosterone-treated group was mediated by altered GH secretion, we calculated the grand mean of 24-hour GH levels obtained from a pool made from equal aliquots from each of the 72 samples withdrawn from the boys in each group. The results are shown in table 2.

TABLE 2. *Mean GH concentration before and during treatment with oxandrolone or testosterone*

	Mean GH concentration (ng/ml)	
	Pre-R_x	2 months on R_x
Oxandrolone treatment	3.4±1.5	3.1±1.6
Testosterone treatment	2.3±1.8	6.4±2.4

NOTE: Measurements reflect the mean ± standard deviation.

There was no significant change in the mean GH level before or during therapy (mean change, -0.25±6 ng/ml; p=.22) in the oxandrolone-treated group. However, in the testosterone-treated group, there was a threefold increase in mean GH concentration (range two- to twelvefold) during treatment with a mean increase of 4.1±1.2 ng/mI (p=.001) (Link et al. 1986). The increases in IGF-I concentrations and growth rates in the testosterone-treated boys reflect the biological relevance of the increase in the mean daily GH concentrations. Similar elevations in IGF-I levels occur during spontaneous puberty in boys (Parker et al. 1984; Link et al. 1986) and further support this effect of augmented testosterone secretion as a mechanism for the pubertal growth spurt. By contrast, as noted above, a rise in serum testosterone level without an increase in GH concentrations does not increase the circulating levels of IGF-I.

If there is but one androgen receptor, why is the anabolic-androgenic steroid oxandrolone ineffective in augmenting GH secretion, although it clearly increases the growth rate of prepubertal boys? Oxandrolone may act directly at the bony epiphysis to augment growth or possibly enhance the bioactivity of the existing circulating GH. We are unaware of data to distinguish either of these mechanisms or others. Perhaps effects of testosterone are mediated after aromatization to 17-ß estradiol, since oxandrolone cannot be aromatized to a biologically effective estrogen. Studies in adults that demonstrate that circulating concentrations of 17-ß estradiol (total or free) are correlated with higher mean GH concentrations indirectly support this hypothesis (Blizzard et al. 1974; Ho et al. 1987). Alternatively, the dose of oxandrolone did not equal that of testosterone in anabolic potency; a greater dose of oxandrolone might show the same effect as the doses of testosterone employed in these studies.

CROSS-SECTIONAL STUDY OF HORMONAL CHANGES AT PUBERTY

To more fully investigate the augmented GH secretion linked to anabolic-androgenic steroids, Mauras and colleagues studied the specific characteristics of pulsatile GH release responsible for the altered mean GH levels previously noted. Serum GH profiles were analyzed for 10 pre- and early pubertal boys and compared to those from 5 boys late in their pubertal development (Mauras et al. 1987). Using a conservative objective pulse detection method, CLUSTER (Veldhuis and Johnson 1986), the investigators noted markedly augmented circulating levels of GH (and IGF-I) in the late pubertal boys compared to the pre- and early pubertal boys (table 3).

TABLE 3. *Cluster analysis of the GH concentration series and circulating IGF-I levels*

| | CLUSTER Analysis | | | |
	Mean GH (ng/ml)	IGF-I (U/ml)	Number of pulses/24 hrs	Amplitude (ng/ml)
Prepubertal boys*	2.7±0.5	0.92±0.10	5.5±0.4	8.6±1.7
Late pubertal boys*	5.4±0.7	1.78±0.24	5.4±0.5	17.1±2.6

NOTE: Measurements reflect the mean ± standard deviation.

SOURCE: Mauras et al. 1987.

These data demonstrate significant augmentation of total GH secretion at the more advanced stages of sexual development. This increase is due entirely to the increased amplitude of the individual GH secretory bursts, since there was no alteration in the frequency of pulsatile GH release. Similar data, i.e., augmented pulse amplitude without change in frequency, were generated upon reanalysis of the previous study in which prepubertal boys were given testosterone treatment (Mauras et al. 1987). The underlying mechanism of altered GH release, whether attributed to an increased sensitivity of the pituitary somatotrophs, the stimulatory effects of GH-releasing hormone, increased amplitude of GH-releasing hormone secretory pulses, decreased inhibitory tone of somatostatin upon the pituitary, or a combination, cannot be determined from these studies. To more fully define altered GH secretion during puberty, Martha and colleagues (1989) performed an extensive study of the mode of pulsatile release of GH in healthy male volunteers of normal stature whose ages and physical development spanned the entire pubertal range, defined as follows: prepubertal (PRE)=Tanner (Marshall and Tanner 1970) stage I physical development; early puberty (EARLY)=pubertal, but pubic hair development no greater than Tanner stage II; late pubertal (LATE)=Tanner stage III or IV pubic hair and hand epiphyses open; postpubertal (POST)=chronological age $\leq$=18 years, but hand epiphyses fully closed; and adult (ADULT)=healthy young men.

Testosterone

Serum testosterone concentrations increased with advancing sexual development (table 4).

TABLE 4. *Morning mean ($\pm$SE) testosterone concentrations (nmol/L) of study subjects*

PRE	EARLY	LATE	POST	ADULT
<0.87	4.8±1.25	14.7±1.14	17.1±1.1	21.3±1.6

Since testosterone levels did not fall in the POST and ADULT groups as did the GH values (see below), serum concentrations did not correlate positively with any of the assessed GH pulse properties or serum IGF-I concentrations. No significant correlations were obtained between the serum testosterone level and the mean number of pulses per 24 hours (r=0.09, p=0.58).

Growth Hormone

Some specific properties of the pulsatile pattern of GH release are shown in table 5.

The size of the serum GH pulses was clearly greater in the late pubertal group, whether assessed as the mean sum of the GH pulse areas (p<0.001), the mean pulse area (p=0.004) or mean GH pulse amplitude (p=0.001). However, as distinguished from many other GH pulse characteristics, the mean number of detectable GH pulses per 24 hours was not distinguishable from the values for any of the other study groups. Figure 1 illustrates the values for the average GH pulse amplitude (panel B) and average number of pulses per 24 hours (panel C) for the study groups. Note the similarity and dissimilarity of panels B and C, respectively, to the profile of the 24-hour mean concentration of GH illustrated in panel A. Plasma values for

TABLE 5. *Properties of pulsatile GH release*

	PRE	EARLY	LATE!	POST	ADULT
24-hour mean concentration (μg/L)	6.7±1.0	4.7±0.7	13.8±2.4	4.4±0.9	3.9±0.5
Mean pulse area (μg/Lxmin)	648±66	615±87	1,288±215[a]	714±216	614±91
Mean pulse amplitude (μg/L)	14.4±1.3	12.8±1.3	22.4±2.8	14.7±39	10.3±1.3
Sum GH pulse increments (μg/L)	104±10.7[a,b]	80±0.8[a,b]	142±18.0[a,b]	82.0±23[a,b]	48.73±60[c]
Number of pulses per 24 hours	8.8±0.7[b]	7.0±0.5[a]	7.8±0.6[a,b]	6.6±0.6[a]	6.1±0.5

NOTE: GH pulse properties were determined using the CLUSTER algorithm (Veldhuis and Johnson 1986). All values are mean ± SE Any two values in the same row that either lack a superscript or are designated by identical superscripts do not differ statistically; otherwise values are distinguishable statistically from one another (p<0.05).

SOURCE: Table based on data after Martha et al. 1989.

IGF-I mirror the mean GH concentrations (data not shown) and correlate positively with the 24-hour mean GH concentration (r=0.48; p<0.001), the mean and sum of GH pulse areas (r=0.39, p=0.002 and r=0.47, p<0.001, respectively), and the mean and sum of GH pulse increments (r=0.42, p<0.001 and r=0.48, p<0.001, respectively). By contrast, there was no correlation of plasma IGF-I concentration and 24-hour frequency of GH pulses (r=.17, p<.2). However, when the analyses were repeated including only those values from subjects whose hand epiphyses remained open, several strong correlations emerged (Martha et al. 1989). Morning serum testosterone concentrations from only the PRE, EARLY, and LATE pubertal boys correlated positively with plasma IGF-I concentration (r=0.68, p<0.001), 24-hour mean GH concentration (r=0.47, p<0.001), and the mean and sum of GH pulse increments (r=0.58, p<0.001 and r=0.47, p<0.001, respectively).

The results of this cross-sectional study indicate that, along with a rise in plasma IGF-I concentrations, mean circulating levels of GH increase during puberty in normally growing boys around the time of the expected midpubertal growth spurt. The levels of testosterone rise continuously during the ascending portion of the GH and IGF-I increases. This and other studies (Link et al. 1986; Mauras et al. 1987; Stanhope et al. 1988; Liu et al. 1987) strongly suggest a central role for the gonadal hormone environment, particularly circulating androgen concentrations, in mediating the pulse amplitude changes. However, circulating testosterone concentrations cannot be the sole determinant of the pubertal increase in GH pulse

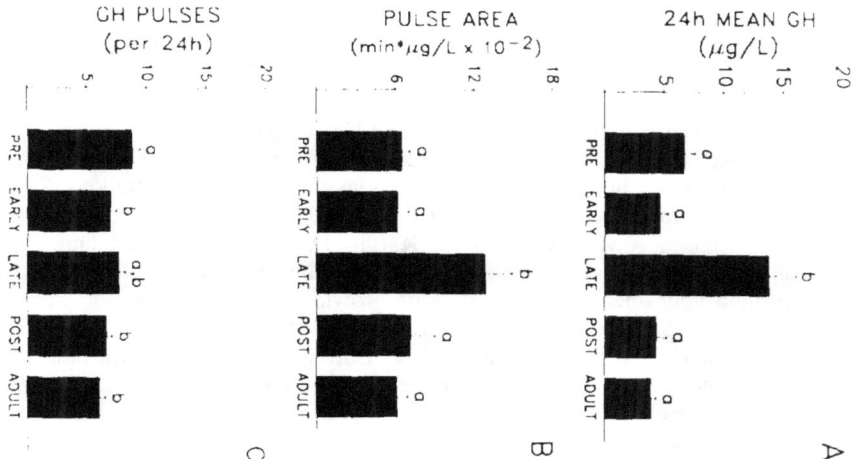

FIGURE 1. *Summary of mean and pulsatile properties of GH release in pubertal boys*

NOTE: Panel A illustrates the mean ±SE 24-hour integrated concentrations of GH for the five study groups. Panel B presents the mean (±SE) area under the GH concentration vs. time curve for individual GH pulses as identified by the CLUSTER pulse detection algorithm. Panel C shows the number of growth hormone pulses (mean±SE) as detected by the CLUSTER algorithm in the 24-hour GH concentration profiles for subjects in the five study groups. In each panel, any two vertical bars not identified by the same letter represent statistically different values ($p < 0.05$) bars sharing a common letter represent statistically indistinguishable values ($p < 0.05$).

amplitude in man, since this pulse parameter decreased in postpubertal boys and young men whose circulating testosterone levels continued to rise.

At all the pubertal stages it is apparent that there is a strong interaction between anabolic-androgenic steroid hormones and GH secretion. What the precise molecular mechanisms are cannot be determined from these results. Further research into the aromatization products (estrogens) and opioid peptide pathways involved may produce new insights, as there is good evidence that the former (Ho et al. 1987) and the latter hormonal products are involved in hypothalamic feedback mechanisms (Veldhuis et al. 1984; Borer et al. 1986).

REFERENCES

Blizzard, R.M.; Thompson, R.G.; Baghdassarian, A.; Kowarski, A.; Migeon, G.J.; and Rodriguez, A. The interrelationships of steroids, growth hormone, and other hormones on pubertal growth. In: Grumbach, M.M.; Gilman, G.D.; and Mayer, F.E., eds. *The Control of the Onset of Puberty.* New York: Wiley and Sons, 1974. 342 pp.

Borer, K.T.; Nicoski, D.R.; and Owens, V. Alteration of pulsatile growth hormone secretion by growth-inducing exercise: Involvement of endogenous opiates and somatostatin. *Endocrinology* 118:844-850, 1986.

Eden S. Age- and sex-related differences in episodic growth hormone secretion in the rat. *Endocrinology* 105:555-560, 1979.

Ho, K.Y.; Evans, W.S.; Blizzard, R.M.; Veldhuis, J.D.; Merriam, G.R.; Samojlik, E.; Furlanetto, R.; Rogol, A.D.; Kaiser, D.L.; and Thorner, M.O. Effects of sex and age on the 24-hr secretory profile of GH secretion in man: Importance of endogenous estradiol concentrations. *J Clin Endocrinol Metab* 64:151-58, 1987.

Link, K.; Blizzard, R.M.; Evans, W.S.; Kaiser, D.L.; Parker, M.W.; and Rogol, A.D. The effect of androgens on the pulsatile release and the twenty-four hour mean concentration of growth hormone in peripubertal males. *J Clin Endocrinol Metab* 62:159-164, 1986.

Liu, L.; Merriam, G.R.; and Sherins, R.G. Chronic sex steroid exposure increases mean plasma growth hormone concentration and pulse amplitude in men with isolated hypogonadotropic hypogonadism. *J Clin Endocrinol Metab* 64:651-656, 1987.

Luna, A.M.; Wilson, D.M.; Wibbelsman, C.J.; Brown, R.C.; Nagashima, R.J.; Hintz, R.L.; and Rosenfeld, R.G. Somatomedins in adolescence: A cross-section study of the effect of puberty on plasma insulin-like growth factor I and II levels. *J Clin Endocrinol Metab* 57:268-271, 1982.

Marshall, W.A., and Tanner, J.M. Variation in the pattern of pubertal changes in boys. *Arch Dis Child* 45:13-23, 1970.

Martha, P.M.; Rogol, A.D.; Veldhuis, J.D.; Kerrigan, J.R.; Goodman, D.W.; and Blizard, R.M. Alterations in the pulsatile properties of circulating growth hormone concentrations during puberty in boys. *J Clin Endocrinol Metab* 69:563-570, 1989.

Mauras, N.; Blizzard, R.M.; Link, K.; Johnson, M.L.; Rogol, A.D.; and Veldhuis, J.D. Augmentation of growth hormone secretion during puberty; evidence for a pulse amplitude-modulated phenomenon. *J Clin Endocrinol Metab* 64:596-601, 1987.

Parker, M.W.; Johanson, A.J.; Rogol, A.D.; Kaiser, D.L.; and Blizzard, R.M. Effect of testosterone on somatomedin C concentrations in prepubertal boys. *J Clin Endocrinol Metab* 58:87-90, 1984.

Rosenfield, R.L., and Furlanetto, R. Physiologic testosterone or estradiol induction of puberty increases plasma somatomedin C. *J Pediat* 107:415-417, 1985.

Stanhope, R.; Pringle, P.J.; and Brook, C.G.D. The mechanism of the adolescent growth spurt induced by low dose pulsatile GnRH treatment. *Clin Endocrinology* 28:83-91, 1988.

Tanner, J.M., and Davies, P.W. Clinical longitudinal standards for height and height velocity for North American children. *J Pediatr* 107:317-329, 1985.

Veldhuis, J.D., and Johnson, M.L. Cluster analysis: A simple, versatile, and robust algorithm for endocrine pulse detection. *Am J Physiol* 250:E486-E493, 1986.

Veldhuis, J.D.; Rogol, A.D.; Samojlik, E.; and Ertel, N.H. Role of endogenous opiates in the expression of negative feedback actions of androgen and estrogen on pulsatile properties of luteinizing hormone secretion in man. *J Clin Endocrinol Metab* 59:580-586, 1984.

ACKNOWLEDGMENTS

Sandra Jackson and her nursing staff at the University of Virginia General Clincial Research Center provided expert patient care. Miss Ginger Bauler, Catherine Kern, and Beth Epstein of the Core Radiological Assay Laboratory performed most of the immunoassays. Data handling and analysis employed the CLINFO system. This work was supported in part by U.S. Public Health Service grant RR 00897 from the National Institutes of Health to the University of Virginia Clinical Research Center.

AUTHORS

Alan D. Rogol, M.D., Ph.D.
Department of Pediatrics and
  Department of Pharmacology

Paul M. Martha, Jr., M.D.
Department of Pediatrics

Robert M. Blizzard, M.D.
Department of Pediatrics

University of Virginia Health Sciences Center
Building MR-4, Room 3037
Charlottesville, VA 22908

Indications of Psychological Dependence Among Anabolic-Androgenic Steroid Abusers[1]

C.E. Yesalis, J.R. Vicary, W.E. Buckley, A.L. Streit, D.L. Katz, and J.E. Wright

INTRODUCTION

Although a great deal of attention has been paid in recent years to adolescent drug use and abuse, it has been only recently that the phenomenon of teen use of anabolic-androgenic steroids (AS) has been documented on a national scale (Buckley et al. 1988). The nonmedical use of AS among adolescents has become an issue for concern because of the potentially harmful physical and psychological outcomes (Haupt and Rovere 1984; Herrmann and Beach 1976; Pope and Katz 1988; Wilson 1988; Wright 1980; Yesalis et al. 1989). Most of the short-term physiologic effects in adult males are transitory (Haupt and Rovere 1984; Wright 1980; Yesalis et al. 1989), but several studies suggest that the biophysical consequences for adolescent males could be more serious (Rosefeld et al. 1982; Strauss 1987; Blether et al. 1984; Wilson et al. 1988). Furthermore, the psychological effects of AS have not been welt documented, and it is in this area that indications of dependence may be evidenced. Taylor (1987) suggests habituation among AS users, although his position appears to be based on user testimonials.

Although AS have been used in the treatment of depression and other mental health disorders (Danziger and Blank 1942; Vogel et al. 1985), serum testosterone levels have also been linked to aggressive behavior with evidence derived from both the literature on animals (Adams 1983; Bouissou 1983) and humans (Ehrenkrantz et al. 1974; Olweus et al. 1980; Perskey et al. 1971; Scaramella and Brown 1978; Susman et al. 1987). Use of AS has been associated with self-reported changes in mood, behavior, and somatic perceptions (Heller 1959; Strauss et al. 1983; Wright, unpublished; Bahrke et al., in press[a]). AS have been shown to elicit electroencephalographic changes similar to those seen with amphetamines and tricyclic

196

antidepressants (Itil et al. 1974; Itil 1976). Case reports of hypomania (Freinhar and Alvarez 1985), schizophrenic, and psychotic episodes have been noted among AS users (Annitto and Layman 1980; Pope and Katz 1987; Pope and Katz 1988), but objective measures (i.e., blind studies) of hostility have not been documented (Bahrke et al., in press[b]).

Other psychological effects of use, that is, increased confidence, euphoria, and enhanced libido (Wright 1980; Haupt and Rovere 1984; Rahrke et al., in press [b]), are powerful reinforcers in their own right. However, these effects, like the physical outcomes, diminish when use is discontinued (Wright 1978; Wright 1982) and may in fact turn into frank depression (Pope and Katz 1988). Such reductions may be associated, therefore, more with a psychological than a physical motivation for continued cyclical use of the drugs. It is possible that the psychological or affective outcomes act as secondary reinforcers, equally as powerful as the primary physical ones.

Several findings from our national study of AS use among adolescent male high school seniors are suggestive of psychological dependence. In this chapter, data from that survey are discussed in relation to psychological rewards of use and the potential for dependence to develop. In particular, the relationships between age of initiation of use, frequency of use, methods of administration, unwillingness to discontinue use, and perceptions of strength, health, and peer use are examined.

BACKGROUND

Current research indicates that, by their senior year in high school, 58 percent of teenagers have tried an illicit drug and that male adolescents are more likely to use illicit drugs (Johnston et al. 1987). It also appears that the development of drug-use patterns, including acquisition and habit formation, for various substances is most likely to occur between 11 and 24 years of age (Pandina et al. 1984). The outcomes of use behaviors, from initiation of use through possible dependence on drugs, are of concern for both their physical and psychological consequences. Adolescence is an age period during which a number of major developmental tasks are addressed (Adelson 1980). While each of these is of importance and potentially affected by drug use, two are of particular relevance to AS use, namely, (1) development and maintenance of physical health care behaviors and (2) development of self-identity, self-esteem, and psychological well-being.

To understand adolescent AS use in a developmental context, it is useful to identify parallels with other teen drug use. Research has shown a variety of factors associated with teen drug use, several of which may be similar to those related to AS use. Recreational drugs, both licit and illicit, generally are expected to provide pleasurable effects for the user, with mood-altering capabilities most valued (Johnston et al. 1987). Although AS do not provide immediate euphoric effects, the physical and psychological outcomes have the potential to affect social status and peer perceptions as well as mood and self-image. Not uncommonly, problems in personal, family, school, and peer domains are identified as causative or contributing to drug use, along with the interactions between these and other contexts, e.g., sociocultural (Huba et al. 1980). Clearly personal and peer values and expectations need to be identified to understand adolescent AS use.

The physiological addictiveness of AS is not known but has been suggested by anecdotal reports of withdrawal symptoms by users (Goldstein, this volume), and two cases of apparent dependence on AS have recently been reported (Brower et al. 1989; Tennant et al. 1988). Although studies to document endogenous opiate levels following AS administration have not been conducted, the potential for physiological dependence on these drugs is strengthened by numerous reports demonstrating the role of opiate peptides in the mediation of sex steroid effects on the central nervous system (particularly hypothalamic hormone secretion) (Bhanot and Wilkinson 1983; Cicero et al. 1979; Ieiri et al. 1979; Mauras et al. 1986; Van Vugt et al. 1982; Veldhuis et al. 1983; Veldhuis et al. 1985; Veldhuis et al. 1984).

Drug treatment programs recognize that physical dependence on most drugs can be relatively easily reduced, but eliminating psychological dependence is more difficult, although necessary for total recovery. Several psychological attitudes associated with AS use among adolescents parallel those associated with drug dependence in general. One such attitude is a tendency to overlook, disbelieve, or argue against the physical risks of drug use and to perceive the benefits as outweighing the risks.

Drug use continues, at various levels, as long as the perceived benefits, often real as well, outweigh the perceived and equally real problems associated with use. Research also indicates that a general tendency to take risks is associated with the development of drug abuse (Crowley 1988).

Adolescent substance users usually overestimate the prevalence and acceptability of use by their peers (Sherman et al. 1983; Chassin et al. 1985). A strong predictor of an individual's use of drugs is reported use by a friend or admired other (Hansen et al. 1987), although it is not always clear whether drug-related friendships follow or precede use. Although many of the problems associated with teen drug use generally are not present with users of AS, there may be some parallel psychological factors related to their use and potential for psychological dependence.

METHODS

Participants for this investigation were 12th-grade male students in both private and public high schools. A sample of schools was drawn from an available nationwide pool of 150 high schools, known to the researchers because these schools employed certified athletic trainers who had recently participated in a sports epidemiology survey (Powell 1987). Only 10 percent of high schools nationwide employ certified athletic trainers. However, there is no evidence to suggest that adolescent AS users who attend high schools with an athletic trainer behave differently than AS users in academic settings without athletic trainers.

The high schools were stratified into eight categories based on general demographic characteristics: (1) urban and rural locale, using the Metropolitan Statistical Area (MSA) designation; (2) large (more than 700 students) and small (fewer than 700 students) enrollment based on school records 1 month prior to survey administration; and (3) sunbelt and nonsunbelt locale. Sunbelt locale was defined as schools in States that were contiguous and bordered any ocean body or Mexico, from Virginia south and west to Texas, Arizona, New Mexico, and California. These strata were selected based upon anecdotal accounts that the rate of AS use is higher among students in large, urban schools in sunbelt States.

The 150 schools were stratified according to the above three characteristics. This produced eight separate categories or "cells" of schools. A random sample, proportional to the national distribution of schools on these characteristics, was drawn from each of these cells, yielding a total of 67 schools the researchers then contacted for the study. The exceptions to this random subsampling were the categories of sunbelt schools with enrollment of less than 700 and rural sunbelt schools with enrollment of more than 700; for these categories, all available schools were used because of the small numbers in the original pool. Based on these characteristics, the schools in our sample are representative of secondary schools across the nation on the stratification characteristics. The schools were treated as clusters of potential respondents, and all male seniors were invited to participate.

The athletic trainer at each school was contacted individually by phone by the principal investigators. The study was described to him or her, and only eight athletic trainers (12 percent) declined to participate. The majority expressed great interest in the study and were eager to help out. In total, 46 of the 67 schools contacted completed the study protocol for a return rate of 68.7 percent. There were 3,403 (50.3 percent) students who participated in the study out of a potential 6,765 male senior students who were eligible from the participating institutions.

An anonymous 23-item questionnaire, generated by the researchers, was employed to collect the data. The majority of athletic trainers, acting as onsite coordinators, had suggested using homeroom teachers to administer the surveys, as this would include the greatest number of students and provide the most routine form of administration. The athletic trainers circulated the surveys to the homeroom teachers, along with the list of the project's administration instructions. The homeroom teachers administered the surveys to all male seniors present that day, after having given them each a copy of the survey's purpose and description and having read it aloud to them. This setting provided a standardized testing environment and was used for all survey completion. The students' confidentiality was further maintained by having the homeroom teachers seal the collection envelope prior to returning it to the athletic trainer, who then forwarded all responses directly to the researchers for scoring and tabulation.

The tabular analysis involved simple frequency counts and percentages. The chi-square statistic was used to test for significant differences between groups at a level of .05. Additional detail regarding the methodology is reported elsewhere (Buckley et al. 1988).

RESULTS

AS drug use was determined by a yes or no response to the question: "Have you ever used anabolic steroids?" Using the school as the analysis unit, the mean rate of AS use was 6.34 (4.61) percent; with the student as the analysis unit, a mean use rate of 6.64 percent (226/3,403) was derived. The results indicated significant variation of AS use among the participating schools, with respondents from seven schools (15 percent) reporting no AS use.

Use levels among respondents included 40 percent of users reporting five or more episodes (i.e., cycles) of use, 44 percent reporting using more than one AS at the same time (i.e., "stacking"), and 38 percent reporting use of injectable AS.

The AS users in this study perceived significant strength and health benefits from their AS use. The majority of adolescent AS users perceive their relative strength to be greater than average and assess their health as very good or excellent (table 1); their self-perceptions of strenglh and health were generally more extreme than those of nonusers (Buckley et al. 1988). The data also indicated that approximately 40 percent of AS users do not want AS use in sports stopped, even if they were assured their competitors were not using the drugs (25 percent of AS users hold this opinion strongly).

Self-reported users were presented with health-risk scenarios related to the use of AS. Again approximately one out of four stated their intentions to continue use regardless of dire health consequences such as liver cancer, heart attack, or sterility. Thus a clear picture of a "hard core" group of AS users who appear to have no intention of discontinuing use emerges. The characteristics of this hard-core group in terms of episodes of use and age at first use are of special interest. Specifically, adolescents who have completed more cycles and who initiated AS use at a younger age are more

TABLE 1. *AS users' perceptions and behaviors (n=226*)*

	Frequency	Percent
1. Use of injectable AS		
Yes	80	38.3
No	129	61.7
2. Use of more than one AS at one time ("stacking")		
Yes	93	43.7
No	120	56.1
3. Personal strength perceptions		
Greater than average	126	57.3
Average	67	30.9
Less than average	13	5.9
4. Personal health perceptions		
Excellent	89	39.7
Very good	71	31.7
Good	39	17.4
Fair	14	6.3
Poor	11	4.9
5. I would like to see the use of AS to improve performance in sports stopped.		
Strongly agree	38	17.0
Agree	25	11.2
Undecided	71	31.7
Disagree	35	15.6
Strongly disagree	55	24.6
6. I would stop using AS if I were absolutely convinced my fellow competitors no longer used them.		
Definitely yes	37	17.0
Probably yes	28	12.8
Unsure	69	31.7
Probably no	33	15.1
Definitely no	51	23.4

TABLE 1. (continued)

	Frequency	Percent
7. I would stop using AS if it was *proven* beyond doubt that they would . . .		
a. lead to permanent sterility		
Definitely yes	69	31.4
Probably yes	48	21.8
Unsure	46	20.9
Probably no	21	9.5
Definitely no	36	16.4
b. greatly increase my risk of liver cancer		
Definitely yes	69	31.1
Probably yes	59	26.6
Unsure	40	18.0
Probably no	26	11.7
Definitely no	28	12.6
c. greatly influence my risk of a heart attack before age 40		
Definitely yes	69	31.5
Probably yes	60	27.4
Unsure	39	17.8
Probably no	21	9.6
Definitely no	30	13.7

*Instances where the number of respondents does not equal 226 is due to nonresponse or an answer of "don't know."

likely to exhibit those behaviors, perceptions, and opinions that are consistent with habituation.

The data in tables 2 and 3 show that the number of episodes of use (i.e., cycles) is significantly and positively correlated with use of injectable AS and with stacking. Likewise "heavy users" (those who reported using five or more cycles) were more likely to assess their strength as being above average, although the relationship approached but did not reach statistical significance (p=.06) (table 4); 86 percent of the heavy users selected the highest category for both their health and their strength (data not shown). Adolescents who reported more than one episode of AS use were much more apt to perceive their health as being excellent than were one-time users (table 5). However, the multi-cycle users (i.e., more than one cycle) were also more likely to have assessed their health as poor (12.5 percent vs.

202

TABLE 2. *Use of injectable AS*

Number of Cycles	Yes (%)	No (%)
1	2.7	97.3
2-4	28.6	71.4
≥5	65.4	34.6

NOTE: p<.0001; χ^2=**23.45** (χ^2 was calculated from the number of adolescents in each cell). Percents are presented for ease of interpretation.

TABLE 3. *Stacking*

Number of Cycles	Yes (%)	No (%)
1	17.9	82.1
2-4	35.9	64.1
≥5	65.4	34.6

NOTE: p<.0001; χ^2 =28.33.

TABLE 4. *Strength perception*

Number of Cycles	Greater Than Average (%)	Average (%)	Less Than Average (%)
1	48.9	46.2	2.6
2-4	59.1	32.2	6.5
≥5	61.2	22.4	7.1

NOTE: p=.06; χ^2= 11.92.

0 percent), and roughly 73 percent of all users who perceived their health as poor were heavy users.

When AS users were asked if they wanted to see the use of these drugs stopped in competitive sports or if they themselves were willing to stop use if everyone else did, the opinions of the heavy users were once again significantly different from other users and were consistent with addictive attitudes (tables 6 and 7). This group of heavy users is also dramatically more

TABLE 5. *Health status perception*

Number of Cycles	Excellent (%)	Very Good (%)	Good (%)	Fair (%)	Poor (%)
1	24.4	41.5	26.8	7.3	0
2-4	45.4	35.1	12.4	4.1	3.1
≥5	41.2	22.3	18.8	8.2	9.4

NOTE: p=.02; χ^2= 18.22.

TABLE 6. *Wish AS use to be stopped*

Number of Cycles	Strongly Agree (%)	Agree (%)	Undecided (%)	Disagree (%)	Strongly Disagree (%)
1	12.5	22.5	35.0	17.5	12.5
2-4	21.4	13.3	37.8	18.4	9.2
≥5	14.1	3.5	22.3	11.8	48.2

NOTE: p<.0001; χ^2=47.64.

TABLE 7. *Willingness to stop if all will*

Number of Cycles	Definitely Yes (%)	Probably Yes (%)	Undecided (%)	Probably No (%)	Definitely No (%)
1	25.6	7.7	38.5	10.3	17.9
2-4	14.4	20.6	33.0	21.7	10.3
≥5	16.1	6.2	27.2	8.6	42.0

NOTE: p<.0001; χ^2= 36.57.

likely to report intentions to continue use regardless of long-term health consequences (table 8).

The data were examined to determine if the length of cycles (measured in weeks) were associated with the number of cycles. As expected, the heavy users of AS repotted longer cycles (table 9).

TABLE 8. *Health risk*

Number of Cycles	Definitely Yes (%)	Probably Yes (%)	Undecided (%)	Probably No (%)	Definitely No (%)
Sterility*					
1	50.0	30.0	17.5	2.5	0
2-4	29.9	32.0	23.7	10.3	4.1
≥5	24.4	4.9	19.5	12.2	39.0
Cancer**					
1	35.0	32.5	22.5	10.0	0
2-4	34.0	33.0	17.5	12.4	3.1
≥5	26.2	15.5	16.7	11.9	29.8
Heart Attack***					
1	35.9	33.3	23.1	5.1	.6
2-4	37.5	33.3	15.6	10.4	3.1
≥5	22.9	16.9	18.1	10.9	31.3

*p<.0001; χ^2=35.82.
**p<.0001; χ^2=39.23.
***p<.0001 .; χ^2=40.35.

TABLE 9. *Length of cycles*

Number of Cycles	6 Weeks (%)	6-9 Weeks (%)	10-12 Weeks (%)	>13 *Weeks* (%)
1	47.5	45.0	7.5	0
2-4	41.2	36.1	18.6	4.1
≥5	37.2	19.2	15.4	28.2

NOTE: p<.0001; χ^2=.6.28.

Lastly, reported users and nonusers were asked to estimate the number of their fellow senior students whom they think have used AS. In keeping with the perceptions of users of other illicit drugs (Johnston et al. 1987), AS users noted a significantly greater prevalence of use than did nonusers, and these perceptions of peer AS use were significantly and positively related to the number of cycles the respondent reported using. That is, 74 percent of nonusers reported peer AS use in the 0-to-10 category, while only 37 percent of users did so. Once more, acknowledged heavy users stood

TABLE 10. *Peer-use perceptions*

	AS Users (%)	Nonusers (%)
How many students in your senior class do you think have ever used AS?		
0	5.8	25.25
1 to 10	31.3	48.75
10 to 20	22.8	16.07
21 to 40	10.7	6.41
over 40	29.5	3.52

NOTE: p<.0001; $\chi^2 = 341.1$.

apart and perceived a greater prevalence of use among their peers; while 29.4 percent of all users believed peer AS use was in the over-40 cateogry, 60.2 percent of the 5-or-more-cycle users perceived this level of peer use (table 11). Whether this difference between heavy user, light user, and non-user perceptions of peer use was a rationalization of use behavior on the part of the heavy users or the result of insider knowledge was tested by applying the survey's approximate 7-percent-use rate to the total number of male seniors enrolled at each high school. This estimate of expected users at each school was then compared to the estimates given by the heavy users at each school. Almost without exception, the nonusers' estimate of peer AS use was closer to the expected number calculated from the 7-per-cent-use rate than was the heavy users'. Heavy users often estimated more than twice the expected number of users. This could suggest that, as the intensity of AS use increases, users start to rationalize their use and engage in denial and projection as a way to justify their behavior (Semeonoff 1976). On the other hand, the high estimates on the part of users could indicate a significant underreporting of AS use in our survey. Alternatively, the heavy users may tend to associate to a greater extent with other AS users, a situation that could influence their perception of total use.

Finally the variables listed in tables 1 through 11 were cross-tabulated with age at time of first use of AS. Not surprisingly, the perceptions of adolescents who initiated their AS use before they were 16 years old were virtually identical in direction and magnitude to those of the heavy user group described above (data not displayed). More important, only 9.5 percent of those students who reported initiating use at age 15 or less reported having used only one cycle; 63 percent of these early starters reported having used more than five cycles.

TABLE 11. *Peer-use perceptions*

Number of Cycles	0 (%)	1-10 (%)	11-20 (%)	21-40 (%)	40+ (%)
1	9.8	43.8	19.5	14.6	7.3
2-4	6.1	38.4	30.3	12.1	13.1
>=5	3.6	14.5	14.5	7.2	60.2

NOTE: p<.0001; χ^2=64.09.

DISCUSSION

Data from our national survey suggest that the admitted use of AS is currently much higher in our male adolescent population than was reported over a decade ago (Corder et al. 1975). It is particularly significant that approximately one-quarter of AS users in the study reported behaviors, *perceptions*, and opinions that are consistent with psychological dependence, in terms of their unwillingness to stop use, their perceptions of risks and benefits of use, and their rationalization of use. The dismissal of health risks, real or perceived, is consistent with other adolescent drug use behaviors as well (Johnston et al. 1987). This hard core group was comprised primarily of adolescents who initiated their AS use at a younger age and who reported a greater number of episodes of use. This is also consistent with outcome research that suggests that earlier and heavier substance users are more likely to have problems associated with use (Brunswick and Boyle 1979; O'Donnell and Clayton 1979).

It is widely recognized that a drug's chemical structure alone does not predict the addictive effect the substance will have on a person. Both individual needs and expectations, for example, have a powerful effect on behavior following administration of a drug (Hansen 1988). These psychological components especially are responsible for possible addictive outcomes. It is interesting to note the similarities in attitudes of heavier AS users with those of other drug-dependent young people, for whom the reinforcement strength of positive affective outcomes is a powerful motivator to continue use. For AS users, feeling good about oneself can result from increased self-esteem and positive peer admiration that may be precipitated by improved appearance and performance. These outcomes are strong reinforcers, as are the altered mood states that have often been reported with higher levels of AS use, e.g., increased self-confidence, feelings of euphoria and of well-being, sometimes to the point of true grandiosity with hypomania or frank mania (Pope and Katz 1988). Such psychological effects may be as strong in their own right as the physical benefits of use.

Several of the findings deserve additional comment. The use of injectable AS indicates an increased level of commitment to this drug behavior for two reasons: (1) few people other than addicts enjoy injections, and (2) since insulin needles are not usually used for these injections, black market, larger gauge needles (larger than 20 gauge) must be obtained. The use of injectable AS could therefore lead to additional health problems associated with reusing or sharing needles, such as AIDS and hepatitis. One case of AIDS in a bodybuilder who shared needles for AS injection has already been noted (Sklarek et al. 1984). More recently, a Florida man's positive test for HIV was attributed to infected hypodermic needles used for injection of AS (U.S. Olympic Committee 1988). On the other hand, the orally active 17α-alkylated AS appears to have the greatest potential for direct health risk due to their hepatotoxiclty and their ability to alter lipid states (Haupt and Rovere 1984; Wilson 1988; Wright 1980; Yesalis et al. 1989).

The fact that AS users perceive their physical strength and health status to be better than that of their nonuser peers does not bode well for intervention strategies. Feeling good and looking good can be psychologically addicting and are obviously not incentives for terminating AS use. It should be noted, however, that AS users were also twice as likely as nonusers to report their health as fair or poor (11.2 percent vs. 5.8 percent, $p<.0001$). This is an inordinately high figure for this age group, four times above the national average (U.S. Department of Health and Human Services 1987). It is not known whether this is a function of extremely high expectations of performance or of actual health problems; 70 percent of users who reported using AS to treat injury reported their health as excellent. The group with the lowest health perceptions were actually those who reported using AS because of peer pressure; 25 percent of these users reported their health as fair or poor. The potential for deleterious health effects among adolescent AS users cannot be overlooked.

What can be done to deal with this problem? Clearly the data indicate that at least a major intervention effort should be directed at early adolescents (junior high students). Programs aiming at youth should determine whether AS prevention is best included in general drug abuse prevention material or should be addressed separately in health and gym classes. Parents, teachers, coaches, and other school officials should also be included in educational programs. They should be made aware of the signs and symptoms associated with recreational drug use in general, and with AS use in particular, e.g., secretive behavior, mood swings, sudden and dramatic weight gain (especially lean mass gain), edema, or gynecomastia (Crawshaw 1985). In addition, unfamiliar pills and paraphernalia such as vials and needles in an adolescent's possession should raise suspicion.

Moreover, all geographic areas should be included, as the study did not detect, contrary to anecdotal reports, any significant differences in use rates between rural and urban or sunbelt and nonsunbelt areas. The only significant difference was between large and small schools; a slightly higher use rate was found among large schools. Surprisingly, the heaviest use, that is, the greatest concentration of 5-or-more-cycle users, was found to be in *rural nonsunbelt* schools, both large and small. It was also found that AS use is not just a high school football problem but that it exists in wrestling, track and field, baseball, and basketball as well (Buckley et al. 1988). Interestingly, high school students participating in sports also use significantly more beer than do nonathletes (Swisher and Hu 1983). Further, users who did not play sports reported using AS for appearance more often than did sports players; sports participants reported using AS to improve athletic performance most often (Buckley et al. 1988). This suggests that prevention campaigns might have to employ different strategies to address each motivation.

Given the apparent dramatic growth in the use of AS among young adults, despite significant informational and drug-testing programs, it is difficult to be optimistic (Cowart 1987; Yesalis and Friedl 1988). However, better educational efforts can be developed, as can other approaches that address the appearance and performance needs of young people.

For this to be accomplished, further research is necessary. First, it will be important to determine the extent of physical or psychological dependence among adolescent AS users, and what, if any, other substances they are using concurrently, e.g. alcohol, marijuana. Studies may begin to identify those young people at greatest risk for developing dependence and ascertain if there are factors similar to those seen in other addictions. It may be possible to build on other drug abuse prevention strategies found to be successful (Hansen et al. 1988), but modified specifically for AS-using teens. Prevention should aim at students both before they begin use and while they are at the experimental-use phase.

We cannot rely on drug testing alone as a deterrent. Announced drug testing at competitive events has had no documented effect on AS use rates (Yesalis et al. 1988). Moreover, drug testing is currently facing legal challenges and is prohibitively expensive at the college and international level, let alone at the high school level (Cowart 1988). In addition, our seeming inability to control the import, distribution, and sale of cocaine does not generate confidence in law enforcement as a potential solution to the problem. To be successful, enforcement of any sort, whether through regulations or testing, must involve schools, coaches, and parents to a much greater degree.

CONCLUSION

The most important strategy, although idealistic, would be to place amateur sports and physical appearance in a more reasonable perspective in society in general, and in each school and community. Our societal fixation with winning and with body image, often shown in parental as well as peer pressures on teens and on teams, help motivate-or pressure-our children (Yesalis and Friedl 1988). Their response in using anabolic-androgenic steroids, often with implied if not tacit adult approval, should alarm but not surprise us.

FOOTNOTES

1. This chapter was adapted from material contained in "Anabolic Steroid Use: Indications of Habituation Among Adolescents" *J Drug Education* 19(2):103-116, 1989.

REFERENCES

Adams, D. Hormone-brain interactions and their influence on agonistic behavior. In: Svare, B., *ed. Hormones and Aggressive Behavior.* New York: Plenum Press, 1983. pp. 223-246.

Adelson, J., *ed. Handbook of Adolescent Psychology. New* York: John Wiley, 1980.

Annitto, W., and Layman, W.A. Anabolic steroids and acute schizophrenic episode. *J Clin Psychiatry* 41(4):143-144, 1980.

Bahrke, M.; Wright, J.; O'Connor, J.; Strauss, R.; and Catlin, D. Selected psychological characteristics of anabolic steroid users. *N Engl J Med,* in press [a].

Bahrke, M.; Yesalis, C.; and Wright, J. Psychological and behavioral effects of endogenous testosterone levels and anabolic-androgenic steroids among males: A review. Sports *Med,* in press [b].

Bhavot, R., and Wilkinson, M. Opiatergic control of gonadotropin secretion during puberty in the rat: A neurochemical basis for the hypothalamic gonadostat? *Endocrinology* 113:596-603, 1983.

Blether, S.; Gaines, S.; and Weldon, V. Comparison of predicted and adult heights in short boys: Effect of androgen therapy. *Pediatr Res* 18(5):467-469, 1984.

Bouissou, M. Androgens, agressive behavior and social relationships in higher mammals. *Horm Res* 18:43-61, 1983.

Brewer, K.; Blow, F.; Beresford, T.; and Fuelling, C. Anabolic-androgenic steroid dependence. *J Clin Psychiatry* 50:31-33, 1989.

Brunswick, A., and Boyle J. Patterns of drug involvement: Developmental and secular influences on age of initiation. *Youth Soc* 11(2):139-162, 1979.

Buckley, W.; Yesalis, C.; Friedl, K.; Adnerson, W.; Streit, A.; and Wright, J. Estimated prevalence of anabolic steroid use among male high school seniors. *JAMA* 260(23):3442-3445, 1988.

Chassin, L.; Presson, C.; and Sherman, S. Stepping backward in order to step forward: An acquisition-oriented approach to primary prevention. *J Consult Clin Psychol* 53(5):612-622, 1985.

Cicero, T.J.; Shainker, B.A.; and Meyer, E.R. Endogenous opioids participate in the regulation of the hypothalamic-pituitary luteinizing hormone axis and testosterone's negative feedback control of luteinizing hormone. *Endocrinology* 104:1286-1291, 1979.

Corder, B.; Dezelsky, T.; Toohey, J.; and DiVito, C. Trends in drug use behavior at ten central Arizona high schools. *Ariz J Health Phys Educ Recreation Dance* 18(1):10-11 1975.

Cowan, V. Some predict increased steroid use in sports despite drug testing, crackdown on suppliers. *JAMA* 257(22):3025-3029, 1987.

Cowart, V. Drug testing programs face snags and legal challenges. *Phys Sportsmed* 16(2):165-173, 1988.

Crawshaw, J. Recognizing anabolic steroid abuse. *Patient Care,* August 15, 1985. pp. 28-47.

Crowley, T. Learning and unlearning drug abuse in the real world: Clinical treatment and public policy. In: Ray, B.A., ed. *Learning Factors in Substance Abuse.* National Institute on Drug Abuse Research Monograph 84. DHHS Pub. No. (ADM)88-1576. Rockville, MD: the Institute, 1988.

Danziger, C., and Blank, H. Androgen therapy of agitated depressions in the male. *Med Ann DC* 11:181-183, 1942.

Ehrenkrantz, J.; Bliss E.; and Sheard, M. Plasma testosterone: Correlation with agressive behavior and social dominance in man. *Psychosom Med* 36:469-475, 1974.

Freinhar J., and Alvarez, W. Androgen-induced hypomania. *J Clin Psychiatry* 46(8):354-355, 1985.

Hansen, W. Theory and implementation of the social influence model of primary prevention. Presented at First National Conference on Prevention Research Findings. Office of Substance Abuse Prevention, Kansas City, MO, March 1988.

Hansen, W.; Graham, J.; Sobel, J.; Shelton, D.; Flay, B.; and Johnson, C.A. The consistency of peer and parent influences in tobacco, alcohol and marijuana use among young adolescents. *J Behav Med* 10:559-579, 1987.

Hansen, W.; Malotte, C.; and Fielding, J. Evaluation of a tobacco and alcohol abuse prevention curriculum for adolescents. *Health Educ Q* 15(1):93-114, 1988.

Haupt, H., and Rovere, G. Anabolic steroids: A review of the literature. *Am J Sports Med* 12(6):469-484, 1984.

Heller, C.; Moore, D.; Paulsen, C.; Nelson, W.; and Laidlow, W. Effects of progesterone and synthetic progestines on the reproductive physiology of normal men. *Fed Proc* 18:1057-1065, 1959.

Herrmann, W., and Beach, R. Psychotropic effects of androgens: A review of clinical observations and new human experimental findings. *Pharmacopsychiatry* 9:205-219, 1976.

Huba, G.; Wingard, J.; and Bentler, P. Framework for an interactive theory of drug use. In: Lettieri, D.; Sayers, M.; and Person, H., eds. *Theories on Drug Abuse.* National Institute on Drug Abuse Research Monograph 30. DHHS Pub. No. (ADM)80-967. Rockville, MD: the Institute, 1980.

211

Ieiri, T.; Chen, H.T.; and Meites, J. Effects of morphine and naloxone on serum levels of luteinizing hormone and prolactin in prepubertal male and female rats. *Neuroendocrinology* 29:288-292, 1979.

Itil, T. Neurophysiological effects of hormones in humans: Computer EEG profiles of sex and hypothalamic hormones. In: Schar, E.J., ed. *Hormones, Behavior, and Psychopathology.* New York: Raven Press, 1976.

Itil, T.; Akpinar, C.; Herrmann, W.; and Patterson, C. "Psychotropic" action of sex hormones: Computerized EEG in establishing the immediate CNS effects of steroid hormones. *Curr Ther Res* 16:1147-1170, 1974.

Johnston, R.; O'Malley, P.; and Bachman, T. *National trends in drug use and related factors among American high school students and young adults,* 1975-1986. DHHS Pub. No. (ADM)87-1535. Rockville, MD: National Institute on Drug Abuse, 1987.

Mamas, N.; Veldhuis, J.D.; and Rogol, A.D. Role of endogenous opiates in pubertal maturation: Opposing of naltrexone in prepubertal and late pubertal boys. *J Clin Endocrinol Metab* 62:1256-1263, 1986.

O'Donnell, J., and Clayton, R. Determinants of early marijuana use. In: Beschner, G., and Friedman A., eds. *Youth Drug Abuse.* Lexington, MA: Lexington Books, 1979. pp. 63-110.

Olweus, D.; Mattsson, A.; Schalling, D.; and Low, H. Testosterone, agression, physical and personality dimensions in normal adolescent males. *Psychosom Med* 42(2):253-269, 1980.

Pandina, R.; Labouvie, E.; and White, H. Potential contributions of the life span developmental approach to the study of adolescent alcohol and drug use: The Rutgers Health and Human Development Project, a working model. *J Drug Issues* 14(2):253-268, 1984.

Perskey, H.; Smith, K.; and Basic, G. Relation of psychologic measures of agression and hostility to testosterone production in man. *Psychosom Med* 33:265-277, 1971.

Pope, H., and Katz, D. Bodybuilder's psychosis. *Lancet* 1:863, 1987.

Pope, H., and Katz, D. Affective and psychotic symptoms associated with anabolic steroid use. *Am J Psychiatry* 145(4):487-490, 1988.

Powell, J. 636,000 injuries annually in high school football. *Athletic Training* 22(1):19-22, 1987.

Rosefeld, R.; Northcraft, G.; and Hentz, R. A prospective, randomized study of testosterone treatment of constitutional delay of growth and development on male adolescents. *Pediatrics* 68(6):681-687, 1982.

Scaramella, R., and Brown, W. Serum testosterone and aggressiveness in hockey players. *Psychosom Med* 40:262-265, 1978.

Semeonoff, B. *Projective Techniques.* London: John Wiley and Sons, 1976.

Sherman, S.; Presson, C.; Chassin, L.; Corty, E.; and Olshavsky, R. The false consensus effect in estimates of smoking prevalence: Underlying mechanisms. *Personality Soc Psychol Bull* 9:197-207, 1983.

Sklarek, H.; Mantovani, R.; and Erens, E. AIDS in a bodybuilder using anabolic steroids. *N Engl J Med* 311(26):1701, 1984.

212

Strauss, R. Anabolic steroids. In: Strauss R., ed. *Drugs and Performance in Sports.* Philadelphia, PA: W.B. Saunders Co., 1987.

Strauss, R.; Wright, J.; Finerman, G.; and Catlin, D. Side effects of anabolic steroids in weight-trained men. *Phys Sportsmed* 11:87-96, 1983.

Susman, E.; Inoff-Germain, G.; Nattelman, E.; Loriaux, D.; Cutler, G.; and Chrousos, G. Hormones, emotional dispositions and agressive attributes in early adolescents. *Child Dev* 58:1114-1134, 1987.

Swisher, J., and Hu, T. Alternatives to drug abuse: Some are and some are not. In: Glynn, T.; Leukefeld, C.; and Ludford, J., eds. *Preventing Adolescent Drug Abuse.* National Institute on Drug Abuse Research Monograph 47. DHHS Pub. No. (ADM)83-1280. Rockville, MD: the Institute, 1983.

Taylor, W. Synthetic anabolic-androgenic steroids: A plea for controlled substance status. *Phys Sportsmed* 75(5):140-150, 1987.

Tennant, F.; Black, D.; and Voy, R. Anabolic steroid dependency with opioid-type features. *N Engl J Med* 319:578, 1988.

U.S. Department of Health and Human Services. *Health United States 1986 and Prevention Profile.* DHHS Pub. No. (PHS)87-1232. Washington, DC: Supt. of Docs., U.S. Govt. Print. Off., 1987.

U.S. Olympic Committee. *Drug Education News.* The Committee, March 1988.

Van Vugt, D.A.; Sylvester, P.W.; Aylsworth, C.F.; and Meites, J. Counteraction of gonadal steroid inhibition of luteinizing hormone release by naloxone. *Neuroendocrinology* 34:274-278, 1982.

Veldhuis, J.D.; Rogol, A.D.; Johnson, M.L.; and Dufau, M.L. Endogenous opiates modulate the pulsatile secretion of biologically active luteinizing hormone in man. *J Clin Invest* 72:2031-2040, 1983.

Veldhuis, J.D.; Rogol, A.D.; Perez-Palacios, G.; Stumpf, P.; Kitchin, J.D.; and Dufau, M.L. Endogenous opiates participate in the regulation of pulsatile luteinizing hormone release in an unopposed estrogen milieu: Studies in estrogen-replaced, gonadectomized patients with testicular feminization. *J Clin Endocrinol Metab* 61:790-793, 1985.

Veldhuis, J.D.; Rogol, A.D.; Samojlik, E.; and Ertel, N.H. Role of endogenous opiates in the expression of negative feedback actions of estrogen and androgen on pulsatile properties of luteinizing hormone secretion in man. *J Clin Invest* 74:47-55, 1984.

Vogel, W.; Klaiker, E.; and Broverman, D. A comparison of the antidepressant effects of a synthetic androgen (mesterolone) and amitriptyline in depressed men. *J Clin Psychiatry* 46(1):6-8, 1985.

Wilson, J. Androgen abuse by athletes. *Endocr Rev* 9(2):181-199, 1988.

Wilson, D.; Kei, J.; Hintz, R.; and Rosenfeld, R. Effects of testosterone therapy for pubertal delay. *AIDC* 142:96-99, 1988.

Wright, J. *Anabolic Steroids and Sports.* Natick, MA: Sports Science Consultants, 1978.

Wright, J. Anabolic steroids and athletics. *Exerc Sport Sci Rev* 8:149-209, 1980.

Wright, J. *Anabolic Steroids and Sports: Volume II.* Natick, MA: Sports Science Consultants, 1982.

Wright, J.; Bahrke, M.; Strauss, R.; and Catlin, D. Psychological characteristics and subjectively perceived behavioral and somatic changes accompanying anabolic steroid usage. Unpublished manuscript.

Yesalis, C., and Friedl, K. Anabolic steroid use in amateur sports: An epidemiologic perspective. In: *Between Calgary and Seoul. Proc US Olymp Acad* 12:83-89, 1988.

Yesalis, C.; Herrick, R.; Buckley, W.; Friedl, K.; Brannon, D.; and Wright, J. Self-reported use of anabolic-androgenic steroids by elite powerlifters. *Phys Sportsmed* 16(12):91-100, 1988.

Yesalis, C.; Wright, J.; and Bahrke, M. Epidemiologic and policy issues in the measurement of the long term health effects of anabolic-androgenic steroids. Sports Med 8(3):129-138, 1989.

AUTHORS

C.E. Yesalis, Sc.D.
Professor of Health Policy and Administration
and Exercise and Sport Science

J.R. Vicary, Ph.D.
Associate Professor of Health Education

W.E. Buckley, Ph.D.
Assistant Professor of Health Education

A.L. Streit, M.H.A.

The Pennsylvania State University
115 Henderson Building
University Park, PA 16802

David L. Katz, M.D.
Lecturer on Psychiatry
Harvard Medical School
McLean Hospital
Belmont, MA 02178
  and
101 North Carolina Avenue, S.E., #203
Washington, DC 20003

J.E. Wright, Ph.D.
Sports Science Consultants
Northridge, CA 91324

Anabolic-Androgenic Steroid-Induced Mental Status Changes

David L. Katz and Harrison G. Pope, Jr.

INTRODUCTION

Testosterone and its analogs, the anabolic-androgenic steroids, have been widely used in athletics for over 35 years, and it appears that their use has continued to escalate recently. Unfortunately, most of the research available on these drugs has involved subjects being administered modest doses in laboratory settings, rather than the large doses used illicitly by actual athletes in the field. As a result, there are limited data available on the medical and psychiatric effects of these drugs under the conditions that they are most commonly used.

Despite the difficulty of studying illicit steroid use, it is critical to acquire further data in this area. One reason for this is that steroid use appears to be increasingly prevalent among young men in the United States. Pope and colleagues (1988), in a mailed questionnaire survey, found that 1.7 percent of male college seniors at three institutions reported using anabolic steroids. Since only about a third of the questionnaires were returned in this study, it is likely that this 1.7-percent figure represents an underestimate and, possibly, a substantial underestimate of the true prevalence of steroid use. Buckley et al. (1988) reported that 6.6 percent of 12th-grade male students had used anabolic steroids. Taylor (1987) estimated that 1 million Americans have used or are using anabolic steroids for physique enhancement. Lombardo (this volume) and others have commented that anabolic steroids have now become virtually mandatory for competition bodybuilders and line positions in professional and college football. These drugs are even becoming increasingly popular among college, high school, and junior high school students who simply want to look better. Indeed, in the survey of Pope et al. (1988), nearly half of the respondents who admitted to steroid use cited personal appearance as one of their reasons for using these drugs. In short, anabolic steroid use appears to be a widespread phenomenon, and the medical and psychiatric side effects of these drugs therefore have major public health significance.

215

Although the medical side effects of anabolic steroids have been fairly extensively documented (Haupt and Rovere 1984), there are few studies available regarding the psychiatric effects of anabolic steroids. This is perhaps curious, given the large amount of common lore among bodybuilders and athletes themselves, who have often considered changes of mood, temperament, and personality to be among the most characteristic effects of these drugs.

PSYCHIATRIC EFFECTS OF STEROIDS

Among the few studies discussing psychiatric effects of steroids, there are several that have investigated subjects receiving replacement doses of steroids for the treatment of hypogonadism. Among these studies, those of Davidson et al. (1979), Salmimies et al. (1981), and O'Carroll and Bancroft (1984) did not report significant mood changes in subjects receiving anabolic steroids as opposed to those receiving placebo. By contrast, similar studies of hypogonadal males, such as those of Luisi and Franchi (1980) Skakkebaek et al. (1981), and O'Carroll et al. (1985) did find significant changes in certain aspects of mood and behavior, including increased energy, aggressiveness, tenseness, and irritability, in subjects receiving steroids. These equivocal results, however, must be viewed with recognition of the fact that they were conducted with physiologic doses of testosterone or synthetic androgens and thus represent a degree of steroid exposure far lower than that of eugonadal athletes using very large doses of anabolic steroids.

In an extensive review, Haupt and Rovere (1984) summarized the findings of 25 well-documented studies of athletes taking anabolic steroids. In this review, it was noted that 32 percent of athletes who were studied for mood changes did report such effects. Perhaps the most common of these was increased aggressiveness. However, the population in these studies was taking an average of only 15 mg of methandrostenolone per day, a dose that is much lower than that usually taken by athletes (Katz and Pope 1988). It should be noted that the above studies involved male subjects or male athletes. In the one available study that exclusively examined women, Strauss and colleagues (1985) found that 80 percent of 10 elite women athletes reported increased aggressiveness in association with steroid exposure.

Turning to the psychiatric literature, a few reports, generally anecdotal, have documented psychiatric changes from anabolic steroids. Wilson et al. (1974) described an attempt to add methyltestosterone to imipramine in treating five men suffering from unipolar depression. Four of the five men developed paranoid delusions, agitation, and severe anxiety in association with methyltestosterone treatment. These symptoms remitted promptly when the drug was discontinued. In another report, Annitto and Layman (1980) described a 17-year-old weightlifter who became psychotic with cognitive dysfunction, paranoia, auditory hallucinations, and depression. However, this individual did not develop psychotic symptoms until about 6 months after his first steroid exposure, making it more difficult to be certain that steroids were a necessary etiologic factor in his symptoms. In another report, Freinhar and Alvarez (1985) described a 27-year-old bodybuilder who developed irritability, decreased desire and need for sleep, increased energy, racing thoughts, and continuous euphoria within 2 days of starting a regimen of anabolic steroids. These symptoms disappeared when he discontinued use of steroids and reappeared when steroids were resumed.

AN ASSESSMENT OF PSYCHIATRIC SYMPTOMS AMONG ATHLETE ANABOLIC STEROID USERS

We became interested in the effects of anabolic steroids when we encountered two patients at McLean Hospital in Belmont, MA, both of whom had experienced prominent psychotic symptoms in association with steroid use. These patients have been described previously (Pope and Katz 1988); both had extensive neuroendocrine, medical, psychosocial, psychological, and laboratory workups that revealed no obvious etiology for their symptoms other than their steroid exposure. Neither patient, for example, had ever suffered any psychiatric disorder prior to steroid use. The first, a middle-aged white male, had received methyltestosterone, 15 mg twice per day, from his local physician for the treatment of impotence. Within 14 days of beginning treatment, he developed major depression, associated with psychotic features such as auditory and visual hallucinations and delusions of reference. The other patient, a 22-year-old construction worker, had taken two courses, each 8 weeks in length, of 15 mg orally per day of methandrostenolone. Although he did not develop any acute psychotic symptoms with methandrostenolone exposure, he developed a syndrome of depression and anxiety following the termination of the second course. Then, some months later, he abruptly developed psychotic symptoms including religious and paranoid delusions, immediately after a brief re-exposure to steroids. Both patients experienced a remission of their affective and psychotic symptoms after withdrawal of anabolic steroids and a few weeks in the hospital. Now, after 3 to 4 years followup, both patients have remained asymptomatic without psychiatric medication; both have remained abstinent from steroids.

On the basis of this experience, we decided to conduct an interview study to assess the prevalence of psychiatric symptoms among athletes using anabolic steroids. To recruit these subjects, advertisements were sent to gymnasiums in the Boston, MA, and Santa Monica, CA, areas, offering $25 for a confidential interview of anyone who had used at least one cycle (course) of steroids. A total of 41 subjects (39 men and 2 women) were recruited. They ranged in age from 17 to 51 years (mean 26.1 years). Their use of steroids had ranged from a single cycle to as many as 30 cycles. The average lifetime exposure to steroids in the sample was 45.1±51.5 weeks. (Total range of lifetime exposure was from 8 to 240 weeks.)

All subjects were interviewed, beginning with a history of anabolic steroids used, including the names of drugs, dosages, and duration. Changes in body weight and athletic ability (for example, changes in the bench press or squat) were recorded for the times before and after steroid use. Medical history on and off anabolic steroids was also included. The subjects were next administered the Structured Clinical Interview for DSM-III-R (SCID) (American Psychiatric Association 1980; Spitzer et al. 1987). This interview has been subjected to a large multicenter test-retest reliability study (Spitzer et al., unpublished data) in which our center, the Laboratories for Psychiatric Research at McLean Hospital, was involved.

In administering the SCID, the questions were asked two times. First, they were posed for the period during which the subject was taking anabolic steroids, referred to as the on-steroid period, and then they were asked again for the period when the subjects were off steroids. The on-steroid period was defined as the period when the subject was actually taking steroids and the 6-month period after steroid exposure (the latter to allow for possible withdrawal effects, such as depression, following the discontinuation of steroid use). The frequency of various psychiatric syndromes in the subjects during the on-steroid period was then compared with the frequency of the same syndromes during the off-steroid period, thus using each subject as his own control.

The findings, which have been presented in our earlier report (Pope and Katz 1988), indicated that affective and psychotic symptoms were significantly more prevalent during the periods of anabolic steroid exposure than during the off-steroid periods. Indeed, about one-third of the subjects developed either a full manic syndrome or a syndrome closely approaching DSM-III-R criteria for a manic syndrome (referred to as subthreshold manic on the SCID). In addition, 5 of the 41 users were found to meet DSM-III-R criteria (American Psychiatric Association 1987) for psychotic symptoms, 4 experienced delusions of various types and another experienced auditory hallucinations. In all cases, the psychotic symptoms disappeared promptly when steroids were discontinued.

It should be noted that DSM-III-R contains an exclusion criterion that states that a manic episode cannot be diagnosed as such if it is drug induced. Thus, these athletes would be technically diagnosed as having an organic affective syndrome under DSM-III-R. However, the symptoms described by the athletes closely resembled those of naturally occurring manic episodes, differing primarily in the fact that most subjects displayed a particularly prominent component of aggressiveness and irritability. As a result, the exclusion criterion has not been used for the purposes of the diagnoses quoted above.

Some case descriptions will illustrate the severity of these symptoms and how they affected the users. One young male bodybuilder bought an old car for $25 and deliberately drove it into a tree at 35 miles per hour, while a friend videotaped him. He reported feeling invincible. Another body-builder, who began using methadrostenolone, bought an expensive automobile that he could not afford. After stopping methandrostenolone, he realized he could not make the car payments and sold the car. Some months later, he began a new cycle of methandrostenolone and impulsively bought another, more expensive car. A third subject on anabolic steroids was driving down Santa Monica Boulevard and became incensed that the driver in front of him had left his right turn signal flashing without making the turn. At the next stoplight, he jumped out of his car, ran up to the driver in front of him, screamed at him for leaving the signal on, and then pulled a road sign out of the dirt and smashed it through the driver's window. As these examples vividly illustrate, affective and psychotic symptoms, particularly increased aggressiveness and impaired judgment, were significantly more common during and immediately after anabolic steroid use than at all other times of the subjects' lives.

THE EFFECT OF ANABOLIC STEROID USE ON PUBLIC HEALTH

What are the public health consequences of this phenomenon? It appears that there may be a greater number of cases of anabolic-steroid-induced psychiatric illness in this country than has been assumed previously, and these effects may pose a danger not only for steroid users themselves, but also for the public at large. The public danger posed by steroids is illustrated by our experience following publication of the initial study. We began to receive telephone calls from lawyers and district attorneys around the country, describing clients who had committed various violent crimes, including several homicides, apparently while under the influence of anabolic steroids. We have now followed up on a number of these individuals charged with criminal activity, and one case description follows.

Mr. X, a 23-year-old single male, began bodybuilding for personal pleasure at age 18. Over the next 3 years, he became increasingly involved with the gym and other bodybuilders and spent more and more of his spare time in the weight room. At age 21, he decided to enter a local bodybuilding contest and, in preparation for this event, began a 5-month cycle of methandro-stenolone, oxymetholone, and testosterone cypionate. He took the three anabolic steroids simultaneously. After a brief lapse of 3 weeks, during which he worked out while taking no drugs, he resumed the same drugs for another 25 weeks. During the last 9 weeks of this second cycle, he ingested oxymetholone, 250 mg per day, and testosterone cypionate, 800 mg per week.

A review of Mr. X's history prior to steroid exposure revealed no evidence of any affective disorder, psychotic illness or symptomatology, anxiety disorder, or eating disorder. Social drinking (two to eight beers over a weekend) was reported as having occurred during a few brief periods of his years in high school. He also reported other times in which he and several others would collectively consume about 1 g of cocaine intranasally (again, only on weekends). He met no DSM-III-R criteria for antisocial personality disorder either prior to or after age 15. His history was negative for violence, and he denied having ideation of committing violent acts. There was no known history of psychiatric illness in his family. In fad, Mr. X's father was a minister, and Mr. X himself had joined the youth ministry and was known as an energetic, active member. Mr. X had worked part time throughout high school, helping with various construction jobs and, after completing a 2-year trade school program, began full-time employment on a construction crew. He was known to be very social, with many friends, and was described as a caring, kindly, religious man.

During his anabolic steroid use, Mr. X noted severe mood changes. Where he had been respectful and obedient prior to his cycles, he now had many arguments with his parents and his temper was shortened incredibly. He remembers "challenging others for no apparent reason," He recalls, and others confirm, that on more than one occasion he tore chunks of aluminum out of cans with his teeth to intimidate bystanders. He also ripped telephones out of the wall on impulse. At this time, he met DSM-III-R criteria for a manic episode (except for the previously mentioned technicality that his affective state was apparently caused by a known substance) with decreased desire and need for sleep, explosive temper, extremely reckless behaviors with a high potential for dangerous and undesirable consequences, continued irritability, and grandiosity that reached delusional proportions.

While out one weekend evening with some friends during the second course of anabolic steroids, the group stopped at a small market. While in the parking lot, Mr. X, without known or observed provocation, suddenly wrapped his arms around the telephone booth, tore it from its base, and threw it across the lot. The group left immediately and soon thereafter saw a hitchhiker on the road. Mr. X told the driver to stop. After the hitchhiker, a stranger to all present, entered the vehicle, Mr. X instructed the driver to drive to a remote spot in the woods. Once there, without instigation, Mr. X beat the victim repeatedly, tied him between two poles, smashed a wooden board over his back, and kicked him. The hitchhiker was found dead the next morning.

Mr. X was arrested and imprisoned. Shortly after his incarceration and the consequent abrupt discontinuation of his steroids, it was noted that he returned to his previous mild-mannered personality. Reports of him during 19 months of imprisonment consistently described him as shy, cooperative, quiet, and still upset and stunned by his behavior and the events of that evening. Our interview with him and reports from his parents and others are in agreement with this impression.

Given these dramatic psychiatric changes that apparently may be induced by steroids in susceptible individuals, what is the mechanism by which steroids produce these effects? One possibility is that anabolic steroids may have corticosteroidlike properties. It has been well documented that some individuals taking corticosteroids have suffered psychiatric side effects, including psychotic symptoms (Lewis and Smith 1983). Alin et al. (1984) observed that athletes ingesting large doses of anabolic steroids had decreased levels of adrenocorticotropic hormone. This observation would favor the hypothesis that anabolic steroids might mimic some of the biologic activities of corticosteroids. However, the mechanism by which corticosteroids, in turn, cause psychotic symptoms is still unknown.

CONCLUSION

In recent years, increased research has focused on neurochemical aspects of aggression, particularly in animal models. Many substances and most known neurotransmitter systems have been implicated at one time or another. Eichelman (1987), in a review of the available literature, pointed out that the noradrenergic, serotonergic, GABAergic, dopaminergic, and acetylcholine systems have all been studied to some extent in this connection. In the review, the author suggests that research on the noradrenergic and serotonergic systems shows particular consistency of findings between animal and human studies. Svare (this volume) describes his research on androgen-induced aggression, particularly in mice, and suggests that dihydrotestosterone and andrastenedione (an aromatized androgen) may act synergistically to promote aggression. In short, research in this area remains highly preliminary, and much further work will be required to elucidate the psychiatric mechanism of action of anabolic-androgenic steroids.

A substantial number of studies have documented the medical side effects of anabolic steroids. However, psychiatric side effects, though apparently common, are little explored. Preliminary research findings indicate that major affective symptoms, particularly increased aggression, irritability, and impairment of judgment, and even psychotic symptoms may occur in some individuals who use anabolic steroids. Such changes in mental status may have profound implications both for the individual and for society at large.

REFERENCES

Alen, M.; Reinila, M.; and Vihko, R. Response of serum hormones to androgen administration in power athletes. *Med Sci Sports Exerc* 17(3):354-359, 1984.

American Psychiatric Association. *Diagnostic and Statistical Manual of Mental Disorders.* 3d ed. Washington, DC: American Psychiatric Association, 1980.

Annitto, W.R., and Layman, W.A. Anabolic steroids and acute schizophrenic episode. *J Clin Psychiatry* 41(4):143-144, 1980.

Buckley, W.E.; Yesalis, C.E., III; Freidl, K.E.; Anderson, W.A.; Streit, A.L.; and Wright, J.E. Estimated prevalence of anabolic steroid use among male high school seniors. *JAMA* 260(23):3441-3445, 1988.

Davidson, J.M.; Cavhargo, C.A.; and Smith, E.R. Effects of androgen on sexual behavior in hypogonadal men. *J Clin Endrocrinol Metab* 48(6):955-958, 1979.

Eichelman, B. Neurochemical and psychopharmacologic aspects of aggressive behavior. In: Meltzer, H.Y., ed. *Psychopharmacology: The Third Generation of Progress.* New York: Raven Press, 1987. pp. 696-704.

Freinhar, J.P., and Alvarez, W. Androgen-induced hypomania. *J Clin Psychiatry* 46(8):354-355, *1985.*

Haupt, H.A., and Rovere, G.D. Anabolic steroids: A review of the literature. *Am J Sports Med* 12(6):469-484, 1984.

Katz, D.L., and Pope, H.G., Jr. Psychiatric effects of anabolic steroids. In: Garrett, W.E., Jr., and Malone, T.R., *eds. Muschle Development: Nutritional Alternatives to Anabolic Steroids.* Columbus, OH: Ross Laboratories, 1988 pp. 41-44.

Lewis, D.A., and Smith, R.E. Steroid-induced psychiatric syndromes. *J Affective Disord* 5:319-332, 1983.

Luisi, M., and Franchi, F. Double-blind group comparative study of testosterone undecanoate and mesterolone in hypogonadal male patients. *J Endocrinol Invest* 3:305-308, 1980.

O'Carroll, R., and Bancroft, J. Testosterone therapy for low sexual interest and erectile dysfunction in men: A controlled study. *Br J Psychiatry* 145(1):146-151, 1984.

O'Carroll, R.; Shapiro, C.; and Bancroft, J. Androgens, behavior, and nocturnal erection in hypogonadal men: The effects of varying the replacement dose. *Clin Endocrinol* 23:527, 1985.

Pope, H.G., Jr., and Katz, D.L. Affective and psychotic symptoms associated with anabolic steroid use. *Am J Psychiatry* 145(4):487-490, 1988.

Pope, H.G., Jr.; Katz, D.L.; and Champoux, R. Anabolic-androgenic steroid use among 1,010 college men. *Phys Sportsmed* 16(7):75-81, 1988.

Salmimies, P.; Kockett, G.; and Pirk, K.M. Effects of testosterone replacement on sexual behavior in hypogonadal men. *Arch Sex Behav* 11(4):345-353, 1981.

Skakkebaek N.E.; Bancroft J.; Davidson D.W.; and Warner, P.M. Androgen replacement with oral testosterone undecanoate in hypogonadal men: A double-blind controlled study. *Clin Endocrinol* 14:49-61, 1981.

Spitzer, R.L.; Williams, J.B.W.; and Gibbon, W. Structured Clinical Interview for DSM-III-R. New York: New York State Psychiatric Institute, Biometrics Research, 1987.

Strauss, R.H.; Liggett, M.T.; and Lanes, R.R. Anabolic steroid use and perceived effects in ten weight-trained women athletes. *JAMA* 253(19):2871-2873, 1985.

Taylor, W.M. Synthetic anabolic-androgenic steroids: A plea for controlled substance status. *Phys Sportsmed* 15(5):140-148, 1987.

Wilson I.C.; Prange, A.J., Jr.; and Lara, P.P. Methyltestosterone with imipramime in men: Conversion of depression to paranoid reaction. *Am J Psychiatry* 131(1):21-24, 1974.

AUTHORS

David L. Katz, M.D.
Lecturer on Psychiatry
Harvard Medical School
McLean Hospital
Belmont, MA 02178
  and
101 North Carolina Avenue, S.E., #203
Washington, DC 20003

Harrison G. Pope, Jr., M.D.
Associate Professor of Psychiatry
Harvard Medical School
Chief, Biological Psychiatry Laboratory
Laboratories for Psychiatric Research
McLean Hospital
Belmont, MA 02178

Anabolic Steroids and Behavior: A Preclinical Research Prospectus

Bruce B. Svare

INTRODUCTION

Steroid hormones secreted by the testes have been long implicated in reproductive physiology and behavior, and a substantial body of literature exists attesting to their prominent role in these functions (Svare 1983; Leshner 1978). The apparent abuse of these hormones by growing numbers of our society may have derived, in part, from our understanding (and misunderstanding in some cases) of the reputed effects and presumed benefit of steroid hormones. The purpose of this chapter is twofold. First, I will review some of the information derived from preclinical research on androgenic steroids and behavior. In particular, androgenic modulation of aggression will be considered. Second, because preclinical research utilizing appropriate animal models will be critical for understanding the causes and consequences of anabolic steroid abuse in humans, I will provide a preclinical research prospectus for future work in this area.

Behavioral side effects of anabolic steroid abuse are little studied but apparently not uncommon. In their review of the literature, Haupt and Rovere (1984) found that 34 percent (52 out of 155) of athletes studied in 13 investigations reported subjective side effects following anabolic steroid administration. Roughly 30 percent repotted increased libido and aggressive behavior (Johnson et al. 1972; Stamford and Moffatt 1974; Strauss et al. 1982). More serious side effects, including psychiatric syndromes, also have been reported following anabolic steroid administration. In one recent study (Pope and Katz 1988), interviews of 41 bodybuilders and football players who had used steroids revealed that 22 percent displayed full affective syndrome and 12 percent displayed psychotic symptoms. Psychiatric syndromes were absent when anabolic steroid use was terminated.

THE ROLE OF ANABOLIC STEROIDS IN ACTIVATING AGGRESSIVE BEHAVIOR

In the past year, two reports in the popular press (Chaikin 1988; Telander and Noden 1989) have documented extreme behavioral alterations following heavy anabolic steroid abuse in two football players (one in high school and one in college). In both individuals, dramatic physiological and behavioral effects were reported. In addition to focusing widespread national attention on steroid abuse for the first time, the above articles have a common thread running through them in that both individuals reported dramatic increases in violence (e.g., "roid rages") and general aggressive behavior.

Changes in behavior, especially those related to aggression, may be a desirable outcome of anabolic steroid abuse for many individuals. In the same way in which anabolics are used by some athletes to promote strength and performance, they also may be used to enhance combativeness, especially in sports such as football where violence and aggressiveness are the norm. If the above reports of elevated aggressive behavior following anabolic steroid abuse are true, then they apparently confirm what we already know to be the case in laboratory animals; that is, androgenic steroid hormones promote aggressive behavior, and they do so with great effectiveness.

It is important to note that, although other hormones secreted from other endocrine glands have at one time or another been implicated in aggression (Svare 1983), androgenic steroid hormones, in particular testosterone, have been repeatedly implicated in the aggressive behavior of a wide variety of mammalian species (Svare 1983). Also, although testosterone is the steroid hormone most involved in aggression, it is also involved in many other behaviors including copulatory behavior, activity, food intake and body weight gain, learning, and sensation and perception (table 1). The data in these areas are no less persuasive than that in the area of steroid hormone involvement in aggressive behavior (Leshner 1978; Svare and Kinsley 1987). In fact, much of it parallels what will be reviewed here for aggression. In this review, attention is focused on aggressive behavior because it seems the most relevant in view of what is strongly suspected to be the case in humans. Namely, that one important outcome of anabolic steroid abuse in humans is the facilitation of aggressive behavior.

The two best known forms of testosterone-modulated aggressive behavior in laboratory animals are intermale aggression and infanticide. Intermale aggression is the fighting behavior exhibited by male rodents toward one another in the establishment of dominance-subordinance hierarchies (Scott 1966). Mice have been most frequently studied in this context because they display an easily quantifiable repertoire of aggressive responses that reliably occur when two adult males confront each other for the first time. The topography of this type of aggression in male mice consists of a series of initial anogenital investigations, followed by episodes of rough grooming.

TABLE 1. *Androgenic steroid hormones are known to influence many different behavioral responses in laboratory animals*

Behavioral Response	Representative Citations
Aggression	Edwards (1968) Svare et al. (1974)
Copulation	Beach and Holz-Tucker (1949) Phoenix et al. (1959)
Activity	Richter (1922) Broida and Svare (1984)
Food Intake and Body Weight Gain	Bell and Zucker (1971) Slob et al. (1973)
Learning	Beatty and Beatty (1970) Chambers (1976)
Parental Care	Gandelman and Vom Saal (1975) Samuels et al. (1981)
Sensation and Perception	Wade and Zucker (1969) Pietras and Moulton (1974)

After several minutes, the behavior escalates into attacks (severe biting and wrestling), with retaliation by each upon the other. The attacks are usually directed at the back and flank area of the male and will continue until one animal assumes a submissive posture.

Infanticide is the killing behavior that male rodents exhibit when they encounter conspecific neonates for the first time. Because postpartum females typically resume cycling once young are removed, it is thought that infanticidal behavior functions to enhance the reproductive success of strange males that encroach upon the nest site of lactating females (Hrdy 1979). Thus, it is to the competitive advantage of the male to eliminate the offspring of others. Mice have been studied most extensively for the biobehavioral factors governing this response. Killing of neonates by males typically consists of a short (less than 2 minutes) attack latency followed by bites to the head, neck, and flank area. Pups frequently are eaten after the initial attack.

Sex Differences

Male mice typically exhibit the aggressive behaviors outlined above, while females do not, and this sex difference, like many others, is controlled by the presence or absence of testosterone during certain critical developmental periods. A model describing these events is referred to as the "organization-activation" model of sexually differentiated behavior. The effects of perinatal hormone exposure during early critical periods of sexual differentiation are called "organizational" effects and are separate and distinct from the so-called "activational" effects that are seen during pubertal and adult life (Phoenix et al. 1959; Grady et al. 1965). Organizational effects of testosterone permanently bias an organism in a masculine fashion as well as defeminize it. They promote aggressive behavior if they are present during early life, while their absence results in an organism that is less responsive to the aggression-activating effects of pubertal and adult testosterone.

In 1968, Edwards reported that male mice were relatively nonaggressive if they were castrated during early life and then were given activational testosterone injections during adult life. He also showed that genetic female mice would become as aggressive as normal males if they were given testosterone both during the early organizational period as well as during the activational period. This finding, as well as many others of a similar nature (Svare and Gandelman 1975), led to the view that females were innately less aggressive than males, primarily because they lacked the underlying neural architecture that was provided by testosterone during early life.

Sex differences in neural architecture have been reported in rodents. For example, male and female rats differ with respect to the size and number of neurons in certain hypothalamic areas, most prominently in the preoptic area (Gorski et al. 1978; Jacobson and Gorski 1981), as well as in the structure of the dendrites in this brain area (Greenough et al. 1977; Raisman and Field 1973). These sex differences can be reversed by neonatal castration in the male and by neonatal testosterone administration in the female (Raisman and Field 1973). In spite of the above-mentioned morphological sex differences, the current view concerning testosterone action on aggression is that females are simply less sensitive to the aggression-promoting quality of adult testosterone exposure, not that they are refractory or insensitive to the steroid (Gandelman 1980).

It is the activational effects of testosterone and other steroid hormones that are of greatest interest to those examining anabolic steroid abuse. Table 2 summarizes the four critical variables involved in modulating the activational effects of androgens on aggressive behavior. Briefly, they are sex; dose, duration, and route of administration; type of androgen; and genotype. Each of these factors is illustrated by research from my own as well as other laboratories.

TABLE 2. *Primary variables modulating the aggression promoting quality of androgenic steroids*

Primary Variables	Representative Citations
1. Sex (i.e., perinatal androgen environment)	Edwards (1968) Barkley and Goldman (1977) Vom Saal et al. (1976a) Svare and Gandelman (1975)
2. Dose, duration, and route of administration	Svare et al. (1974) Owen et al. (1974) Svare (1979) Vom Saal et al. (1976b)
3. Type of androgen (i.e., aromatizable or 5α reduced)	Luttge and Hall (1973a) Svare (1979) Finney and Ecpino (1976) Luttge et al. (1974)
4. Genotype	Selmanoff et al. (1977) Luttge and Hall (1973b) Svare et al. (1984) Simon and Whalen (1986)

There is little doubt that pubertal and adult exposure to testosterone activates aggressive behavior in mice. In males, the development of intermale aggressive behavior and infanticide corresponds to the increase in circulating testosterone around the time of puberty (McKinney and Desjardins 1973; Gandelman 1973). Castration in adulthood reduces these behaviors, while testosterone administration restores it (Beeman 1947; Gandelman and vom Saal 1975). The postcastration decline in intermale aggression is modulated by previous fighting and copulatory experience; male mice with considerable pregonadectomy fighting or sexual experience persist in their aggressive behavior following castration much longer than naive animals (Schecter and Gandelman 1981; Palmer et al. 1984).

Female mice also exhibit aggressive behaviors following adult (activational) testosterone administration but generally are less sensitive to the steroid than are males (Svare et al. 1974; Barkley and Goldman 1977). For example, in one study (Barkley and Goldman 1977), female mice were subcutaneously implanted with either a 0.3- or 10-mg silastic implant of testosterone. Three weeks following exposure to the implant, the 10-mg testosterone implant produced levels of intermale aggression in the females almost identical to that of normal males, while the 0.3-mg steroid implant, which restored aggression in castrated males, produced little aggression. Testosterone also is capable of promoting infanticidal behavior in female mice. For example,

228

some studies show that virtually 100 percent of female mice will switch from parenting to killing following the administration of daily injections of 500 μg testosterone propionate (TP) a day for 20 days (Samuels et al. 1981; Svare et al. 1984).

Why females are less responsive to the aggression-activating effects of testosterone is not well understood. However, in addition to the aforementioned sex differences in the morphology of the brain (Raisman and Field 1973), the weaker response is probably related to qualitative and quantitative differences between the sexes in steroid uptake and binding and in the distribution of steroid receptors in central neural tissue (Whitsett et al. 1972).

The dose of testosterone exposure is also a critical variable in the effectiveness of the steroid in activating aggressive behaviors, with high doses more effective than low doses. For example, research conducted in my laboratory a number of years ago documented dose-response relationships between testosterone exposure and the stimulation of intermale aggressive behavior and infanticide in female mice. In one study (Svare et al. 1974), adult female mice were injected daily for 42 days with 10, 200, or 500 μg TP, the results showed that 20, 50, and 80 percent of the animals, respectively, exhibited aggressive behavior. In another study (Svare 1979), adult female mice were injected daily for 6 days with 125, 250, 500, or 1,000 μg of testosterone; the results showed that 5, 35, 35, and 75 percent of the animals, respectively, exhibited infanticide. Similar findings in castrated male mice have been reported by a number of different researchers (Brain 1983).

Dose, Duration, and Route of Administration

The effectiveness of testosterone in stimulating aggressive behavior also is influenced by the duration of testosterone exposure. Simply put, the greater the duration of testosterone exposure, the greater the probability that aggressive behavior appears. In work conducted in my laboratory (vom Saal et al. 1976a; vom Saal et al. 1976b), castrated male mice were given daily subcutaneous injections of TP (500 μg) and were assessed every other day for 44 days for intermale aggressive behavior. Roughly 10 percent of the animals fought following 4 injections, 50 percent exhibited aggression following 10 injections, and 100 percent fought following 40 injections. Similar findings for testosterone arousal of infanticide have been reported; 58 percent of females exhibit killing behavior following 5 injections of 500 μg TP, 79 percent exhibit the behavior following 15 injections, and 100 percent kill young following 25 injections (Samuels et al. 1981).

The route of testosterone administration also is an important variable in determining the effectiveness of the steroid in activating aggressive behavior. Intracranial testosterone implants (10 μg TP) promoted intermale aggressive behavior in almost 100 percent of castrated male mice within about 8 days (Owen et al. 1974). In comparison, castrated males receiving daily subcutaneous injections (500 μg TP) of the steroid required 40 days of treatment before 100 percent of animals fought (vom Saal et al. 1976a; vom Saal et al. 1976b), while castrates receiving subcutaneously implanted silastic capsules of testosterone (0.3 mg) required 28 days of steroid exposure before 100 percent of the animals exhibited aggressive behavior (Barkley and Goldman 1977). Clearly, these differences can probably be overridden by dosage variables. However, the important point is that the rapidity with which testosterone gets to neural tissue determines the steroid's behavioral effectiveness in promoting aggression. It is appropriate to assume that testosterone works on neural tissue very rapidly upon intracranial administration, while absorption and uptake of the hormone into the brain following subcutaneous injection or implant requires more time.

Data on intracranial testosterone administration is also helpful in understanding just where in the brain testosterone acts to promote aggressive behavior. Intracranial septal and preoptic area testosterone implants promoted intermale aggressive behavior in castrated male mice, while implants in other brain areas (amygdala, olfactory bulbs, cortex, and medial reticular formation) were ineffective (Owen et al. 1974). These findings support other data in both mice and rats showing that these areas are rich in androgen receptors and that they selectively concentrate testosterone (Luttge 1983). Although similar experiments have not as yet been conducted for infanticide, it is strongly suspected that the same brain sites also will be found to mediate testosterone's effects on this form of aggressive behavior.

Type of Androgen

Another important variable determining the effectiveness of androgenic steroids in promoting aggressive behaviors is whether or not the steroids are of the aromatizable or 5α-reduced variety. In central tissue, testosterone is metabolically converted to other steroids. On the one hand, testosterone can be reduced enzymatically to dihydrotestosterone, while, on the other hand, it can be aromatized to estrogen. Some reports suggest that aromatization of testosterone to estrogen may be important for the stimulation of aggressive behaviors. For example, in mice, estrogen and androstenedione (an aromatizable steroid), but not androstandione (a nonaromatizable androgen), have been found to maintain fighting behavior in castrated males and to stimulate infanticide in females (Luttge 1972; Luttge and Hall 1973a; Svare 1979). Also, administration of antiandrogens does not block testosterone-maintained intermale aggression (Clark and Nowell 1980), although systemic administration of aromatase blockers does attenuate testosterone-maintained fighting (Bowden and Brain 1978). In contrast, other reports suggest that the reduction of testosterone to dihydrotestosterone may be more important for maintaining intermale aggressive behavior. This follows from findings showing that dihydrotestosterone alone can maintain intermale aggression and infanticide (Schecter et al. 1981; Svare 1979) and that antiestrogens are ineffective in suppressing testosterone-maintained intermale fighting behavior (Simon et al. 1981). Several reports indicate that the combined treatment of dihydrotestosterone and estrogen is effective in stimulating intern-tale aggression and infanticide (Finney and Erpino 1976; Svare 1979), suggesting of course that both aromatization and reduction may be important for maintaining aggressive behaviors in mice.

Genotype

A variable of major significance in determining testosterone's effectiveness in promoting aggressive behavior is genotype, and there are many research reports attesting to this fact. For example, castrated CF-1 male mice are responsive to the intermale aggression-promoting properties of either androgens or estrogens, castrated CFW males are sensitive only to estrogenic hormones, and CD-1 males fight only in response to relatively high doses of androgens and are insensitive to estrogens (Simon and Whalen 1986). Also, with respect to intermale aggression, castrated C57BL/10 males are responsive to both hyper- and hypophysiological silastic implants of testosterone; castrated DBA/2 males show reduced aggression in response to a hypophysiological implant and increased aggression scores to hyperphysiological implants (Selmanoff et al. 1977). Finally, male and female mice of the C57BL/6 and DBA/2 strains are differentially sensitive to the infanticide-promoting property of adult testosterone exposure. In contrast to DBA/2 animals, more C57BL/6 animals respond to the hormone by exhibiting killing behavior, and the latter require fewer testosterone injections to exhibit infanticide in comparison to the former (Svare et al. 1984). Strain differences in the morphology of androgen-sensitive hypothalamic brain areas have been detected (Robinson et al. 1985), suggesting that genetic variation in the propensity to respond to the aggression-activating effects of testosterone may be neural in origin.

Other than the few anecdotal reports of anabolic steroid promotion of human rage and violence, systematic research examining androgenic steroid hormone involvement in human aggressive behavior is very limited and generally only correlative in nature. Studying normal male volunteers, Persky et al. (1971) reported a positive relationship between circulating levels of testosterone and measures of hostility, aggressive behavior, and social dominance, but Brown and Davis (1975) showed no relationship. In a widely cited study, Kreuz and Rose (1972) found that prisoners with histories of violent crime during adolescence tended to have significantly higher levels of plasma testosterone compared to prisoners without the same adolescent histories. In another widely cited study, Ehrenkranz et al. (1974) measured circulating testosterone levels in prison convicts separated into three different categories. One group consisted of men that were socially dominant (they had asserted themselves into prestigious jobs in the inmate hierarchy) but nonaggressive, a second group consisted of prisoners that were chronically aggressive (continued acts of aggression and threats while in prison), and a third group consisted of convicts that were neither dominant nor aggressive. The socially dominant but unaggressive group and the chronically aggressive group, although not differing from each other in plasma testosterone levels, exhibited significantly higher levels of the hormone than did the nondominant, unaggressive group. Finally, castrated sex criminals with records of violent are are less likely to commit these acts in the future (LeMaire 1956), and antiandrogen treatment, e.g., medroxyprogesterone, of aggressive individuals and sex offenders is known to make these individuals placid (Bell 1978; Money 1980; Laschet 1972; Blumer and Migeon 1975; O'Connor and Baker 1983).

The foregoing selective survey indicates that androgenic steroids promote species-typical aggression in laboratory animals. The survey also suggests that some forms of human dominating and aggressive behaviors also may be modulated by steroid hormones, though more research is clearly needed to strengthen this statement. The important question at this point is how might this information be useful for understanding the causes and consequences of anabolic steroid abuse in humans? A preclinical research agenda for this growing problem clearly emerges from the data reviewed here as well as from other findings in the field of behavioral endocrinology. A prospectus for future research is elucidated in the remainder of this chapter (table 3).

TABLE 3. *Key questions for future preclinical research on the causes and consequences of anabolic steroid abuse*

Question	Test
1. Do the commonly abused anabolic steroids promote aggressive behavior (and other androgen-dependent behaviors) in laboratory animals?	Animal models of steroid-facilitated aggression (and other androgen-dependent behaviors).
2. Do the commonly abused anaolic steroids produce physical dependence?	Signs of physical dependence such as withdrawal symptoms (the abstinence syndrome) following the termination of chronic treatment; reversal of withdrawal symptoms following steroid administration.
3. Do the commonly abused anabolic steroids produce behavioral dependence?	Signs of behavioral dependence such as the production of pleasurable "subjective" states, with such states having the potential to control behavior.

PROSPECTUS FOR FUTURE RESEARCH

First, we need to know whether or not and to what extent the commonly abused anabolic steroids do in fact promote aggressive behavior as well as other androgen-dependent behaviors. This can easily be done by exploring the effects of anabolic steroids in the context of the aforementioned animal models of species-typical aggressive behaviors.

An important question pertaining to the recommendation raised above is why anabolic steroids have not already been extensively studied in laboratory animals for their potential behavioral effects (Svare 1988)? In 1983, I edited what many considered to be an authoritative volume summarizing the current state of knowledge on hormones and aggressive behavior. The book, entitled *Hormones and Aggressive Behavior,* included an exhaustive analysis of hormone involvement in the aggressive behavior of many vertebrate and invertebrate species from humans to insects. However, an analysis of the contents of the book reveals that it does not contain a single reference to the aggression-promoting effects of anabolic steroids in either humans or subhumans. This was not a case of oversight or omission; there simply was no data base to draw upon. The fact that we continue to know so little about anabolic steroids and aggressive behavior is partly a reflection of the relative newness of the problem of anabolic steroid abuse. However, at least two other factors have contributed to our relative ignorance in this area. First, the original goal in making anabolics was to promote the tissue-building effects of testosterone without its androgenic (masculinizing) qualities. Thus, drug companies that created anabolic steroids probably have focused primarily upon morphological changes in their screening and testing procedures and have given scant attention to potential behavioral effects. Second, basic researchers considering behavioral endpoints generally have not been interested in studying the effects of the synthetic (anabolic) versions of testosterone but rather have focused their interests on the so-called naturally produced (masculinizing) androgens. In view of the fact that anabolics were created so as to provide a hormone that would promote the tissue-building effects of testosterone without its masculinizing (androgenic) qualities, it makes sense then that behavioral endocrinologists were simply not interested in studying hormones that were thought to be devoid of behavioral (masculinizing) properties to begin with.

Significantly, we now know that none of the anabolic steroids available are completely free of androgenic (masculinizing) properties (Gilman et al. 1985), and abusers routinely self-administer extremely large doses of the hormone (or hormones) for long periods of time (Katz and Pope 1988; Haupt and Rovere 1984). Thus, increasingly it appears that anabolic-steroid-induced behavioral change, especially alteration in aggression and violence, may be one of the more reliable outcomes of this form of drug abuse (Katz and Pope 1988).

Second, we need to know more about the similarity (or lack thereof) of anabolic steroids to other drugs of abuse, in terms of physical dependence. It is clear that anabolic steroids can produce a form of psychological dependence in that abusers like their appearance much in the same way that an anorexic likes his or her appearance. But, we must also ask whether or not anabolic steroid abusers continue to use these hormones because they also enjoy the physiological and psychological effects produced by their use, in the same way in which an addict craves the pleasurable effects of heroin or cocaine.

Preclinical research with laboratory animals is critical to answering the above question. First, we must know whether anabolic steroids (indeed, steroids in general) produce physical dependence. That is, when injected acutely, as well as chronically, do anabolics produce predictable changes in physiological and behavioral parameters typically seen with other drugs of abuse? For example, changes in activity, sleep cycles, circadian rhythms, meal patterns, core temperature changes, stereotypies, reflexive changes, etc. Second, when anabolics are removed, do they produce an abstinence syndrome in animals in which distinct behavioral changes are detected? Is it also possible to produce reversal of the abstinence syndrome by readministration of anabolics? These questions are not difficult ones to answer, since behavioral pharmacologists have already laid the groundwork in this area. AU one needs to do is to employ anabolic steroids in some of the commonly used screening tests that scientists typically have employed in the past for other drugs of abuse.

A more difficult but potentially fruitful research question concerns whether or not anabolic steroids produce subjective states in the same way that other drugs of abuse do. Clinical work and anecdotal reports indicate that it is virtually impossible to conduct double-blind studies with anabolic steroids, since human subjects report that they know when they are and when they are not being administered the steroid (Haupt and Rovere 1984). This suggests that anabolic steroids are capable of producing a subjectively discriminable state in human beings.

The problem of subjective states is one that strikes to the very heart of the field of behavioral endocrinology. Scientists have for years speculated as to whether or not hormones produced states that could in fact serve as internal cues for the organism. Determining the presence of a subjective state cannot be done by using the techniques typically employed by behavioral endocrinologists. However, it can be elucidated with the aid of an approach commonly used by the behavioral pharmacologist. The approach is a very simple one. If a substance produces a subjective state, then that state must be regarded as a stimulus. The stimulus, under appropriate conditions, should then serve to control a given behavior. To be specific, the stimulus could also serve a discriminative function, and, theoretically, it could be either negative or positive in its ultimate effects upon behavior. This

234

approach to the assessment of the stimulus properties of pharmacological agents in general and drugs of abuse in particular has been used very successfully by workers in the field of behavioral pharmacology (Thompson and Shuster 1964; Phillips and LePiane 1982).

Research in my laboratory has started to use the above approach to examine the extent to which steroid hormones can produce negative and positive subjective states that can control behavior. In one series of studies (Miele et al. 1988) we utilized the steroid hormone estradiol benzoate as an unconditioned stimulus in a conditioned taste aversion paradigm. Simply put, conditioned taste aversion learning involves coupling a novel highly preferred taste such as sugar water with a stimulus that is unpleasant to an organism. Typically, an intraperitoneal injection of lithium chloride is used because it temporarily makes animals ill, but any drug can be used to examine whether or not it too has negative consequences for the animal. Following this pairing, animals usually avoid the formerly preferred substance because it has been associated with the negative effects of the lithium chloride.

We conducted experiments with mice in which we paired saccharin exposure with an injection of very low doses of estradiol benzoate. The doses of the hormones were ones that produced activation of hormone-dependent behavior in mice such as female sexual responding (lordosis reflex). Even though there were no observable signs of illness in the animals, they avoided the saccharin on subsequent days and instead drank mostly water when given a two-bottle preference test with saccharin in one bottle and water in the other. The higher the dose of estradiol benzoate, the greater the aversion, and males seemed to be more affected than females. The important result of this work is that the steroid apparently produced a negative subjective state that, to our knowledge, first demonstrated the use of a steroid hormone as an unconditioned stimulus. It is significant to note that other drugs of abuse are effective unconditioned stimuli when used in a conditioned taste aversion paradigm (Horowitz and Whitney 1975).

Of equal interest is the possibility that steroid hormones also may have pleasurable (rewarding) consequences for the organism. Thus, organisms may seek out situations that are associated with the hormone or may actively work to gain access to administration of the hormone. Clearly, a finding like this would have dramatic implications for classification of steroid hormones as potential drugs of abuse.

Although the investigation is in the preliminary stages at the present time, we have started to explore this possibility in our laboratory by using an apparatus called a place-preference chamber. The chamber has a middle or start area and two sides that can be entered through small doors. One side is white, while the other side is black. Mice are placed in either the white or black side on the first day approximately 90 minutes following a single subcutaneous injection of a steroid hormone. This corresponds to the time at which the steroid is probably peaking in plasma. The door is shut, and the animal remains there for 30 minutes. The next day the animal is placed in the center portion of the box, both doors are opened, and the animal can freely explore either side for 30 minutes. The amount of time spent on either side is automatically recorded. If the animal prefers the "state" of steroid hormone exposure and associates that state with contextual cues (white or black), then it should spend most of its time on the side that it had been exposed to when it received the steroid hormone. Place-preference tests have been successfully used by behavioral pharmacologists to explore the potential hedonic value of drugs of abuse (Phillips and LePiane 1982).

Finally, utilization of operant conditioning techniques is another obvious approach to examining the potential rewarding effects of anabolic steroids. Operant conditioning has been used with great success in establishing that certain drugs of abuse have powerful pleasurable consequences for the organism (Thompson and Schuster 1964). In this situation, an animal must depress a bar to receive an injection of a drug. If the drug in question is reinforcing, then the animal should readily learn to depress the bar to receive the drug. We have not begun pilot work in this area at present because of anticipated problems associated with steroid solubility and with temporal delay between response and reinforcer. For example, injected steroids take time before absorption, circulation, and behavioral and physiological effects, and it is well known from the operant conditioning literature that delays between response and reinforcer cannot be too long or learning will not proceed. For these reasons, it would seem that the aforementioned classical-conditioning-oriented place-preference tests would be more productive.

CONCLUSION

Anabolic steroid hormone abuse is a growing problem for increasing segments of our society. Such abuse is associated with adverse effects upon behavior including increased incidence of violence, aggression, and psychiatric syndromes such as psychotic reactions. Androgenic steroid hormones are known to promote aggressive behavior in laboratory animals, but systematic studies examining the aggression-promoting quality of anabolic steroid hormones have not been conducted. Moreover, the extent to which anabolic steroids are similar to other common drugs of abuse has not been explored. In particular, research examining signs of physical and psychological dependence as well as the hedonic (rewarding) value of these substances has not been conducted. Therefore, preclinical research using animal models will be necessary for determining the causes and consequences of anabolic steroids abuse in humans.

236

REFERENCES

Barkley, M.S., and Goldman, B.D. Testosterone-induced aggression in adult female mice. *Horm Behav* 9:76-84, 1977.

Beach, F.A., and Holz-Tucker, A.M. Effects of different concentrations of androgen upon sexual behavior in castrated male rates. *J Comp Physiol Psychol* 42:433-441, 1949.

Beatty, W., and Beatty, P.A. Hormonal determinants of sex differences in avoidance behaviors and reactivity to electric shock in the rat. *J Comp Physiol Psychol* 73:446-455, 1970.

Beeman, E.A. The effect of male hormone on aggressive behavior in mice. *Physiol Zool* 20:373-405, *1947.*

Bell, R. Hormone influences on human aggression. *Ir J Med Sci* 147:5-9, 1978.

Bell, D.D., and Zucker, I. Sex differences in body weight and eating: Organization and activation by gonadal hormones in the rat. *Physiol Behav* 7:869-871, 1971.

Blumer, D., and Migeon, C. Hormones and hormonal agents in the treatment of aggression. *J Nerv Ment Dis* 160:127-137, 1975.

Bowden, N.G., and Brain, P.F. Blockade of testosterone-maintained intermale fighting in albino laboratory mice by an aromatization inhibitor. *Physiol Behav* 20:543-546, 1978.

Brain, P.F. Pituitary-gonadal influences on social aggression. In: Svare, B., ed. *Hormones and Aggressive Behavior.* New York: Plenum, 1983. pp. 3-26.

Broida, J., and Svare, B. Genotype modulates testosterone-dependent activity and reactivity in male mice. *Horm Behav* 17:76-85, 1984.

Brown, W., and Davis, G. Serum testosterone and irritability in man. *Psychosom Med* 37:87-97, 1975.

Chaikin, T. The nightmare of steroids. *Sports Illustrated* 69:82-102, 1988.

Chambers, K.C. Hormonal influences on sexual dimorphism in rate of extinction of a conditioned taste aversion in rats. *J Comp Physiol Psychol* 90:851-856, 1976.

Clark, C.R., and Nowell, N.W. The effect of the nonsteroidal antiandrogen flutamide on neural receptor binding of testosterone and intermale aggressive behavior in mice. *Psychoneuroendocrinology* 5:39-45, 1980.

Edwards, D.A. Mice: Fighting by neonatally androgenized females. *Science* 161:1027-1028, 1968.

Ehrenkranz, J.; Bliss, E.; and Sheard, M. Plasma testosterone: Correlation with aggressive behavior and social dominance in man. *Psychosom Med* 36:469-475, 1974.

Finney, H.C., and Erpino, M.J. Synergistic effect of estradiol benzoate and dihydrotestosterone on aggression *in* mice. *Horm Behav* 7:391-400, 1976.

Gandelman, R. The development of cannibalism in male Rockland-Swiss and the influence of olfactory bulb removal. *Dev Psychobiol* 6:159-164, 1973.

Gandelman, R. Gonadal hormones and the induction of intraspecific fighting in mice. *Neurosci Biobehav Rev* 4:133-140, 1980.

Gandelman, R., and vom Saal, F.S. Pup-killing in mice: The effects of gonadectomy and testosterone administration. *Physiol Behav* 15:647-651, 1975.

Gilman, A.G.; Goodwin, L.S.; Rall, T.W.; and Murad, F., eds. *The Pharmacological and Physiological Basis of Therapeutics.* New York: Macmillan, 1985. 1,843 pp.

Gorski, R.A.; Gordon, J.H.; Shryne, J.E.; and Southam, A.M. Evidence for a morphological sex difference within the medial proptic area of the rat brain. *Brain Res* 148:333-346, 1978.

Grady, K.L.; Phoenix, C.H.; and Young, W.C. Role of the developing rat testis in differentiation of the neural tissues mediating mating behavior. *J Comp Physiol Psychol* 59:176-182, 1965.

Greenough, W.T.; Carter, C.S.; Steerman, C.; and DeVoogd, T.J. Sex differences in dendritic patterns in hamster preoptic area. *Brain Res* 126:63-72, 1977.

Haupt, H.A., and Rovere, G.D. Anabolic steroids: A review of the literature. *Am J Sports Med* 12:469-484, 1984.

Horowitz, G.P., and Whitney, G. Alcohol-induced conditioned aversion: Genotypic specifity in mice *(mus musculus). J Comp Physiol Psychol* 89:340-346, 1975.

Hrdy, S.B. Infanticide among animals: A review, classification, and examination of the implications for the reproductive strategies of females. *Ethol Sociobiol* 1:13-40, 1979.

Jacobson, C.D., and Gorski, R.A. Neurogenesis of the sexually dimorphic nucleus of the preoptic area in the rat. *J Comp Neurol* 196:519-529, 1981.

Johnson, L.C.; Fisher, B.; and Silvester, L.J. Anabolic steroid: Effects on strength, body weight, oxygen uptake and spermatogenesis upon mature males. *Med Sci Sports* 4:43-45, 1972.

Kreuz, L., and Rose, R. Assessment of aggressive behavior and plasma testosterone in a young criminal population, *Psychosom Med* 34:321-332, 1972.

Laschet, U. Antiandrogen in the treatment of sex offenders: Mode of action and therapeutic outcome. In: Zubin, J., and Money, J., eds. *Contemporary Sexual Behavior: Critical Issues in the 1970s.* Baltimore: Johns Hopkins University Press, 1972. pp. 311-320.

LeMaire, E. Danish experiences regarding the castration of sexual offenders. *J Crim Law Criminol Pol Sci* 47:294-310, 1956.

Leshner, A.I. *An Introduction to Behavioral Endocrinology.* New York: Oxford, 1978. 361 pp.

Luttge, W.G. Activation and inhibition of isolation induced intermale fighting behavior in castrate male CD-1 mice treated with steroidal hormones. *Horm Behav* 3:71-81, 1972.

Luttge, W.G. Molecular mechanisms of steroid hormone actions in the brain. In: Svare, B., *ed. Hormones and Aggressive Behavior.* New York: Plenum, 1983. pp. 247-312.

Luttge, W.G., and Hall, N.R. Androgen-induced agonistic behavior in castrate male Swiss-Webster mice: Comparison of four naturally occurring androgens. *Behav Biol* 8:725-732, 1973a.

Luttge, W.G., and Hall, N.R. Differential effectiveness of testosterone and its metabolites in the induction of male sexual behavior in two strains of albino mice. *Horm Behuv* 4:31-43, 1973b.

Luttge, W.G.; Hall, N.R.; and Wallis, C.J. Studies of the neuroendocrine, somatic, and behavioral effectiveness of testosterone and its reduced metabolites in Swiss-Webster mice. *Physiol Behav* 13:553-561, 1974.

McKinney, T.D., and Desjardins, C. Postnatal development of the testis, fighting behavior, and fertility in the house mouse. *Biol Reprod* 9:279-294, 1973.

Miele, J.; Rosellini, R.; and Svare, B. Estradiol benzoate can function as an unconditioned stimulus in a conditioned taste aversion paradigm. *Horm Behav* 22:116-130, 1988.

Money, J. *Love and Love Sickness.* Baltimore: John Hopkins, 1980. 311 pp.

O'Connor, M., and Baker, H.W.G. Depo-medroxy progesterone acetate as an adjunctive treatment in three aggressive schizophrenic patients. *Acta Psychiatr Scand* 67:399-403, 1983

Owen, K.; Peters, P.J.; and Bronson, F.H. Effects of intracranial implants of testosterone propionate on intermale aggression in the castrated male mouse. *Horm Behav* 5:83-92, 1974.

Palmer, R.K.; Hauser, H.; and Gandelman, R. Relationship between sexual activity and intraspecific fighting in male mice. *Aggres Behav* 10:317-324, 1984.

Pet-sky, H.; Smith, K.; and Basu, B. Relation of psychologic measures of aggression and hostility to testosterone production in man. *Psychosom Med* 33:265-277, 1971.

Phillips, A.G., and LePiane, F.G. Reward produced by microinjection of (D-ala$_2$)-met5enkephalinamide into the ventral tegmental area. *Behav Brain Res* 5:225-229, 1982.

Phoenix, C.H.; Goy, R.W.; Gerall, A.A.; and Young, W.C. Organizing action of prenatally administered testosterone propionate on the tissues mediating mating behavior in the female guinea pig. *Endocrinology* 65:369-382, 1959,

Pietras, R.J., and Moulton, D.G. Hormonal influences on odor detection in rats: Changes associated with the estrous cycle, pseudo-pregnancy, ovariectomy, and administration of testosterone propionate. *Physiol Behav* 12:475-491, 1974.

Pope, H.G., and Katz, D.L. Affective and psychotic symptoms associated with anabolic steroid *use. Am J Psychiatry* 145:487-490, 1988.

239

Raisman, G., and Field, P.M. Sexual dimorphism in the neurophil of the preoptic area of the rat and its dependence on neonatal androgens. *Brain Res* 54:1-29, 1973.

Richter, C.P. A behavioral study of the activity of the rat. *Comp Psychol Monogr* 1 (No. 2), 1922.

Robinson, S.M.; Fox, T.O.; and Sidman, R.L. A genetic variant in the morphology of the medial preoptic area in mice. *J Neurogenet* 2:381-388, 1985.

Samuels, 0.; Jason, G.; Mann, M.; and Svare, B. Pup-killing behavior in mice: Suppression by early androgen exposure. *Physiol Behav* 26:473-477, 1981.

Schecter, D., and Gandelman, R. Intermale aggression in mice: Influence of gonadectomy and prior fighting experience. *Aggres Behav* 7:187-193, 1981.

Schecter, D.; Howard, S.M.; and Gandelman, R. Dihydrotestosterone promotes fighting behavior in female mice. *Horm Behav* 15:233-237, 1981.

Scott, J.P. Agonistic behavior of mice and rats: A review. *Am Zool* 6:683-701, 1966.

Selmanoff, M.K.; Abreu, E.; Goldman, B.D.; and Ginsburg, B.E. Manipulation of aggressive behavior in adult DBA/2/Bg and C57BL/10/Bg male mice implanted with testosterone and silastic tubing. *Horm Behav* 8:377-390, 1977.

Simon, N.G.; Gandelman, R.; and Howard, S.M. MER-25 does not inhibit the activation of aggression by testosterone in adult Rockland-Swiss mice. *Psychoneuroendocrinology* 6:131-137, 1981.

Simon, N.G., and Whalen, R.E. Hormonal regulation of aggression: Evidence for a relationship among genotype, receptor binding, and behavioral sensitivity to androgen and estrogen. *Aggres Behav* 12:255-266, 1986.

Slob, A.K.; Goy, R.W.; and van der Werff ten Bosch, J.J. Sex differences in growth of guinea pigs and their modification by neonatal gonadectomy and prenatally administered androgen. *J Endrocrinol* 58:11-19, 1973.

Stamford, B.A., and Moffatt, R. Anabolic steroid: Effectiveness as an ergogenic aid to experienced weight trainers. *J Sports Med* 14:191-197, 1974.

Strauss, R.H.; Wright, J.E.; and Finerman, G.A.M. Anabolic steroid use and health status among forty-two weight-trained male athletes. *Med Sci Sports* 14:119, 1982.

Svare, B. Steroidal influences on pup-killing behavior in mice. *Horm Behav* 13:153-164, 1979.

Svare, B., ed. *Hormones and Aggressive Behavior.* New York: Plenum, 1983. 595 pp.

Svare, B. Steroid use and aggressive behavior. *Science* 242:1227, 1988.

Svare, B.; Davis, P.; and Gandelman, R. Induction of fighting behavior in female mice following chronic androgen treatment during adulthood. *Physiol Behav* 12:339-343, 1974.

Svare, B., and Gandelman, R. Aggressive behavior of juvenile mice: Influence of androgen and olfactory stimuli. *Dev Psychobiol* 8:405-415, 1975.

Svare, B., and Kinsley, C.H. Hormones and sex-related behavior: A comparative analysis. In: Kelley, K., ed. *Females, Males, and Sexuality: Theories and Research.* Albany: SUNY-Press, 1987. pp. 13-58.

Svare, B.; Kinsley, C.H.; Mann, M.A.; and Broida, J. Infanticide: Accounting for genetic variation *in* mice. *Physiol Behav* 33:137-152, 1984.

Telander, R., and Noden, M. The death of an athlete. *Sports Illustrated* 70:68-78, 1989.

Thompson, T., and Schuster, C.R. Morphine self-administration, food reinforced and avoidance behavior in rhesus monkeys. *Psychopharmacologia* 5:87-94, 1964.

vom Saal, F.S.; Gandelman, R.; and Svare, B. Aggression in male and female mice: Evidence for changed neural sensitivity in response to neonatal but not adult androgen exposure. *Physiol Behav* 17:53-57, 1976a.

vom Saal, F.S.; Svare, B.; and Gandelman, R. Time of neonatal androgen exposure influences length of testosterone treatment required to induce aggression in adult male and female mice. *Behav Biol* 17:391-397, 1976b.

Wade, G.N., and Zucker, I. Taste preferences of female rats: Modification by neonatal hormones, food deprivation, and prior experience. *Physiol Behav* 4:935-943, 1969.

Whitsett, J.M.; Bronson, F.H.; Peters, P.J.; and Hamilton, T.H. Neonatal organization of aggression in mice: Correlation of critical period with uptake of hormone. *Horm Behav* 3:11-21, 1972.

AUTHOR

Bruce Svare, Ph.D.
Professor of Psychology
State University of New York at Albany
1400 Washington Avenue
Albany, NY 12222

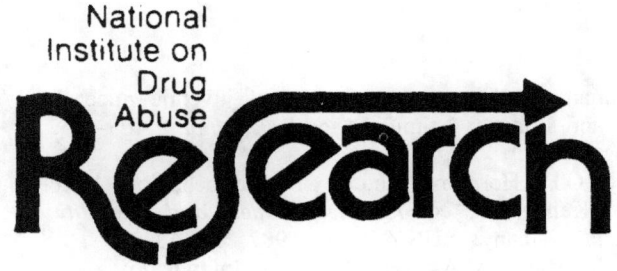

National
Institute on
Drug
Abuse

Research

monograph series

While limited supplies last, single copies of the monographs may be obtained free of charge from the National Clearinghouse for Alcohol and Drug Information (NCADI). Please contact NCADI also for information about availability of coming issues and other publications of the National Institute on Drug Abuse relevant to drug abuse research.

Additional copies may be purchased from the U.S. Government Printing Office (GPO) and/or the National Technical Information Service (NTIS) as indicated. NTIS prices are for paper copy; add $3.00 handling charge for each order. Microfiche copies are also available from NTIS. Prices from either source are subject to change.

Addresses are:

NCADI
National Clearinghouse for Alcohol and Drug Information
P.O. Box 2345
Rockville, MD 20852

GPO
Superintendent of Documents
U.S. Government Printing Office
Washington, DC 20402

NTIS
National Technical Information Service
U.S. Department of Commerce
Springfield, VA 22161
(703) 487-4650

For information on availability of National Institute on Drug Abuse Research Monographs 1 through 24 (1975-1979) and others not listed write to NIDA, Community and Professional Education Branch, Room 10A-54, 5600 Fishers Lane, Rockville, MD 20857.

25 BEHAVIORAL ANALYSIS AND TREATMENT OF SUBSTANCE
ABUSE. Norman A. Krasnegor, Ph.D., ed.
GPO out of stock   NCADI out of stock
                                        NTIS PB #80-112428/AS $31

26 THE BEHAVIORAL ASPECTS OF SMOKING. Norman A. Krasnegor,
Ph.D., ed. (Reprint from 1979 Surgeon General's Report on Smoking and
Health.)
GPO out of stock   NTIS PB #80-118755/AS $23

30 THEORIES ON DRUG ABUSE: SELECTED CONTEMPORARY
PERSPECTIVES. Dan J. Lettieri, Ph.D.; Mollie Sayers; and Helen W. Pearson,
eds.
GPO Stock #017-024-00997-1   NCADI out of stock
                                        Not available from NTIS

31 MARIJUANA RESEARCH FINDINGS: 1980. Robert C. Petersen, Ph.D.,
ed.
GPO out of stock   NTIS PB #80-215171/AS $31

32 GC/MS ASSAYS FOR ABUSED DRUGS IN BODY FLUIDS. Rodger L.
Foltz, Ph.D.; Allison F. Fentiman, Jr., Ph.D.; and Ruth B. Foltz.
GPO out of stock   NCADI out of stock
                                        NTIS PB #81-133746/AS $31

36 NEW APPROACHES TO TREATMENT OF CHRONIC PAIN: A
REVIEW OF MULTIDISCIPLINARY PAIN CLINICS AND PAIN CENTERS.
Lorenz K.Y. Ng, M.D., ed.
GPO out of stock   NCADI out of stock
                                        NTIS PB #81-240913/AS $31

37 BEHAVIORAL PHARMACOLOGY OF HUMAN DRUG DEPENDENCE.
Travis Thompson, Ph.D., and Chris E. Johanson, Ph.D., eds.
GPO out of stock   NCADI out of stock
                                        NTIS PB #82-136961/AS $39

38 DRUG ABUSE AND THE AMERICAN ADOLESCENT. Dan J. Lettieri,
Ph.D., and Jacqueline P. Ludford, M.S., eds. A RAUS Review Report.
GPO out of stock   NCADI out of stock
                                        NTIS PB #82-148198/AS $23

40 ADOLESCENT MARIJUANA ABUSERS AND THEIR FAMILIES.
Herbert Hendin, M.D.; Ann Pollinger, Ph.D.; Richard Ulman, Ph.D.; and
Arthur Carr, Ph.D., eds.
GPO out of stock   NCADI out of stock
                                        NTIS PB #82-133117/AS $23

42 THE ANALYSIS OF CANNABINOIDS IN BIOLOGICAL FLUIDS.
Richard L. Hawks, Ph.D., ed.
GPO out of stock   NTIS PB #83-136044/AS $23

44 MARIJUANA EFFECTS ON THE ENDOCRINE AND REPRODUCTIVE SYSTEMS. Monique C. Braude, Ph.D., and Jacqueline P. Ludford, M.S., eds. A RAUS Review Report.
GPO out of stock   NCADI out of stock
                                    NTIS PB #85150563/AS $23

45 CONTEMPORARY RESEARCH IN PAIN AND ANALGESIA, 1983. Roger M. Brown, Ph.D.; Theodore M. Pinkert, M.D., J.D.; and Jacqueline P. Ludford, M.S., eds. A RAUS Review Report.
GPO out of stock   NCADI out of stock
                                    NTIS PB #84-184670/AS $17

46 BEHAVIORAL INTERVENTION TECHNIQUES IN DRUG ABUSE TREATMENT. John Grabowski, Ph.D.; Maxine L. Stitzer, Ph.D.; and Jack E. Henningfield, Ph.D., eds.
GPO out of stock   NCADI out of stock
                                    NTIS PB #84-184688/AS $23

47 PREVENTING ADOLESCENT DRUG ABUSE: INTERVENTION STRATEGIES. Thomas J. Glynn, Ph.D.; Carl G. Leukefeld, D.S.W.; and Jacqueline P. Ludford, M.S., eds. A RAUS Review Report.
GPO Stock #017-024-01180-1 $5.50   NCADI out of stock
                                    NTIS PB #85159663/AS $31

48 MEASUREMENT IN THE ANALYSIS AND TREATMENT OF SMOKING BEHAVIOR. John Grabowski, Ph.D., and Catherine Bell, M.S., eds.
GPO Stock #017-024-01181-9 $4.50   NCADI out of stock
                                    NTIS PB #84-145184/AS $23

50 COCAINE: PHARMACOLOGY, EFFECTS, AND TREATMENT OF ABUSE. John Grabowski, Ph.D., ed.
GPO Stock #017-024-01214-9 $4   NTIS PB #85-150381/AS $23

51 DRUG ABUSE TREATMENT EVALUATION: STRATEGIES, PROGRESS, AND PROSPECTS. Frank M. Tims, Ph.D., ed.
GPO Stock #017-024-01218-1 $4.50   NTIS PB #85-150365/AS $23

52 TESTING DRUGS FOR PHYSICAL DEPENDENCE POTENTIAL AND ABUSE LIABILITY. Joseph V. Brady, Ph.D., and Scott E. Lukas, Ph.D., eds.
GPO Stock #17-024-01204-1 $4.25   NTIS PB #85-150373/AS $23

53 PHARMACOLOGICAL ADJUNCTS IN SMOKING CESSATION. John Grabowski, Ph.D., and Sharon M. Hall, Ph.D., eds.
GPO Stock #017-024-01266-1 $3.50   NCADI out of stock
                                    NTIS PB #89-123186/AS $23

54 MECHANISMS OF TOLERANCE AND DEPENDENCE. Charles Wm. Sharp, Ph.D., ed.
GPO out of stock   NCADI out of stock
                            NTIS PB #89-103279/AS $39

55 PROBLEMS OF DRUG DEPENDENCE, 1984: PROCEEDINGS OF THE 46TH ANNUAL SCIENTIFIC MEETING, THE COMMITTEE ON PROBLEMS OF DRUG DEPENDENCE, INC. Louis. S. Harris, Ph. D., ed.
GPO out of stock   NCADI out of stock
                            NTIS PB #89-123194/AS $45

56 ETIOLOGY OF DRUG ABUSE: IMPLICATIONS FOR PREVENTION. Coryl LaRue Jones, Ph.D., and Robert J. Battjes, D.S.W., eds.
GPO Stock #017-024-01250-5 $6.50   NTIS PB #89-123160/AS $31

57 SELF-REPORT METHODS OF ESTIMATING DRUG USE: MEETING CURRENT CHALLENGES TO VALIDITY. Beatrice A. Rouse, Ph.D.; Nicholas J. Kozel, M.S.; and Louise G. Richards, Ph.D., eds.
GPO Stock #017-024-01246-7 $4.25   NTIS PB #88-248083/AS $23

58 PROGRESS IN THE DEVELOPMENT OF COST-EFFECTIVE TREATMENT FOR DRUG ABUSERS. Rebecca S. Ashery, D.S.W., ed.
GPO Stock #017-024-01247-5 $4.25   NTIS PB #89-125017/AS $23

59 CURRENT RESEARCH ON THE CONSEQUENCES OF MATERNAL DRUG ABUSE. Theodore M. Pinkert, M.D., J.D., ed.
GPO Stock #017-024-01249-1 $2.50   NTIS PB #89-125025/AS $23

60 PRENATAL DRUG EXPOSURE: KINETICS AND DYNAMICS. C. Nora Chiang, Ph.D., and Charles C. Lee, Ph.D., eds.
GPO Stock #017-024-01257-2 $3.50   NTIS PB #89-124564/AS $23

61 COCAINE USE IN AMERICA: EPIDEMIOLOGIC AND CLINICAL PERSPECTIVES. Nicholas J. Kozel, M.S., and Edgar H. Adams, M.S., eds.
GPO Stock #017-024-01258-1 $5   NTIS PB #89-131866/AS $31

62 NEUROSCIENCE METHODS IN DRUG ABUSE RESEARCH. Roger M. Brown, Ph.D., and David P. Friedman, Ph.D., eds.
GPO Stock #017-024-01260-2 $3.50   NCADI out of stock
                                      NTIS PB #89-130660/AS $23

63 PREVENTION RESEARCH: DETERRING DRUG ABUSE AMONG CHILDREN AND ADOLESCENTS. Catherine S. Bell, M.S., and Robert J. Battjes, D.S.W., eds.
GPO Stock #017-024-01263-7 $5.50   NTIS PB #89-103287/AS $31

64 PHENCYCLIDINE: AN UPDATE. Doris H. Clouet, Ph.D., ed.
GPO Stock #017-024-01281-5 $6.50   NTIS PB #89-131858/AS $31

65 WOMEN AND DRUGS: A NEW ERA FOR RESEARCH. Barbara A. Ray, Ph.D., and Monique C. Braude, Ph.D., eds.
GPO Stock #017-024-01283-1 $3.50   NTIS PB #89-130637/AS $23

66 GENETIC AND BIOLOGICAL MARKERS IN DRUG ABUSE AND ALCOHOLISM. Monique C. Braude, Ph.D., and Helen M. Chao, Ph.D., eds.
GPO Stock #017-024-01291-2 $3.50   NCADI out of stock
                                      NTIS PB #89-134423/AS $23

68 STRATEGIES FOR RESEARCH ON THE INTERACTIONS OF DRUGS OF ABUSE. Monique C. Braude, Ph.D., and Harold M. Ginzburg, M.D., J.D., eds.
GPO Stock #017-024-01296-3 $6.50   NCADI out of stock
                                      NTIS PB #89-134936/AS $31

69 OPIOID PEPTIDES: MEDICINAL CHEMISTRY. Rao S. Rapaka, Ph.D.; Gene Bamett, Ph.D.; and Richard L. Hawks, Ph.D., eds.
GPO Stock #017-024-1297-1 $11   NTIS PB #89-158422/AS $39

70 OPIOID PEPTIDES: MOLECULAR PHARMACOLOGY, BIOSYNTHE-SIS, AND ANALYSIS. Rao S. Rapaka, Ph.D., and Richard L. Hawks, Ph.D., eds.
GPO Stock #017-024-1298-0 $12   NTIS PB #89-158430/AS $45

71 OPIATE RECEPTOR SUBTYPES AND BRAIN FUNCTION. Roger M. Brown, Ph.D.; Doris II. Clouet. Ph.D.; and David P. Friedman, Ph.D., eds.
GPO Stock #017-024-01303-0 $6   NTIS PB #89-151955/AS $31

72 RELAPSE AND RECOVERY IN DRUG ABUSE. Frank M. Tims, Ph.D., and Carl G. Leukefeld, D.S.W., eds.
GPO Stock #017-024-01302-1 $6   NTIS PB #89-151963/AS $31

73 URINE TESTING FOR DRUGS OF ABUSE. Richard L. Hawks, Ph.D., and C. Nora Chiang, Ph.D., eds.
GPO Stock #017-024-01313-7 $3.75   NTIS PB #89-151971/AS $23

74 NEUROBIOLOGY OF BEHAVIORAL CONTROL IN DRUG ABUSE. Stephen I. Szara, M.D., D.Sc., ed.
GPO Stock #017-024-1314-5 $3.75   NTIS PB #89-151989/AS $23

75 PROGRESS IN OPIOID RESEARCH. PROCEEDINGS OF THE 1986 INTERNATIONAL NARCOTICS RESEARCH CONFERENCE. John W. Holaday, Ph.D.; Ping-Yee Law, Ph.D.; and Albert Herz, M.D., eds.
GPO Stock #017-024-01315-3 $21   NCADI out of stock
                                    Not available from NTIS

76 PROBLEMS OF DRUG DEPENDENCE, 1986. PROCEEDINGS OF THE 48TH ANNUAL SCIENTIFIC MEETING, THE COMMITTEE ON PROBLEMS OF DRUG DEPENDENCE, INC. Louis S. Harris, Ph.D., ed.
GPO Stock #017-024-01316-1 $16   NCADI out of stock
NTIS PB #88-208111/AS $53

77 ADOLESCENT DRUG ABUSE: ANALYSES OF TREATMENT RESEARCH. Elizabeth R. Rahdert, Ph.D., and John Grabowski. Ph.D., eds.
GPO Stock #017-024-01348-0 $4   NTIS PB #89-125488/AS $23

78 THE ROLE OF NEUROPLASTICITY IN THE RESPONSE TO DRUGS. David P. Friedman, Ph.D., and Doris H. Clouet, Ph.D., eds.
GPO Stock #017-024-01330-7 $6   NTIS PB #88-245483/AS $31

79 STRUCTURE-ACTIVITY RELATIONSHIPS OF THE CANNABINOIDS. Rao S. Rapaka, Ph.D., and Alexandros Makriyannis, Ph.D., eds.
GPO Stock #017-024-01331-5 $6   NTIS PB #89-109201/AS $31

80 NEEDLE SHARING AMONG INTRAVENOUS DRUG ABUSERS: NATIONAL AND INTERNATIONAL PERSPECTIVES. Robert J. Battjes, D.S.W., and Roy W. Pickens, Ph.D., eds.
GPO Stock #017-024-0134.5-5 $5.50   NTIS PB #88-236138/AS $31

81 PROBLEMS OF DRUG DEPENDENCE, 1987. PROCEEDINGS OF THE 49TH ANNUAL SCIENTIFIC MEETING, THE COMMITTEE ON PROBLEMS OF DRUG DEPENDENCE, INC. Louis S. Harris, Ph.D., ed.
GPO Stock #017-024-01354-4 $17   NTIS PB #89-109227/AS
Contact NTIS for price

82 OPIOIDS IN THE HIPPOCAMPUS. Jacqueline F. McGinty, Ph.D., and David P. Friedman, Ph.D., eds.
GPO Stock #017-024-01344-7 $4.25   NTIS PB #88-245691/AS $23

83 HEALTH HAZARDS OF NITRITE INHALANTS. Harry W. Haverkos, M.D., and John A. Dougherty, Ph.D., eds.
GPO Stock #017-024-01351-0 $3.25   NTIS PB #89-125496/AS $23

84 LEARNING FACTORS IN SUBSTANCE ABUSE. Barbara A. Ray, Ph.D., ed.
GPO Stock #O17-024-01353-6 $6   NTIS PB #89-125504/AS $31

85 EPIDEMIOLOGY OF INHALANT ABUSE: AN UPDATE. Raquel A. Crider, Ph.D., and Beatrice A. Rouse, Ph.D., eds.
GPO Stock #017-024-01360-9 $5.50   NTIS PB #89-123178/AS $31

86 COMPULSORY TREATMENT OF DRUG ABUSE: RESEARCH AND CLINICAL PRACTICE. Carl G. Leukefeld, D.S.W., and Frank M. Tims, Ph.D., eds.
GPO Stock #017-024-01352-8 $7.50   NTIS PB #89-151997/AS $31

87 OPIOID PEPTIDES: AN UPDATE. Rao S. Rapaka, Ph.D., and Bhola N. Dhawan, M.D., eds.
GPO Stock #017-024-01366-8 $7   NTIS PB #89-158430/AS $45

88 MECHANISMS OF COCAINE ABUSE AND TOXICITY. Doris H. Clouet, Ph.D.; Khursheed Asghar, Ph.D.; and Roger M. Brown, Ph.D., eds.
GPO Stock #017-024-01359-5 $11   NTIS PB #89-125512/AS $39

89 BIOLOGICAL VULNERABILITY TO DRUG ABUSE. Roy W. Pickens. Ph.D., and Dace S. Svikis, B.A., eds.
GPO Stock #017-022-01054-2 $5   NTIS PB #89-1255201AS $23

90 PROBLEMS OF DRUG DEPENDENCE, 1988. PROCEEDINGS OF THE 5OTH ANNUAL SCIENTIFIC MEETING. THE COMMITTEE ON PROBLEMS OF DRUG DEPENDENCE, INC. Louis S. Harris, Ph.D., ed.
GPO Stock #017-024-01362-S $17

91 DRUGS IN THE WORKPLACE: RESEARCH AND EVALUATION DATA. Steven W. Gost, Ph.D., and J. Michael Walsh, Ph.D., eds.
GPO Stock #017-024-01384-6 $10   NTIS PB #90-147257/AS $39

92 TESTING FOR ABUSE LIABILITY OF DRUGS IN HUMANS. Marian W. Fischman, Ph.D., and Nancy K. Mello, Ph.D., eds.
GPO Stock #017-024-01379-0 $12   NTIS PB #90-148933/AS $45

93 AIDS AND INTRAVENOUS DRUG USE: FUTURE DIRECTIONS FOR COMMUNITY-BASED PREVENTION RESEARCH. C.G. Leukefeld, D.S.W.; R.J. Battjes, D.S.W.; and Z. Amsel, Ph.D., eds.
GPO Stock #017-024-01388-9 $10   NTIS PB #90-148941/AS $39

94 PHARMACOLOGY AND TOXICOLOGY OF AMPHETAMINE AND RELATED DESIGNER DRUGS. Khursheed Asghar, Ph.D., and Errol De Sousa, Ph.D., eds.
GPO Stock #017-024-01386-2 $11   NTIS PB #90-148958/AS $39

IN PRESS:

95 PROBLEMS OF DRUG DEPENDENCE, 1989. PROCEEDINGS OF THE 51ST ANNUAL SCIENTIFIC MEETING. THE COMMITTEE ON PROBLEMS OF DRUG DEPENDENCE, INC. Louis S. Harris, Ph.D., ed.

96 DRUGS OF ABUSE: CHEMISTRY, PHARMACOLOGY, IMMUNOL-OGY, AND AIDS. Phuong Thi Kim Pham, Ph.D., and Kenner Rice, Ph.D., eds.

97 NEUROBIOLOGY OF DRUG ABUSE: LEARNING AND MEMORY. Lynda Erinoff, ed.

98 THE COLLECTION AND INTERPRETATION OF DATA FROM HIDDEN POPULATIONS. Elizabeth Y. Lambert, M.S., ed.

DHHS Publication No. (ADM) 91-1720
Alcohol, Drug Abuse. and Mental Health Administration
Printed 1990